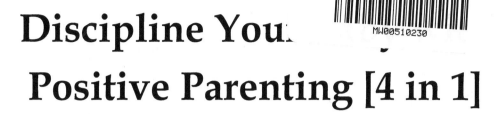

Discipline You...
Positive Parenting [4 in 1]

A Practical Guide to Building Cooperation and
Connecting with Your Child

By

CALEMA DUMONT

Table of Contents

Montessori First-time

Montessori Toddler Disciplines

Potty Training in A Weekend

Potty Training for Newborn Superheroes

Montessori First-time

First-Time Mom? You Need the Modern Toddler Approach with Disciplines Using Easy Baby-Led Weaning, No-Cry Baby, Deep Sleep and Potty Trainings for Your Kids (Age 0-6)

By

CALEMA DUMONT

Table of Contents

Introduction

Infants are born incomplete at conception. It is our given role as adults to help our children in the formidable task of nesting their own human formation. Only in this manner, our children will become fully trained adults and achieve the ability they are able to attain from birth. For both the adult human and his human child, the degree of this challenge sets humans apart from all other species. However, their task is pre-programmed largely by their genes, and their instincts follow a narrowly limited developmental path. Given the care required for their species by the plan of creation, they need only time to grow larger and mature into adulthood. They pay the price though for their existence's predetermined nature. Their adaptation to their environment has limited versatility. Foal and calf, for example, are destined for eating grasses and grains; tiger and lion cub, small mammals. The ways they face certain challenges of life are also programmed: their fur keeps them dry, they are protected by horns and sharp teeth, swift legs take them from danger, and so forth.

On the other hand, the human child is born with no set pattern of instinctive behavior to satisfy its basic survival needs; its options are limitless. No predetermined response limits our ability to identify ways to meet our core food, shelter, clothing, transportation, and defense needs. We are given propensities to certain actions rather than the specific instructions of instincts. Though we are born naked and defenseless without a means of shelter and without instinctual knowledge of what is safe and right for us to eat, we have more than survived through these propensities; our behavioral tendencies account for the development and growth of all the varied civilizations from prehistoric people to the modern era of telecommunications throughout the ages; To help us appreciate how children react to the world in which they are raised, Montessori offered a summary of these propensities. She has no intention of restricting or actually refusing any set of behaviors. No doubt anyone of us will come up with our own different list.

In comparison to conventional teacher-centric teaching, Montessori teaching focuses on empowering kids to guide their own thinking. Teachers direct and give guidance to the students while allowing students to select their assignments and determine how to tackle each difficulty better. Children entering Montessori schools are learning to respect teamwork, keeping inside the guidelines, and worrying about how their behaviors affects others. Students maintain their imagination because of their enjoyment of learning and their own innate interest and drive themselves to succeed. Montessori children are taught how to incorporate a more comprehensive perspective into their knowledge over and above traditional school topics and are motivated to be interested and imaginative pupils. This book will act as a complete guide for you if you are new to the Montessori approach and have difficulty deciding whether to send your child to a Montessori school.

Chapter 1: Introduction to the Montessori Approach

When researching your child's Montessori schooling, it is important to learn a little about Montessori is past and how the approach came to be. Established approximately ten centuries ago, the Montessori Approach was the result of years of work undertaken by Dr. Maria Montessori, the renowned Italian psychiatrist, innovator, and educationist.

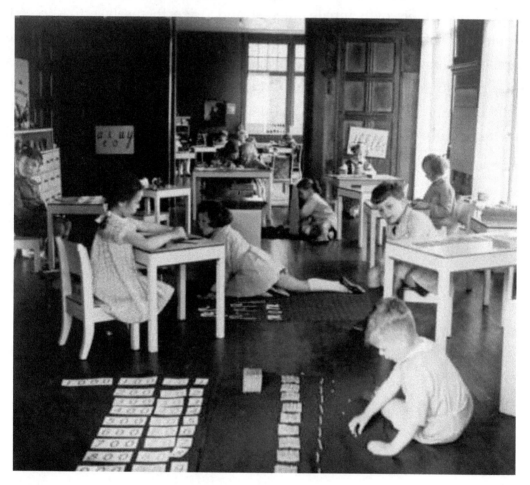

1.1 The History of Montessori

The Montessori education approach aims at the best potential growth of the child, training him ideally for the many rich encounters of life. Complemented by her scientific, developmental, and anthropological experience, Dr. Maria Montessori (1870 – 1952) formulated her teaching theory based on the empirical experiences of children.

Who was Maria Montessori?

Maria Montessori is often called 'before her time.' She is best regarded as the initiator of this famous method known as Montessori today. She was a woman wise beyond her years, determined and unwavering toward the conventions of society.

Born to her parents in Italy in 1870, Maria Montessori later moved to Rome with her parents in her early years, at the age of five in 1875. Maria was determined and curious for learning as a young child, and her mother encouraged her to achieve her academic endeavors, despite the fact that her father did not want her to continue education after her secondary school. While her father Alessandro supported conventional views of education for women, it was her mother's more radical approach, Renilde Montessori that inspired Maria Montessori to pursue her natural ability to know, irrespective of the social constraints imposed on women in today's men-dominated society. By doing so, Renilde took an important part in the education of her daughter, and thus, the whole theory of what is commonly regarded as the "Montessori Approach." At age 13, Montessori attended a vocational school for all-boys in order to pursue engineering. She continued following technical school to pursue her vision of becoming an engineer. She then entered La Sapienza High School at the University of Rome, earning a degree in medicine. Montessori's toughest struggle in medical college was constantly belittled by her colleagues in a male-dominated profession and required to study cadavers by themselves at night (because of university rules). Montessori stay consisted and eventually became Italy's first female scientist. She would be working in different areas that shaped her future: psychiatry wards and pediatrics clinics (one for kids) hospitals.

After Montessori graduated from the Rome University, she worked in the clinical department of the institution, also accompanying children in Rome's insane general asylums. During such experiences, she became persuaded that even such babies, deemed "mentally defective" and ignored by the normas, could be taught. During her period, her involvement in children's growth developed – first from her encounter with autistic children and the deplorable condition of their welfare at the period, then with mentally ill children in her welfare. When she benefited from the research of those already achieved in the area of early childhood education, she developed her own hypotheses, incorporating concepts, insights, and approaches in all fields, and she had studied.

Maria Montessori then created the foremost Casa Dei Bambini, or "Children's Home," in 1906, at the age of 36, for working-class children of the industrial revolution in one of the worst slum districts in town. With some 60 kids in her charge, Maria Montessori launched their education by teaching the older kids how to help with everyday chores. Knowing tools she had already created was added, and Montessori learned, to her delight, how small children instinctively adjusted and loved doing daily activities. The job environment and positive interaction brought the kids a sense of self-worth, which they had never felt before.

One of the first big obstacles Dr. Montessori encountered in changing these children's life was done by convincing parents to realize that their kids were unique and of tremendous importance. The Montessori Approach evolved from this respect for human appearance and potentiality. Via her findings, they established crucial stages in early childhood growth, and the approach developed to tackle these phases through age-appropriate learning materials and activities. Further advancement of the approach followed what Montessori defined as "cosmic schooling" – where the atmosphere and direction for children will be provided to become the peacekeepers of the future, residing in equilibrium with all living things in a prosperous universe.

The common philosophy of the day was that infants were "clean slates" and willing to learn from a parent or older child by clear guidance. In comparison, Montessori claimed that children had an inherent ability for learning and exploring — and were, in reality, motivated to do so. The educator's job, then, was to cultivate this inner ability, examine each child carefully, and provide him or her with activities that would enable him or her to learn the information and skills necessary for their developmental stage. Montessori said they do not need to be pushed to know when children are presented with appropriate resources in a safe, organized environment; yes, they are willing to learn.

In tumultuous times, Maria Montessori followed her values. Living through conflict and international instability encouraged her to complement the Montessori program with peace education. Yet she could do nothing to stop becoming involved in incidents across the globe. Traveling to India in 1940, she was forced to remain in exile for the duration of the war after wars broke out between Italy and Great Britain. She used the chance of her system to educate teachers there.

Maria Montessori expanded her research from this period until her death in 1952 and was generally known and accepted in the United States, Europe, and Asia. She has taught and established training sessions on these continents, set up a research institute in Spain and built training centers for Montessori in the Netherlands and London. Maria has advocated actively, as a public official, on behalf of women's rights. She often wrote and talked on the need for greater equality for women, and was known as a prominent feminist voice in Italy and beyond.

She returned to Europe towards the conclusion of the war and lived her final years in Amsterdam. She died peacefully, on May 6, 1952, in a friend's backyard. Maria Montessori had been a three-time Nobel Peace Laureate winner – in 1949, 1950, and 1951. The campaign she had established in 1907 had dropped out of favor at the time and in the United States was practically non-existent. The Montessori system, however, encountered a resurgence in the US after Dr. Nancy McCormick Rambusch, an early childhood education pioneer, started campaigning for it. She managed to open two Montessori schools, helped establish the American Montessori Society and published a book named: Learning How to Learn: An American Montessori Approach.

How the Montessori Method Evolved

During the year 1896, Montessori gave a speech on her observations from dealing with these special kids at the Educational Congress in Torino. The Education minister was interested and fascinated by the observations of Montessori named her as the head of an organization called Scuola Ortofrenica which was mainly made for the treatment and academics of the developmentally disabled. Montessori called her professional teaching, studying the girls, evaluating ideas, and constructing supplies for her two years there. She concluded, "I think there was nothing peculiarly restrictive about the techniques that I used to teach fools about them. I assumed that the ideals of education were more logical than in practice, much more, indeed, that an inferior mindset might evolve and thrive through its means. This thought, as profound in the form of an emotion, was my guiding concept after I was no longer in my school for shortcomings and, gradually, I was persuaded that identical approaches adapted to regular children would improve or activate their personalities in a marvelous and unexpected fashion." -The Montessori Way, Maria Montessori

Montessori noticed that and felt that if such approaches took children with intellectual disorders to the stage of regular children, after which she understood if that would improve typical children's ability. She got her opportunity to investigate that early. Only a short period after this finding was public, Montessori was approached to open a school which was located in a Rome housing estate. The children played easily and, when their guardians were at work because they were sometimes abusive. The planners used Montessori as a way to rein down the poor children and preserve their residential scheme.

In January 1907, the school in San Lorenzo began and was known as Casa dei Bambini, as well as Children's Home. Montessori provided the children and chance to think about puzzles as well as more, other fascinating meaningful things by teaching them daily tasks. The time Montessori stayed in Casa dei Bambini added in helping her to learn and refine her system further.

Montessori developed a natural world for the children, a world in which "there are no barriers to a their progress, they are eliminated and everything fits his or her age and maturity, and where he or she is allowed means to practice his developing ability" (Lillard and Montessori: A New Method, n. 4).

Montessori's philosophy stated that learning can no longer only express information, but rather follow a different direction, trying to unleash individual potentialities. Montessori was shocked by how pleased and fulfilled the children were as they worked on a subject of importance, often repeating it. Children learnt to do it themselves, to fix their faults and mistakes, to have the right to choose their jobs and resources, and not to seek a praise or penalty for their actions. She found the students were not much concerned about rewards, and often even did not pay attention to the prize or distributed it to someone else if they were rewarded. She claimed that the children wanted a feeling of human integrity and felt it in the workplace.

She has observed that children enjoy discipline, ethical awareness, real-life jobs using actual resources, peaceful jobs, and socially appropriate personal treatment. She admired the person and trusted in his potential. As the reports of the school's performance spread around, more people became increasingly involved in Montessori and her system. Therefore, Montessori began offering seminars, publishing pamphlets and subsequently books, additionally even teacher training in the process. Montessori sought to innovate in her theory, to explore the desires and talents of children and to build an atmosphere and resources that will bring in the maximum ability of the infant.

Montessori travelled widely across countries like the India and from Europe to America in her later years, offering classes, conducting training and workshop courses, going to different colleges, and exhibiting her classrooms at exhibits. She has won numerous awards, and has been nominated three times for the famous Nobel Peace Prize. She has also won various awards and titles in all of Europe. She conducted her last and final teacher-training session in the year before her death and presented at the International Council of Montessori (IMC), lived during two wars several of her sessions centered on teaching children to grow in harmony. Montessori showed the society a modern way of raising girls, a form in which schooling offered life and exploration.

Montessori & Educational Theory

Situating Montessori in Montessori's Educational Philosophy analysis of mental disorders in children inspired her to research education as a far more general field. She agreed that in curriculum foundations, she wanted to seek research that is more specialized. She headed to the University of Rome, where she studied psychology, sociology, history of education and theory, and concepts of pedagogy.

At the start of the twentieth century, the field of educational philosophy that Montessori joined was itself experiencing radical reconstruction. Although textbooks and recitations often controlled school teaching, intellectual thinkers like Rousseau, Pestalozzi, and Froebel had offered fresh insights into the essence of childhood and the schooling of girls.

Throughout his seminal work, Emile, the French philosopher Rousseau expounded a philosophy of natural education under which children were liberated from restrictive societal conventions. Notwithstanding Rousseau's insistence on the independence of children, Montessori considered much to be doubted in the theories of Rousseau, particularly his romantic belief that children learn better by pursuing their desires and urges in an unstructured natural world. Swiss educator Johann Heinrich Pestalozzi (1774–1827) established an instructional philosophy that encouraged classrooms to be turned into homely environments where children feel socially comfortable and learned with the use of their senses through specially crafted interactive lessons. Pestalozzi's focus on learning by experience and engaging with objects was a precursor in Montessori's emphatic practice. Of the three educators, Montessori was more frequently associated and contrasted with the kindergarten author, the German educator Friedrich Froebel (1782–1852).

Like Montessori, Froebel had introduced the notion that early childhood education would take place in a specially designed environment, kindergarten, or "child's garden." According to Froebel, a follower of idealistic theory, children were born with inner divine forces that flourished in an educational setting that promoted learning through self-activity and the unique use of perfect tools. By advocating the integrity and equality of children, she noticed that Rousseau, Pestalozzi, and Froebel had focused on a spiritual understanding of youth rather than an empirical one. They had deduced what it is like to be an infant by introspecting their childhood memories and had extended these beliefs to include all of childhood. Wild romanticism by Rousseau had overlooked the need for a formal learning atmosphere for the boy. The focus Pestalozzi put on utilizing objects as the foundation for learning was too rigid, repetitive, and automatic, though on the right track. Froebel's nursery was so steeped in metaphysical idealism that it was not rooted in contemporary psychology and research. Although acknowledging the achievements of her contemporaries, Montessori will correct their deficiencies by shifting clinically for her theories on the instructional approach to the direct evaluation of children. Around the same period as Montessori had agreed to establish a science-oriented pedagogy in Italy, educators were gaining fresh ideas into schooling elsewhere in the world. In the U.S., innovative educators have been implementing modern teaching approaches.

While Dewey's theory was focused on relativism, Montessori concentrated on universals. The prominent radical William Heard Kilpatrick (1871–1965) became an early and staunch opponent of Montessori.

Kilpatrick adapted Dewey's analytical theory to his widely famous system of projecting. Kilpatrick would fault Montessori for being out-of-date and ineffective in the socializing and imagination areas of the kid. In early childhood education, these radical educators — Parker, Dewey, Kilpatrick — who would become influential forces in American educational philosophy were following a different direction than Montessori's. The socialists tended to emphasize the school as an emerging, socially responsible community in which children studied in a permissive setting utilizing the empirical method. The progressives, calling enthusiastically for democracy in education, denied the role of absolute principles and urged freedom and activity. Montessori's philosophy of schooling will vary from that of the American progressives, with its focus on studying in a formal setting using didactic content.

Even Europe has developed yet another significant way of looking at childhood. In Vienna, Sigmund Freud (1856–1939), through his formulation of psychoanalytic psychology, began to understand the role performed by the abnormal through human growth and development.31 Like Rousseau, Pestalozzi, and Froebel had proposed, youth, Freud realized, was more than accidental liberation and imitative play. It was more than an opportunity to become political actors in an open-ended culture, as advocated by Dewey, Kilpatrick, and the American progressives. Freud's theories have begun to reshape the creation of the existence of babies. To him, early childhood was a period of erotic desires and social deprivation that formed the mind of the human being and had implications for the identity of adults. The "Oedipus complex" was a Freud hypothesis established regarding infant anatomy, in which the child wished to own the opposite sex parent. Freud claimed children are moving through a series of phases of psychosexual development. When at some single period, the infant became over gratified or repressed, so at that point the attitude would become set. The way needs were fulfilled or prevented had implications for the self-esteem of the individual and financial, social, and sexual relationships. Lingering unresolved issues and disputes that arise throughout the developmental phases may trigger issues of internal health and transition during a person's existence. Psychoanalytical treatment was a process by which the problem was established, embedded in the subconscious, and brought to awareness. The individual may identify the problem in this way, analyze it and solve it.

There were several similarities in their career choices, which Freud and Montessori took. Like Montessori, Freud was a pediatric student who then went on to psychiatry, treating psychiatric disorders and specialized in neurology. Montessori and Freud also have come up with a philosophy on infant growth. Freud schooled in the United States, as did Montessori.

Freud and Montessori were mindful of the opinions on early childhood within themselves. While both Montessori and Freud called for the liberation of infants, their creation philosophies were very different. Montessori dismissed Freud's views about child identity and the long-term importance of subsequent psychological, interpersonal conflict.32 A Biography and Review 13 Around 1904 and 1908; Montessori started to create her own position in the world of education. She lectured on the application of sociology and genetics to education at the University of Rome's Pedagogical Level.

Montessori's push into the world of physiological anthropology was part of a broader growth of science and social science of Italy at the time. In Italy, Cesare Lombroso and Giuseppe Sergi founded the area of physical anthropology. Montessori was acquainted with Lombroso's work on criminal anatomy, which included taking unlawful measures, in particular the size and form of the head and neck, and seeking to generalize the illegal sort to any conclusion. She was most inspired by Sergi, who created the University of Rome's Institute of Experimental Psychology, and with whom she worked. Physical anthropology reflects on the human being's biological research as a natural organism; it utilizes analytical methods to calculate, chart, and analyze individual anatomical and morphological differences. The subfield, anthropometry, tests the physical features of people using different instruments.

Montessori expanded schooling into the area of physiological anthropology. In particular, she emphasized the significance of taking accurate physical measurements of children's height, weight, head, pelvis, and limbs as well as identifying some sort of malformations. Such metrics were to be documented regularly as an individualized scientific database, a biographical map to be held for each boy. She focused her lectures on the topics of the empirical approach to pedagogy, the proper methods of scientifically studying both dysfunctional and average children, the science evidence collection and analysis techniques, and how this anthropological knowledge could be used to generalize instructional approaches.

Montessori, a renowned educator, established a reputation among the learners because of her strongly inspired and enthusiastic presentations. Because she was able to draw from a range of fields, from nursing to sociology to psychology, she offered her students an extraordinary multidisciplinary scope of knowledge at the time. Drawing from her history resources in nursing, neuroscience, and (their new interest) sociology. She presented her lectures as L'Antropolgia Pedagogica (Pedagogical Anthropology), a book that incorporates concepts from clinical science, infant psychology, and cultural anthropology and extended them to the growth and education of children. What was starting to arise at this point in Montessori's creation as an instructional thinker was a systematic philosophy of schooling derived from various academic areas. She demonstrated her habit of taking a holistic and multidisciplinary approach to teaching by drawing components from her background in medicine, psychology, and anthropology (their latest interest).

About Casa Die Bambini

The Casa Dei Bambini, a significant opportunity in the profession of Montessori, came in 1907 when Edoardo Talamo requested her to create a school in Rome's slum town. At the time, Talamo was managing director of the Istituto Romano di Beni Stabili (the Strong Building Association), a charitable organization founded to enhance poor people's housing conditions. The association bought and remodeled run-down, overcrowded, and unsanitary tenements in the area. It has been engaged in housing reconstruction in the quarter of San Lorenzo, a part of Rome plagued by violence. The invitation Talamo made to Montessori was an effort to address a very realistic question. When parents who resided in redeveloped housing went to college, their children were left alone and unsupervised in kindergarten. For these babies, the association agreed to create the school as some kind of daycare center.

Nevertheless, Montessori has already had the ability to build a school that will act as a classroom for exploring her theories. John Dewey, too, was researching his theoretical theories at the University of Chicago Laboratory

School is much more desirable conditions. In both educators' situations, such educational studies will create their identities as leading educators.

On January 6, 1907, Montessori founded her first kindergarten, the Casa Dei Bambini, or Children's Home, in a large property on Via Dei Marsi 58, in the poverty-ridden district of San Lorenzo, Rome. Her first pupils were fifty students, between the ages of three and seven, whose families resided in the house. The district of San Lorenzo, a deprived slum town, was similar to those found in Europe and America's growing big cities. Just like Montessori, on the west side of Chicago, Jane Addams, the influential American social worker, had designed a settlement house for the needy, Hull Home. The Casa Dei Bambini and the Hull House were but two of the attempts by philanthropic and educational means to relieve the suffering of the needy.

In post-Risorgimento Italy, internal migration brought to cities like Milan and Rome, in pursuit of jobs, large flowing waves of former peasants. Tenement districts emerged in these cities to accommodate the urban underclass. This subset in an urban environment was ill prepared for life. Montessori named the squalid conditions — crime and vice — they witnessed a dark "land of darkness" in the San Lorenzo district. Despite such modern solutions to urban schooling as the American "Project Head Start" for approximately one hundred years, Montessori recognized the critical significance that early childhood education provided for eventual progress. In the case of children impacted by poverty, they needed to receive the kind of knowledge, which could bring them out of the cycle of deprivation. She found the school to be the original microcosmic history and a 15th Study attempt at a greater endeavor to bring about societal change by way of schooling. Montessori's broad awareness of the essence of social progress and its connection to education put her among the early twentieth century's leading social reformers.

Montessori was driven in establishing the Casa Dei Bambini by the sociological and educational goals she had set throughout the different stages of her life. Located inside the tenement, in which the families of the children stayed, the school was to serve as a crucial organic bridge between schooling and community, embodied by the teachers. Not only was her approach a way of teaching children more humanely and efficiently, but it was meant to help the poor inhabitants of San Lorenzo recover socially. Unlike Jane Addams, Montessori argued that in contemporary life, like in the earlier traditional definition of welfare, help should no longer be in the way of providing alms to the needy.

In the past, assistance was provided to support the victims of deprivation and sickness through well-intentioned people. Montessori argued in the modern era, with its rapid urbanization and industrialization, that the idea of private charity had to be rethought and developed into a more systematic and oriented effort to bring about social reform. If more extensive, more organized, and expected efforts were made to eliminate poverty sectors such as San Lorenzo, Montessori worried that there would be a great divide in modern society, a wide chasm dividing rich and poor. Unless the pattern persisted, the disadvantaged would be trapped in poverty-ridden ghettoes, which Montessori named "islands of the oppressed." The principles of welfare had to be rebuilt in the new period not just to bring temporary relief to the needy, but also to alleviate the circumstances that induced social and economic deprivation. By establishing existing programs to deter sickness, enhance health and sanitation, inform children and adults, and transform culture, human welfare had to be socialized. Montessori believed that such government institutions will boost the standard of living, be more productive than unorganized community actions, promote economic growth, and render citizens autonomous of the dole.

The Children's House was built educationally to be a school-home, an educational entity in near proximity to the families of infants. In reality, it was in the house where the kids lived. Montessori said, "We brought the school inside the building. The school would lead to the socialization of the family and the household, which would in effect, bind the household with the greater community. The real geographical proximity of the children's home to the school had a social aspect linked to Montessori's concept of the "modern woman" of the twentieth century. Casa Dei Bambini was situated in a region of the working class where the majority of mothers employed in the emerging factories of Italy. However, Montessori proposed that in the future, not only working-class women should be hired outside the home, but also more people of all social backgrounds should enter the workplace. The guiding force in bringing about this shift in women's employment was industrialization and technical progress. Schools, as educational bodies, had to recognize this technology-driven transition to cater for working mother children. Schools like the Casa Dei Bambini would encourage mothers to leave their children comfortably and "begin their research with a feeling of great relief and independence." Despite the change in working habits and places, Montessori suggested that mothers would still have a greater obligation for the physical and moral treatment of their children. The Casa Dei Bambini would assist them in serving these parental duties when finding work and leisure beyond their home.40 Montessori then had many reasons in mind while creating the Casa Dei Bambini, the precursor of all present Montessori schools: first, the social and economic motivations of social reform, in particular, the enhancement of the working class's condition; second, third, the social and economic motives of social change; The Casa Dei Bambini, however, was mainly a venue for the education of children; establishing a social utopia was not a concept, nor was it merely a hub for daycare of children for working mothers. It provided schooling, as the new school for the modern age, based on the principles of scientific pedagogy.

One of Montessori's key pedagogical ideals was that instruction with children in a disciplined and organized setting was best accomplished. She requested that any specific rules extend to children attending her school and their guardians. The children were supposed to come to school with clean bodies and clothing, no matter how dirty they were. They must have been given a white dress or apron. Believing schools were most successful when closely related to the families and homes of the students, parents were encouraged to be involved in and endorse the education of their children and attend regular conferences, called "parent-directress" meetings (to be discussed below).

Like John Dewey from the University of Chicago Experimental School, Montessori made sure that the practical structures, desks, seats, and apparatuses of the school were tailored to the needs of children rather than adults. She did not want to limit the freedom of expression of the children in the classroom and its furniture, as it did in traditional schools. Tables and chairs were designed to match the heights and weights of the students. Washstands were placed for smaller children to reach. Classrooms were filled with small cupboards where kids could quickly access didactic materials and be liable for taking them back to their proper location. The Montessori school was built to foster the sensory sensitivity and manual ability of children, give them a degree of option within a controlled atmosphere, create a climate of order, and improve independence and self-assurance in performing skills.

Montessori's understanding of the teacher's position differed from conventional schools. While teachers in traditional elementary schools dominated the middle of the instructional stage as the focal point for the interest of the students, Montessori called her instructor a "directress" who was to lead the students while they learned themselves to understand. The director, a properly trained instructor in the Montessori system, was to instruct the children in their own self-development.41 Skilled in children's health assessment and science pedagogy, the director was to be attentive to infant preparation and developmental phases. With its correct apparatus and resources, she was to develop the prepared atmosphere and cooperate in the self-education of the children.

1.2 Need of Montessori & Its Benefits

Before this chapter discusses the need of Montessori and why it was important for it to form, below is a brief introduction of what the Montessori is about.

From The American Montessori Society: The Montessori Philosophy of Schooling, founded by Dr. Maria Montessori, is an instructional methodology focusing on children from infancy to maturity focused on empirical findings. Dr. Montessori's Approach has been studied over decades, with more than 100 years of global popularity in different societies.

It is a perception of the individual as one who is instinctively excited about the information and willing to facilitate learning in a positive, thoughtfully planned learning environment. This is a philosophy that respects the human soul, and the entire child's development — physical, financial, mental, cognitive.

Montessori schooling provides resources for our children to grow their talents when they venture out into the world when dedicated, knowledgeable, conscientious, and compassionate people with awareness and reverence that learning is for life.

Any child is regarded as a unique adult. Montessori teaching acknowledges that children work in many contexts, and adapts to these forms of learning. Students are often able to study at their own rate, always moving when they are ready through the program, directed by the instructor, and an individualized learning plan. Montessori students start at an early age and build discipline, communication, focus, and freedom. Classroom architecture, facilities, and day-to-day activities help the evolving "self-regulation" of the person (capacity to teach one's self, and care about what one is learning), by adolescents. Students are part of a community that is close and caring. A family dynamic is re-created by the multi-age classroom — typically lasting three years. Older students value status as leaders and role models; newer pupils feel encouraged by the obstacles ahead and develop trust. Teachers are demonstrating empathy, love kindness, and a belief in the successful settlement of the dispute. Students of Montessori practice equality inside the limits. Operating under guidelines established by their professors, students are actively interested in determining what their learning emphasis should be. Montessorians believe that intrinsic happiness stimulates the imagination and excitement of the infant and results in happy, life-long learning that is lasting. Students are motivated to become successful aspirants of information. Teachers have areas in which students are granted the opportunity and opportunities to answer their own concerns.

Self-correction or self-assessment form an integral part of the Montessori approach to the classroom. When students mature, they continue to look objectively at their work and learn from their experiences and understand, evaluate, and improve. Montessori students are positive, active, self-directed learners with the freedom and encouragement to inquire, to explore deeply, and to create connections. They should think creatively, function collaboratively, and behave courageously — an ability set for the 21st century.

1.1   The Traditional Method vs. Montessori Method

Montessori is distinct from conventional education in areas relevant to the future Mainstream Curriculum promotes a one-size-fits-all method to instruction, which sees the infant as a blank canvas to compose on.

The instructor offers the learners information. Rote memorization of information is prevalent in many mainstream classrooms, where kids are sitting at a desk gleaning whatever info they can from the instructor standing at the front of the room. The classroom at Montessori is a "prepared atmosphere," which promotes individual development and learning. Kids will travel across the space to select from a wide variety of crafted materials placed on well-organized shelves. We develop practical and analytical skills by independently studying vocabulary, arithmetic, geography, astronomy, painting, music, and more. Parents new to Montessori's environment often remember how peaceful the classroom is, how great it sounds, and how centered the kids are. This is because they are focused on the learning "job."

So, among the first questions that pop up with many parents when selecting their children's nursery or daycare is whether they will go for one that follows the Montessori system or one that incorporates a play-based methodology. Here are some of the main differences — and what else you can think before you make your choice.

Maria Montessori dig upon the Montessori Theory of Education in the early 1900s. Montessori has a deep belief in human development. She created a modern approach to education focused on her study of children from diverse ethnic, religious, and socioeconomic backgrounds. It was fast expanding too many nations and continents. The First Montessori School in Canada began in 1912, and there are more than 500 in the world today.

Montessori schools believe play is the job of a child. Their services are geared at adolescents, promoting positive, self-paced, individualized learning. Children pick tasks for continuous periods, focused on their preferences and "jobs." Teachers monitor and chart their development, to allow their usage of resources simpler. Via this strategy, children are assumed to become more comfortable, more autonomous, more self-regulated, and more self-disciplined.

Whereas, play-centered traditional schools are focused on the idea that children learn better by practice. Although the playtime is open-ended and unfocused, these pre-schools can be more teacher-directed. Children engage in a broad range of activity-based events, including pretending to play, and teachers respond with learning lessons. In fact, children are improving their problem-solving, teamwork, dispute management, and social skills.

Both Montessori and play-based pre-schools should provide cultures that are inclusive and carefully planned. Usually, Montessori pre-schools are split into five learning areas: English, arithmetic, daily life, sensory, and cultural. Play-oriented centers may often be grouped into events or themes centered areas or stations.

Carol Anne Wien, a retired Montessori instructor and professor emeritus from the School of Education at York University in Toronto, states a significant institutional difference: "Modern school settings seem to be strongly time-oriented — whether you realize what time it's, you realize what the kids are doing — but it's poorly spatially oriented. Montessori is the reverse: very spatially organized and poorly defined in time. When you know where the kids are in the house, you know what they are doing, so it is free time. Teachers prefer to switch between making the kids play and performing instructional exercises in play-based childcare. "Montessori settings appear to be simpler, calmer, and less intense than activity-based settings, which some kids might consider too noisy, bright, or high-stimulus, Wien says. She says, "Look for a peaceful atmosphere, one in which the color comes from the kids and their games and drawings, no matter what sort of pre-school you want. Be very vigilant of an atmosphere overflowing with red, yellow and blue, and big, heavy amounts of print or animated figures, and so on, as they are very physically disturbing for the infant and can wear the infant out.

The Advantages

A major advantage for Montessori is that the child is engaged at his own speed and time, "says Wien, adding the children can are overwhelmed in a convention." Kids often appear to become strongly self-regulated in Montessori systems. That's a major benefit, as it's called, at this point, a huge requirement for school success — not intellect but the capacity to self-regulate. "(Self-regulation implies how easily an individual returns to a stable state after experiencing stress.)

In play-based environments, Wien says, children's imaginations can really thrive, and so their social skills can thrive, such as creating friendships and working through things. "These are both all good stuff. I might suggest that Montessori had little likelihood of tolerating abstract or creative activity. In a play-based child care facility, which is also a successful path to self-regulation, you can have more socio-dramatic activity. "The temperament and attitude of your child will affect your choice. Some kids do best at one or the other environment. "When you have a really busy little boy who likes to play aircraft and create with bricks, I will place him in a play-based system," Wien says. "When you have a timid kid that holds back, and you're not sure what they're involved in, I'd place them in a Montessori system where they have this warm, warm setting that will bring them out in ways you haven't seen before." Making the decision Note, both Montessori and play centers help children train for kindergarten and cultivate a love of learning, so they both have to stick with the laws. All ideologies may also deliver excellent systems and poor ones — you cannot judge only by theory.

In reality, Wien would not prescribe that parents automatically chose between nursery or daycare based on play and Montessori. "The key criteria is to go to the core to search for the consistency of the relationships between educators to adolescents, the educators and each other, and the parents, of course," she says. "It is going to inform the parent whether they choose to put their child in the system."

Differences between Montessori and Pre-school

It is a huge choice to determine the right way to take your kid to nursery or kindergarten. When you want to determine where he or she is most likely to succeed, there are one million things to weigh. Education choices and styles vary in certain places, rendering the choice more complicated, in several respects. A Montessori School is one way out there. However, how precisely is a school like a Montessori renowned for its radical practices separate from a conventional kindergarten or pre-school? Below are some of the key variations.

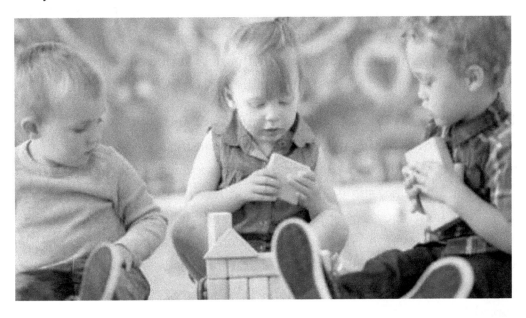

Mixed-age classroom

In a conventional kindergarten, by a certain cutoff date (typically September 1), each infant in the classroom should have had his or her fifth birthday, which ensures that at the beginning of the year every kid in the classroom should be 5, with some turning six throughout the school year.

Montessori colleges also, though, have mixed generation classes. A school for kindergartens involves children aged 3-6. She is the Fountainhead Montessori School Coordinator in Dublin, California. She has worked with Montessori for six years and takes her children to a Montessori school. According to her, one advantage of the mixed-age classroom is that it offers an opportunity for older children to be members. "On a regular basis, I see older students saying 'stand back and wait' to younger students and the older student talking to the younger student." Besides the trust that this would certainly offer the older pupil, it is also a means of showing knowledge of the material and ensuring it has been maintained. The younger child is confident hearing from someone they can respond easily to.

Individualization

Individualized schooling is today one of the buzzwords of the curriculum. About every education-from the most conservative to the most modern-claims to deliver individualized instruction, but it does not often happen in reality. In addition, individualization differs in degree.

However, Montessori schools are built on, and stick to, a belief in individualization in education. All is handled at the speed of the infant with the idea that any kid on his or her own period reaches milestones. "We are bringing a kid as he/she is at present and having them navigate a growth path," says her. "They develop their abilities at their own rate." In a place of their choosing, even a child will understand. "You should sit at the desk here, lie on a mat, or walk about the classroom easily," She says. "There are resources accessible to support children to discover what makes them feel relaxed."

Hands-On

There would be hands-on exercises in a typical nursery or kindergarten classroom because educators understand the desire to include children. Yet as to the degree to which hands-on instruction is used, Montessori varies from conventional schooling. According to her, "Everything is really real and hands-on in a Montessori [classroom]." There is the intention to include as many senses as possible in learning. The hands-on learning in a pre-school or kindergarten in Montessori may look more like playing and or having fun to the kid, but it is purposive.

Therefore, Which One is Right for Your Child

Although she says that every child with a Montessori capacity will succeed, she refers to inspiration as providing a boost to the students. "The students who are performing especially well are inspired emotionally," she says.

Certain characteristics also improve the likelihood of a pupil at a Montessori school to excel. Children of a Montessori school would want to cooperate, socialize, and work on their own continue to perform well. When it comes to kindergarten students, standards about these kinds of items are fewer. "Younger students at our school are also forming the characteristics that will benefit them, and they get more support than those at the upper grades," She says. "At the end of the day, the Montessori curriculum is intended to function best for all children because it is child-friendly." The Bottom Line While a Montessori school is distinct from a conventional system; certain common concepts do apply. Those involve a passion for studying, the inculcation of knowledge to help children excel, and moral accountability. The expectations revolve around four characteristics at a Montessori school: discipline, focus, teamwork, and freedom. "When such characteristics can be inculcated by children, they will adapt them to everything that they do and be effective," says her.

Understanding that there are several choices when you decide what sort of school to send your child too. You will find a system with persistence and dedication that will encourage your kid to achieve his / her ability.

How to Choose Between Montessori and Preschool:

If you have all the details before you, the problem then is, what pre-school is right for your child? Although many parents assume that school is a one-size fit all incentives, the fact is that each child has various talents, various shortcomings and all should value specific forms of learning that. Montessori's similarities over conventional education are numerous. However, in educational theory alone, the option, which is right for a single child, does not always lie. Ask yourself these questions while trying to distinguish between a conventional pre-school classroom and a Montessori classroom:

1. What Was The Purpose Of My Sending To Pre-School?

The target for some parents is to find childcare, which also requires necessary social and academic skills such as counting, colors, and sharing. It is a feature in other typical classes at the nursery. Pre-school is an opportunity for other parents to recognize and develop a passion for learning and adventure that can take them into their academic years. Such guardians, in other terms, perceive the nursery as the gateway to years of academic achievement. That is where childhood Montessori fits in.

2. What kind of environment will benefit my child?

Modern classrooms in the nursery are also noted for vivid colors, lights, and the hustle and bustle of large children's groups at play. Colors become more subdued in a Montessori classroom, and natural light provides the children with the "hot" feeling when they know. Children's play is their "job" in both instances, although the conventional pre-school stresses imaginative play as a way of learning and development. At the same time, Montessori encourages creative tasks that are often intellectual, such as blocks of the wooden alphabet or learning to tie a shoe.

3. Who I Have My Child Attend Before Preschool Of School?

The Montessori approach of education is structured for the expectation that children should arrive at age 3 — or perhaps earlier — and then develop through many years through the curriculum. While certain schools may welcome older children, Montessori schools usually avoid enrolling high school-age children in their systems because they did not first take part in a pre-school Montessori curriculum. This is because it is harder for younger learners who have no previous learning encounters to adjust to the Montessori way of doing stuff.

On the other side, a conventional pre-school classroom is arranged to mimic the typical classes that would be met by children during their college life, irrespective of the school they attend. A traditional nursery, unlike Montessori, is not suitable for educating children before they enter primary school.

4. What Does My Child Need?

The last question welcomes the views and opinions on the three previous issues. There are benefits and drawbacks to all styles of services that it boils down to the kids. All certified, credible pre-school services share the aim of developing your child, training her for kindergarten, and fostering a love of learning. They are governed by the government of the State and responsible for the requirements it establishes.

Every kid has multiple talents, specific difficulties, and different learning styles. What encourages and encourages one child may annoy or shame another child. Although the mainstream curriculum is built with a one-size-fits-all mindset, no one-size-fits-all child exists. Stop and look around when you are trying to decide between Montessori or the traditional pre-school. Where do you want your child to thrive? And what would be of more value to them as they grow? The response to that query is, in the end, everything you need.

Montessori Teachers

One of the most noticeable distinctions between Montessori teachers and conventional teachers is the tremendous trust Montessori teachers put in the children's cognitive ability. To "follow the kid" requires an enormous amount of confidence. It is so much better to tell the kids, follow where I am going so that no one gets lost. Nonetheless, with close monitoring and preparation, Montessori instructors are continuously alert to growing child's progress and are working diligently to help them excel.

Teachers at Montessori are not the object of concern in the classroom. Their job centers on planning and arranging learning resources to match the Montessori children's needs and interests. The emphasis is on educating students, not training teachers.

As a mentor and facilitator, the Montessori instructor develops a well-prepared Montessori setting and an environment of learning and inquisitiveness intended to shift pupils from one experience and stage to the next. An instructor from Montessori also stands back as the kids work, encouraging them to benefit from their own experiences and come to their conclusions. Instead of presenting solutions to students, the Montessori instructor tells them if they can fix the issue, effectively engage students in the learning process, and develop clear thinking skills. For certain situations, rather than the tutor, children learn primarily from the environment, often from other youngsters.

Dr. Montessori claimed the instructor would concentrate on the infant as an individual rather than on the preparations for the everyday classes. While for each child, the Montessori instructor schedules regular lessons, she must be alert to shifts in the child's motivation, development, attitude, and actions.

The topics are interwoven, and the instructor of Montessori must be simple to explain and appreciate the works of literature, poetry, music, education, astronomy, zoology, botany, chemistry, physical geography, writing, physics, geometry, and physical existence. The tutor at Montessori is qualified to give one-on-one or small community lessons and to spend less time delivering big group lessons. The lectures are short and precise, designed to inspire children's minds such that they can come back and know all about themselves. Montessori lectures rely on the most critical knowledge, which the children need to perform the work:

- the name of the products

- where they can be placed in the classroom and on the table
- how to use the items
- In addition, what to do with them.

Teachers at Montessori become kid technology observers. They do not use bonuses and penalties for positive or weak jobs. Teachers at Montessori never criticize or intervene with the education of a pupil. It is only in a comfortable environment that the personality of a child has space to develop. Children must have the right to select their hobbies and experience unlimited conduct. Dr. Montessori assumed that this was a specific task and that the kid should show his / her true self after he/she had found a position demanding complete focus. In The Absorbent Mind (pp. 277-81), Maria Montessori, in the Montessori classroom, gave several basic standards of behavior to students. The teacher is an atmosphere keeper and custodian. She attends to that rather than being disturbed by the restlessness of the babies. All the equipment is carefully kept in place, in good shape, elegant and polished. This means the instructor must always be orderly and safe, calm, and dignified. Thus, the first responsibility of the instructor is to look over the community, so this takes priority over the others. Its impact is indirect, so there can be no successful and lasting consequences of any sort, physical, mental, or spiritual unless it is performed correctly.

In A Way of Learning (1973), Anne Burke Neubert identified the following elements in the Montessori teacher's specific role:

- Montessori teachers are the relational connection between the children and the Prepared Environment.

- They track their students regularly and perceive their needs.

- They continually explore, change the atmosphere to fulfill their expectations of the needs and desires of each child, and critically mention the outcome.

- They plan an atmosphere intended to promote the individuality of children and the freedom to openly choose work we consider appealing, select tasks that would cater to their preferences and maintain the setting in good shape, attach to it and withdraw materials when appropriate.

- Every day, they systematically examine the quality of their research and environmental architecture.

- They track and appraise the individual development of a growing boy.

- They admire the freedom of their pupils and defend it. They need to learn when to reach in to impose boundaries or offer a helping hand, and when it is in the better interest of a child to stand back and not intervene.

- They are welcoming, giving increasing child comfort, protection, security, and non-judgmental acceptance.

- They promote children's contact and help children understand how to express their feelings to adults.

- For parents, school workers, and the neighborhood, they view the success of the children and their performance in the classroom. They provide the children with straightforward, engaging, and valuable lessons. They seek to stimulate the child's curiosity and concentrate on environmental lessons and practices.

- They model positive behavior for the students, observing the class's ground rules, demonstrating a sense of calmness, integrity, dignity, and courtesy and displaying consideration for each child.

- They are the educators of harmony, working diligently to teach courteous attitudes and confrontation.

- They are diagnostic practitioners who can categorize patterns of growth, development, and behavior to better understand the children and make required referrals and suggestions for parents.

Have Trust

Montessori teachers recognize that parents will be "in the know" without needing to be at the forefront through diligent study and properly planned settings.

One of Montessori's most significant contrasts with conventional teachers is the direction the instructor perceives the infant. You may have learned that Montessori instructors "ignore the kid." Yet what you do not know is the degree of confidence (in the infant) it takes to step in and allow the child to truly take the lead. With youngsters, it is the normal tendency of the individual to assume a leadership position. Like little ducklings following our guide, we want to hold children in line securely. This way, we learn (or think we know) where everyone is and what they do. Yet Montessori instructors recognize that adults will stay "in the know," without needing to be at the forefront, through diligent attention and an adequately planned setting.

Teachers at Montessori are not the subject of the classroom. The emphasis is then on the kid getting the best experiences and resources to improve his or her learning. It is known and acknowledged in a Montessori classroom that a child will and should relax and focus until he seeks the correct "job." As Montessori put it, "the instructor will assume that this child can demonstrate his true nature to her when he discovers a piece of work that interests him. In addition, what would she have to watch out for? "This is the inventor's or discoverer's work, the explorer's valiant actions" This is not to imply that the Montessori instructor does not play an essential role in the education of the child. On the opposite, the position of the teacher as a guide is essential. I think of the instructor of Montessori as a Sherpa, a mentor whose indispensable help helps every little adventurer to achieve his unique zenith.

"But when work is the product of an inherent inner emotion; it takes a different form. Such research is exciting, addictive, and elevates man beyond deviations and contradictions inside. This is the inventor or discoverer's job, the explorer's valiant actions, or the artist's creations, that is, the work of people born with such remarkable strength that they may rediscover the characteristics of their race in the forms of their own uniqueness. ~D. Maria Montessori: The Childhood Code.

The Montessori instructor plans the environment (i.e., the classroom) based on each child's diligent and consistent observations. Therefore, the classroom offers learning resources that involve the infant in a developmentally acceptable way. The instructor can step back, enabling them to learn at their own speed, while the children are engaged in their activity of choice. At this level, the instructor does not need to have inspiration. The children are motivated by a desire to learn inside themselves.

"And then we learned that teaching is not something that the instructor does but a normal phenomenon that naturally occurs in the human person. This is not learned by listening to phrases, but by interactions through which the infant acts on his or her surroundings. The responsibility of the teacher is not to speak, but to plan and organize a set of reasons for cultural interaction in a specific atmosphere that is designed for the infant. "~ Dr. Maria Montessori, The Absorbent Mind

The first step is so frail, so delicate that contact will cause it to vanish again, like a soap bubble, and with it, all goes the Teachers from small group lessons as they pass across the classroom, and not just one lesson in front of the whole class. Lessons are realistic, simple, and designed to engage the child in order to pursue the exploration on its own. The Montessori instructor stands back after the child is engaged, and refrains from criticizing, complimenting, or even intervening in any way.

1.3 Montessori Education Today

It's been about 100 years that Dr. Maria Montessori began interacting with kids, but the research and impact of her career has changed our view of the kids and how they interact with the environment around them. Today, licensed Montessori schools around the globe are following the mission of Dr. Montessori, filled by Montessori-certified educators named 'guides' They strive to serve the entire child, helping children become competent, confident, interactive learners at all stages of growth. About a century later, the experience and ideology of her life help us appreciate how children are the secret to a more tranquil planet.

Luckily the Montessori process has survived over time, also included in numerous colleges. This supports games and children's freedom and individuality, as well as engagement to awaken fascination with varied components. In brief, it reaps the innate tendency of children for games and enjoyment, rendering it the key instructional motor.

However, the panorama shifts as we immerse ourselves in modern primary education. Kids spend hours paying proper attention to their instructors, getting disciplined for not communicating (or being criticized for doing so), being reluctant to talk, and trying to be vigilant for lengthy stretches. One class comes ahead of another. This specializes in stripping away all underlying learning incentives.

Several schools have opted for the Montessori system. Given all that, there is always some uncertainty. Is the Montessori approach not accessible to children aged between 0 and 6? While several schools still provide this approach even to this age range, the reality is that it was developed by Maria Montessori so that it could be implemented before she was 12 years old. Also, implement the Montessori approach can, however, at a high school level. Maria Montessori did leave some proven guidelines for the steps to be followed with older children, although she did not have time to plan and refine it entirely for this level. The existing method of schooling depends a lot on the classes. Therefore, a lot of responsibility is exerted on students to accomplish assignments that would contribute to a desirable final score. The reverse is what the Montessori approach wants. There are no tests and no assignments since the key aim is to know and not get the highest score. The evidence shows us that the schooling following primary school unsettles the pupils. Far from making them excited, it lets them realize that going to school is pointless. This condition will have an opportunity to rethink the way we teach. Competitiveness is nurtured today. Students of degrees mark as incompetent or wise. The primary aim, however, is to make students feel inspired to learn the environment around them.

Chapter 2: Understanding Montessori Curriculum for Raising Responsible & Curious Toddlers

The Montessori Philosophy of Schooling, founded by Dr. Maria Montessori, is an instructional methodology focusing on children from infancy to maturity focused on empirical findings. Dr. Montessori's Approach has been studied over decades, with more than 100 years of global popularity in different societies.

It is a perception of the individual as one who is instinctively excited about the information and willing to facilitate learning in a positive, thoughtfully planned learning environment. This is a philosophy that respects the human soul, and the entire child's development — physical, financial, mental, cognitive. Montessori schooling provides resources for our children to grow their talents when they venture out into the world when dedicated, knowledgeable, conscientious, and compassionate people with awareness and reverence that learning is for life.

2.1 The Montessori Curriculum

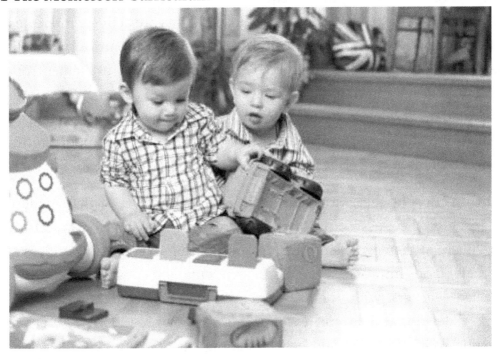

Every child is regarded as a unique adult. Montessori teaching acknowledges that children work in many contexts, and adapts to these forms of learning. Students are often able to study at their rate, always moving when they are ready through the program, directed by the instructor, and an individualized learning plan. Montessori students start at an early age and build discipline, communication, focus, and freedom. Classroom architecture, facilities, and day-to-day activities help the evolving "self-regulation" of the person (capacity to teach one's self, and care about what one is learning), by adolescents.

Students are part of a community that is close and caring. A family dynamic is re-created by the multi-age classroom — typically lasting three years. Older students value status as leaders and role models; newer pupils feel encouraged by the obstacles ahead and develop trust. Teachers are demonstrating empathy, love kindness, and a belief in the successful settlement of the dispute.

Students of Montessori practice equality inside the limits. Operating under guidelines established by their professors, students are actively interested in determining what their learning emphasis should be. Montessorians believe that intrinsic happiness stimulates the imagination and excitement of the infant and results in happy, life-long learning that is lasting. Students are motivated to become successful aspirants of information. Teachers have areas in which students are granted the opportunity and opportunities to answer their own concerns.

Self-correction or self-assessment form an integral part of the Montessori approach to the classroom. When students mature, they continue to look objectively at their work and learn from their experiences and understand, evaluate, and improve. Montessori students are positive, active, self-directed learners with the freedom and encouragement to inquire, to explore deeply, and to create connections. They should think creatively, function collaboratively, and behave courageously — an ability set for the 21st century.

Montessori Philosophy: Put Children First

On the theory of Montessori, they are not simply little people. They are young, and they deserve consideration in their own way and for whom they belong. This indicates, among other aspects, that they will be given the ability to read and gain trust in doing so, in developmentally acceptable ways. Maria Montessori has conducted hundreds of children's work. This ignited some observations in the way they trained. And, over time, it prompted her to believe that children would be put at the education center.

Since conception to age six, the Curriculum Children develop the foundation and identity they will have for the remainder of their lives. Because in this growth, creativity and fantasy play key roles, children require actual, factual facts to construct the framework and character with. Of that purpose, the program of Fountainhead Montessori is focused on fact. That ensures teachers use realistic — also science — vocabulary and resources as much as practicable. Animals are researched within their natural habitats, for example. They are not behaving to people, and they are not wearing clothing. Literature may be enjoyable and amusing, sometimes crazy, but it does not have fairies or super-heroes. Fantasy at Fountainhead can come from the imagination of a child, but the instructor should not force it on the boy. Beliefs and a legacy of customs and legends are valued as things better left to the kin. The Montessori Approach program involves realistic life activities, tactile tools, language (writing and reading), mathematics, and cultural topics.

Realistic Life Experiments ("Help Me Do It by Myself")

Realistic Life activities are the cornerstone of the Montessori educational theory. They include the "motifs for action" that constructively canalize the normal stimulation need of the infant. Practical life experiments are discrete units of research consisting of resources that the infant is likely to encounter in the usage of the everyday world. Each human job must be colorful, appealing, and linked to one of four key fields of its use: Motion control and coordination. Environmental care lessons to learn how to pump, hold, fold, carve, paint, talk, sit, and drive gracefully, etc. Sweeping drills, dusting, cleaning desks, removing drops, watering trees, and so on. Individual love. Exercises to know how to wash faces, shoes, and undress (buttons, zippers, ties, buckles, lacings, bands, safety pins, loops, and eyes), shower, nose blowing, etc. Identified also as Beauty, and Courtesy. Learning to be respectful and compassionate to others, listening to and reacting to other children and adults, taking turns as appropriate, and mirroring the appreciation their teachers and fellow students give them. Even having to walk, stand, and sit respectfully, respectfully preparing things such as meals and demonstrating reverence for the world and those in general.

Realistic life activities include the basic goals of discipline, focus, teamwork, and liberty. As the child is exposed to each operation, executes it by continuous usage, and masters the ability or idea built into the job, these four fundamental elements are simultaneously created. Mastering these skills creates self-confidence by accomplishment pride, and ensures initiative growth.

Dr. Montessori's Sensorial Materials (Educating the Senses) found that by their senses, small children learn knowledge regarding their environment. However, mainstream schooling has traditionally neglected reading or the teaching of the senses. To counter this, Montessori created different apparatuses and practices. Today researchers continue to keep up with Montessori in their debates on the value of sensory integration.

Of such terms as long or short, soft, or light, adults may quickly draw up a visual picture. Children create these abstract comparisons for themselves by using, for example, the red rods, which increase in length from 10 to 100 cm. Dr. Montessori said, "the purpose of the sensory materials is not to provide the infant with new experiences (of scale, form, color, etc.) but to put structure and framework through the numerous experiences that he has already acquired and is still obtaining." In addition to arranging all these sensory impressions, the sensory materials help to organize these impressions. It is incredible to see a four-year-old kid order colorful tiles from deepest red to palest pink because an individual rarely notices the variations in these color gradations. Via this training of the senses, which involves fine motor regulation and hand-eye coordination, and the tactile stimuli along with real-life lessons, the infant is equipped for learning, reading, and mathematics.

Writing and Reading

Dr. Montessori's Language found that children would first begin to write before they learn to read. By breaking down the writing into short, developmentally appropriate activities, young children will quickly learn to write and read. The actual process of writing requires several aspects and is dynamic. The three fingers that support it must carefully balance the writing device; the hand must be able to travel gently over the page, and flexibility must be established to enable the mind to guide the hand to travel accurately. Many of the tasks in the physical existence and tactile fields include as an underlying aim the training of the hand to compose: gripping the knobs of the firm cylinders with the three compose digits, contacting as gently as necessary the rough and smooth surfaces, drawing along the edges and bases of the geometry cabinets, etc. The infant follows the sandpaper letters subtly as he hears the sound of each word, thereby understanding the word phonetically and visually, and transferring it via the sensory mechanism of his muscle memory. He should start constructing basic phonetic words using the mobile alphabet when he learns many letters (a type of mechanical writing — the child normally cannot understand what he has developed at this early stage yet). The other steps involved with writing planning usually accompany writing. It also happens explosively, as the kid accidentally figures out that the letters he has put together really shape a phrase he knows — "f-r-o-g are a frog. I can only understand it! "Then a lengthy time of devouring any term insight accompanies this exploration.

Children at a very early age quickly learn conceptual principles when they are introduced to materials that clearly explain the abstractions they depict. The number rods display the characteristics of "one" to "ten" that no other materials have yet been able to do; sandpaper numbers enable the child to track and understand numerals visually, verbally, and in the muscular-tactile meaning, just as with the letters from the sandpaper. Such things slowly introduce the infant into series numbering; knowing odd and even numbers; the decimal system; principles of addition, subtraction, multiplication, and division; skip numbering (counting in multiples of two, three, etc.); and fractions. In the materials of mathematics, the connection between arithmetic, geometry, and algebra is continually stressed. This base helps children to recognize the role of higher mathematics in later life more readily, and hence they begin to realize its importance for their own lives.

The Children of Sciences have an insatiable interest in the environment around them. The instructor takes advantage of this great learning opportunity by using physiology, zoology, physics, geology, geography, and various world cultures and also history as jumping-off points for environmental and content planning. If the children find a roly-poly bug on the playground, the instructor set up a terrarium with a magnifying glass for a short period to examine the bug before returning it to its natural habitat. From there, the kids might create booklets that explain the roly-poly pieces in exact science terms. This work would combine workflow competencies, design, and writing abilities. Another thing may be to create roly-poly templates in paper or clay. These activities may lead to studying about the variations between roly-polies, which are insects. The instructor may use insect templates for sorting, marking, and counting. And the objects of society are a part of the entire world.

Creativity

The idea of liberty inside boundaries is central to the Montessori process. In this atmosphere, innovation will thrive as children feel secure, valued, and welcomed. A child can explore the possibilities of any material so long as it is used in a manner that does not harm it and is also healthy and respectful of the needs of others.

Knowing the right usage for content stimulates imagination instead of inhibiting it. Much as an artist learns on guitar to create music, and does not use the instrument like a hammer or shield, a child uses red pins, gold beads, scissors, or markers — each object for its own purpose. The professional Montessori instructor is pleased to see a child using a fresh, imaginative content in a meaningful way. Music, sculpture, rhythm, and imagination, excel in each school, along with the Montessori content. Many tasks include different places and hours during the day, but when a child operates "alone, under guidelines," it is also the best time and place for curiosity.

Discipline

Being in a room of many kids and instructors rather than parents provides a child with several different obstacles. In reality, learning to get along in a scenario like this is part of why school is important for young people.

Demonstrate accountability to society by assuming sole responsibility for their actions. In this way, even the principle of justice is created. The children themselves resolve disagreements among children to the fullest degree practicable on the basis of the rules of behavior at school. The teachers will not use corporal punishment, and physical violence by children is not permitted. Teachers work with the implications of an event in both cases, rather than make a judgment about the behavior of the pupil. For example, a conflict about who gets a right to certain content is resolved by the theory that the individual who first chooses the research has the right to use it when completed, without interruption. The instructor may say, "It is now changing to Alice. You could get a change when she puts away the job. Can I give you another piece of work while you wait? "If a child has hurt another infant, he or she is liable for trying to repair the injury to any possible extent — for example, by trying to clean and bandage a wound or by supplying ice for a bruise. The instructor might say, "I can see that Billy is injured. Should we support him? "When an infant makes a mistake, he is liable for clearing it up. The instructor may initially point out the mess and recommend how to clean it up — placing a project back in the box where it belongs or using a sponge to wash a spill. Later, a feeling of obligation in the infant itself triggers the requisite response. The children and teachers express concern for the group by taking moral accountability for their acts.

Development Planes

Montessori's development plans integrated those ideas into a philosophy of child development. Kids advance through four planes during creation, each with distinct physical and psychological evolutions. Consequently, each plane needs the atmosphere to adapt appropriately to deliver suitable learning experiences. The Montessori approach is formulated accordingly based on where the infant is placed in the developmental planes.

Infancy (birth-6 years)

This period is marked by the Sensitive and Absorbent Brain Periods. Those two things function together, creating an unprecedented learning ability. Training is quick and informative. In what is called an involuntary Absorbent Environment, children know through their senses during the first three years of life. Through positive hands-on training, children grow actively throughout the second three years. Learning happens when they can do something alone.

As Dr. Montessori researched the spontaneous engagement of children, she found that children passed through intermittent phases in which they became keenly involved in very particular environmental elements. When children begin increasing stage of growth, new sensitivities emerge and during the first three-year period increase in strength and focus; however, over the next three years, they slowly slip away before the sensitivities of a next phase take over.

Such cycles of heightened attention, or critical times, in the Montessori tradition signify the emergence of opportunities of developmental potential. Kids continue to center their concentration on individual items and events during these intermittent phases of heightened concern, thus avoiding certain environmental factors. -- specific motivation becomes so strong that ' it causes its possessor to conduct a certain set of acts with an incredible outpouring of energy for us' (Montessori in 1949.)

When heightened attention in the midst of a stressful time causes a child to concentrate on the part of the world, Dr. Montessori found the random interaction that resulted to entail a huge amount of effort. In addition, the child is fully integrated into the interaction. If kids are left free to pursue this exercise for as long as they wish, they look relaxed, confident, and content when they are done, rather than drained. Where some people may define this form of child interaction as play, it is considered child labor in the Montessori culture.

When a new vulnerability occurs, if children want to develop the associated 'task' in an appropriate fashion, they need to identify something in their world that is the object of their attention and behavior. If the environment may not encourage a young child to leverage a developmental opportunity indicated by a vulnerable time, the chance will be missed, and it will be far more challenging for the child to achieve the same developmental phase at a later date.

Montessori instructors strive to develop experiences that suit children's needs at critical cycles and thereby promote the development of children at times when their ability to produce the associated accomplishment is at its best, quickly and naturally.

Neuroscientists are also revisiting the concept of the developmentally impaired cycles of infancy and early adolescence. Work tends to support the presence of these cycles, but the consequences for early education remain to be explored. Montessori educators may suggest that crafting a learning experience to a specific level and carefully monitoring the voluntarily chosen behavior of a child within the setting appears to be the strongest approach to draw decisions about whether to address the specific needs, sensitivities, and desires of a particular person.

The Psychic Embryo

The 'psychic embryo' is the term Dr. Montessori used to characterize the post-natal phase. Much as an embryo requires a different, secure atmosphere to 'construct' any of the structures that will eventually work to support existence after conception, newborns require a caring, secure atmosphere to make up any psycho-social 'cell' they will later require to operate in the human community's social and mental existence into which they are raised. For example, the development of the eyes and ears of a child before conception is mirrored by the growth of the visual and aural senses of a child in the immediate period after conception. Whether the psycho-social roles of an adult infant grow relies on the relationship between the extraordinary capacity of the infant to understand and recall, and the content and social atmosphere created by the carers and culture of the child. Children build themselves from the tools available in the world.

The Absorbent Mind

In Dr. Montessori's concept, the 'absorbent mind' is portrayed as a special and effective way small children understand and recall. Small children, she suggests, 'absorb' experiences from the world, and these perceptions shape the internal structure of the under-constructed mind and intelligence. What's more, young people are studying and recalling without realizing they are only doing so because of living without needing more commitment than feeding or breathing! (Montessori, 1949/1982). The absorbent mentality helps the children to adjust to the particular time and position they are born into.

Childhood (6-12 years)

Having learned much of the fundamental skills he would require, this period is marked by consistency. Children develop out of their Absorbent Brain, and through logical thought and creativity know. Children are expected to consider the environment that affects them, how things function, and why. This is the period to identify the most accurate knowledge, as adolescence brings in a reduction in this learning force. The age group's critical time focuses on societal recognition and the creation of a culture of meaning.

Adolescence (12-18 years)

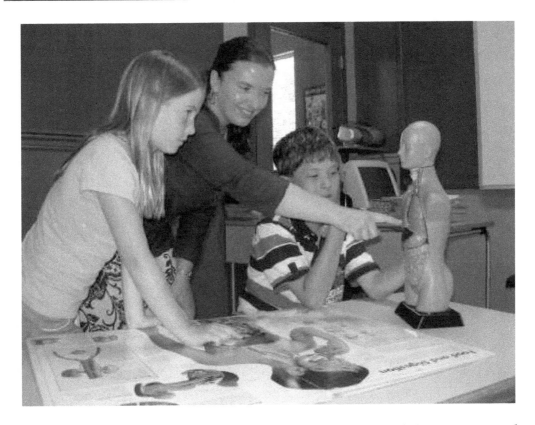

Teenagers show a decrease in motivation at this stage and do not want to be bombarded with knowledge regarding learning. Therefore, schooling will be applied to real-life skills. While Montessori never transformed this stage into a realistic learning method, she conceived of developing schools that were, in reality, self-sustaining families, where learning can arise spontaneously by research on tasks such as cultivating their food, preparing meals, constructing houses and designing clothes. By being autonomous and having to function in peace with others, teenagers will thereby become better able to transition to the adult environment.

Transition into adulthood (18-24 years)

This phase is marked by work development and job beginnings. If, in the preceding stages, the person has acquired the requisite cognitive and social skills, then he would be able to make exact and rewarding career choices.

2.2 Is Montessori A Constructivist Model of Learning

If you are still confused between Montessori and The Traditional Constructivist model of learning, read this chapter for detailed elaboration.

Constructivism is 'a theoretical philosophy that keeps people to actively construct or render their own understanding, and that truth is defined by the learner's interactions' (Elliott et al., 2000, p. 256). Arends (1998) notes in elaborating constructivist theories that constructivism believes in the learner's personal creation of meaning by practice, and that meaning is shaped by the interplay of existing awareness and new experiences.

What are the Constructivist principles?

Knowledge is created, rather than natural, or automatically ingested, the core concept of Constructivism is that human understanding is developed, that learners create new information on the basis of prior experience. This prior knowledge influences what new or modified knowledge an individual will build from new experiences in learning (Phillips, 1995). Learning is an active method. The second idea is that studying is more an involved phase than a passive. The passive view of teaching views the learner as 'an empty vessel' to be filled with knowledge, whereas constructivism states that only through active engagement with the world (such as experiments or real-world problem solving) do the learners build meaning.

Knowledge may be obtained passively, but comprehension can not be, as it must come from making meaningful associations between prior knowledge, new knowledge, and learning processes. Everything knowledge is socially formed learning is a collective task, rather than an abstract idea (Dewey, 1938), something we do together in connection with each other. Vygotsky (1978), for example, believed that the community plays a central role in the "making meaning" process. For Vygotsky, the atmosphere in which children grow up will influence how they think and what they think. So all teaching and learning are about sharing and negotiating knowledge that is socially constituted. For example, Vygotsky (1978) states that cognitive development stems from social interactions of guided learning as children and the co-constructing knowledge of their partner within the proximal development zone.

The aim of traditional Constructivist method is to transmit the already established information, abilities, and expectations of behavior so it can train the children for the potential obligations of the future. The instructor is mainly the significant person in the classroom and offers the stimulus; the setting and resources play another similar function. The program is detached from daily life and does not have conceptual meaning. Students are required to "read" this knowledge, also referred to as "empty slates" or "empty/blank vessels," and bring it back to show that they have become a master at the content. The imaginative, initial thinking is provided very little attention, and performance is strongly dealt in terms of memorized data. Students are inspired by incentives or penalties, which are believed to make learning simpler.

There's a flaw with the definition, however. Since students essentially need to look back at the program, we can say it barely contributes itself to higher-level cognitive skills growth. Since there is never any student involvement in the content being learned, students, for the most of it, merely memorize information to get ahead in the exam and then forget them easily.

Montessori vs. Constructivism

The constructivist philosophy, as suggested by "father of progressive education," John Dewey, is an effort to fix the errors of the old traditional instructive method (i.e., understanding all capitals of the state). The constructivist teacher's job is to guide students articulate their own queries and views and to help students analyze and evaluate their study findings. Constructivists view the process of learning as a cycle of three stages: exploration, implementation of concepts, and application of concepts.

Constructivist philosophy has five main tenants:

- The lessons are constructed over a question that "sparks their interest," which the children make up a hypothesis about.

- The lessons should be of the child's relevance.

- The lessons build on the idea that "less is better."

- Learning starts with simple principles (whole picture), rather than with the specifics. The students form their individual interpretation in such a way that they it understand best.

- Adults view and respect the perspective of their pupils. The constructivist philosophy encourages teachers to practically show a knowledge of the comprehension of the students by answering questions, focusing on to the responses, and answering for detailed elaboration. It is different and in contrast to the previous, old conventional teaching model, which implies that there are correct and incorrect answers (some are supposed to win and some lose) while studying for rote memory and that it is easier to be correct, rather than have intriguing ideas.

- The syllabus and course related tasks are tailored to address the assumptions of the students. There has to be a set dialog with alignment between the queries the students have and what it is they are capable of understanding cognitively for learning to occur. Teachers, instead of teaching and evaluating mediate and review. Authentic assessment inside the constructivist theory framework questions like, "what you know about it," and "what have you actually understood about it?" It encourages interdisciplinary exploration that allows large and questions which are mainly open-ended to be addressed.

The infant begins communicating as the creation causes it to act so. The kid is not growing, but he needs to make use of such inventions. The child will not think that way: "If I want to move from this place to the other, I must begin to improve my walking ability to do so." He will not suggest, "I want to learn language because I can demand for my meal when I am craving it." Nope. The development process comes first, and the human person uses this creation only for a corresponding time. There is also a whole-time where the infant does it itself without the intention of performing the exercise in itself, and this type of exercise involves an immense deal of work on the child's part. And, gradually over time, when the infant grows his thinking capacity, he often gains the willingness to utilize his imagination;

the two items go alongside; when his logic progresses, he implements this growth of the capacity of thinking.

Hence we can conclude that the great distinction [between mainstream schooling and Montessori schooling] resides in the personality, vivacity, curiosity, and excitement that the child displays while attempting the work, as well as the ability and approachability along with which he is studying. (Addressed in 1913 by Maria Montessori.) Like Dewey, Maria Montessori became a vital component of what is regarded as the movement of cognition development. Her research as a physician and science expert set the tone for her hypotheses regarding children's "growth schedules" and "active times." She also felt and recognized that there was a need for cognitive stimulation for repeated behavioral (emotional and motor), along with the role that the atmosphere plays in promoting the intellectual growth and wellbeing of children. Like stated in the quotation above, at the moment, Montessori found it pointless to attempt to improve the growth of a child beyond its potential.

Just like Dewey, Dr. Montessori emphasized that experiencing things is not merely passive reactions to the different stimuli present (lessons). "In schools like that, the students are fastened, like butterflies fixed on sticks, separately on his position, the bench, spreading the worthless wings of pointless intelligence that they have gained" (1964, Dr. Montessori). Indeed, her beliefs also foreshadow those of constructivist supporters: "What is known is formed as a complicate set of ideas in the child. Aggressively developed by the individual child itself through a sequence of psychological processes reflecting an inner development, psychological growth. (Montessori, 1965). The theory of Montessori is focused on both biology and concepts of psychology. She introduced many of the concepts.

Montessori along with Jean Jacques Rousseau assumed:

- Knowledge is the basis of learning

- Non-artificial outcomes are mistake management

- The infant is intrinsically pleasant and wants to do research

Montessori and John Locke believed:

- thoughts arise from basic experiences that occupy the blank slate mind of the newborn

- The sensory system works to establish a bond between the two.

- Children in this developmental plane are motivated to set themselves up and immersed in the abilities that push them toward freedom. As they understand to handle their independent lives, learning is guided inward.

At age 6, infants become most involved in language roots and the theoretical universe surrounding them. They want elegant artifacts and fabrics which are aesthetically pleasing. At this point, children are forming their creativity, morals, and critical thinking skills. They would like to know what position they stand in the global universe, hence the concept of Cosmic Education given by Montessori. She strongly assumed it would be inspired by a message that stimulated the child's mind and have consequences that last much longer. She claimed there's a newfound sense of independence, and students are able to make their own choices over what things to pick from. The areas of interest they select prompt them to ask a lot of questions and investigate, and to make new comments. Having several items in the classroom at Montessori enables the learner to develop their own syllabus and curriculum.

2.3 Montessori Lesson Plans

Montessori educators define the task voluntarily chosen by the children as their work. The phrase 'work' implies an arduous task performed to create some form of the finished product, so it might seem out of position in our age were playing, not working, is known in early childhood as 'the basis for all learning' (Waller and Swann, in 2009). If children in our period are free to create via play, it is in no small portion thanks to the work of social intellectuals like Maria Montessori, who advocated for the abolition of child labor at the turn of the twentieth century. Therefore, it is worth exploring what precisely Dr. Montessori intended when she described the children's spontaneous activity as their work.

Dr. Montessori was very specific about the task that she did not consider was the work of girls. For one, she was horrified by the schoolrooms' 'sorry show' that originated after the Industrial Era, and that proceeded to plague the lives of countless small children long into the twentieth century. Huge numbers of children were 'condemned' in such schoolrooms, in her opinion, to sit on uncomfortable benches in dusty rooms, listening to the instructor for a long period. Furthermore, according to Dr. Montessori, the teachers of 'prizes and rewards' used to make children give attention to 'barren and pointless information' lead in 'unnatural' and 'induced' actions (Montessori, 1912/1964). That, Dr. Montessori concluded, was a type of 'slavery' from which kids wanted emancipation. So, the practice Montessori educators term the job of children is definitely not controlled practice. It is essentially a form of practice that many adult people might consider play; however, with two distinguishing characteristics (Montessori.)

• A lot of purposeful work and focus is required.

• It is targeted to potential milestones.

Using the term 'work' to define this kind of practice is a reflection of the importance it gets in schools of Montessori. Montessori instructors discourage something that may disturb or interrupt a functioning child as often as possible since the initiative and attention of the child are known to be reactions to the heightened concern of critical time and, therefore, a symbol of positive growth. Montessori educators claim the word 'job' gives the practice with which children create the value it owes to the adults of the future. After all, this operation can be seen as the most important contribution that every community gives to society

Prepping a Montessori atmosphere for an Infant Group

The household is the first setting for newborns. The bond developed in the first weeks of existence while the baby is snuggled and fed, and the affection that the baby gets from parents and guiders establishes the foundation of confidence and stability in which the entire future of the infant lies. Montessori Assistants to Infancy offer many ideas for parents to establish order and routine within the home, to give the child as much free movement and autonomy as possible, and to set up everyday activities so that the child can join and contribute. For the first time, a little one journeying away from home will enter any of the two Montessori environments designed for children under three years of age.

• For babies with working parents, a Montessori daycare program for infants aged 2 to 12 months is accessible in the Nido or nest.

• When children start moving, they will attend the Montessori Baby Group for children aged 1-3.

The surroundings of Nido and Infant Community are not anything like the more familiar environment of daycare or playgroups. Like the Children's House, a Montessori environment for infants is a miniature world, this time to the scale of even younger kids. Like the Children's House, it is designed to give exciting activities to these very young children and as much autonomy, freewil and independence as available.

The Infant Group atmosphere, like all Montessori settings, is bright and airy, clean and healthy, orderly, and lovely, with plenty of room for children to walk around freely. Since babies and babies use their perceptions to discover the world, there are several textures, such as bricks, wood, glass, and cloth. For their sensory application as well as for security and practicality, fabrics used for soft furnishings such as rugs, quilts, pillows, and cushions are chosen. At the children's height, there are room mirrors and stunning mobiles that capture the attention. Furniture and artifacts are actual, matching the children's size and their strength and ability. There are stairs to ascend, and objects to grip and push to develop balance and gross motor skills. There's a dedicated area for increasing operation to add to the order, whether it's meal preparing, feeding, or changing nappy. Both events are planned, and these tiny children require as little support as possible for parents. Floor beds encourage kids to sleep anytime they want to, and walk about again anytime they awaken, without having to get assistance from an adult. Parents are advised to give children clothing they may put on and take off on their own. Pre-measured portions carefully help the children make meals individually or in cooperation with adults. The emphasis is on letting the kids reveal what they can do on their own. For starters, if children can move, they are not carried; whether children can rise, as they are moved, they are not required to sit down; although children are yet unwilling to take a spoon, parents will not push food into their mouths but leave the spoon in reach so they can pick as and how much to consume. The Infancy Assistant is actively watching, often able to change the atmosphere to enable growing children to discover new opportunities and obstacles and to ensure that the children are not disturbed, excessively-stimulated, or overloaded.

Movements and mind

So far, we have seen Montessori educators perceive the freely selected, simultaneous activity of a child as the work of the child. That research often requires some sort of movement. In the Montessori perspective, human action is a manifestation of the human spirit.

Equality, purposeful activity, and early childhood focus Dr. Montessori contrasted the production of activity in human infants to that of small animals. When young animals, such as rabbits or horses, are born, they approximate the coordination and agility of the species' adults quickly, sometimes almost immediately. In comparison, premature babies have little of the adult strength, agility, and flexibility. Human infants continue to develop mastery of movement through their prolonged infancy. This involves attempts and monotonous practice, whereby children simultaneously impose themselves both mentally and physically. Children make this attempt in pre-school years as they find such gestures as the preceding so interesting:

• lifting, walking and juggling, in other words, rotating the whole body with balance

• engaging individually in the everyday events of the modern society they see around them

• use the hand with consistency and precision

Dr. Montessori stated that while children participate in voluntarily chosen goal-oriented play, intellectual energy and physical action become organized and focused. Over time, if children use their minds regularly to direct their motion, they demonstrate the ability to control both their movements and their thoughts, willingly and independently. In other terms, when their bodies develop the strength they acquire strength over their brains. Children who can monitor their minds can, on a voluntary basis, focus their attention for prolonged times; that is, they have the ability to focus. In Montessori words, this is how they free themselves of their own needs from becoming captives.

More and more children are empowered to get their actions and behavior under voluntary regulation, that is, the more they will guide and govern themselves, the fewer they need to be controlled and governed by others, and the freer and more autonomous they can become. Children take the first initiative down this journey of growth by selecting things that they consider naturally fascinating, that is, a plan that suits the responsive cycles of their era. Once children are on the road, the practice moves them to self-regulation, focus, and independence.

Teaching Social Skills

Every toddler's parent knows that teaching them social skills is not straightforward. That's because even if babies want healthy, enjoyable experiences with others — their own anxieties and expectations get in the way. They can't help wondering — is that child going to grab its toy? Will they bring the truck in front of the other? When the other kid is forced off the cycle and speeded off, can they get away with it?

And the first move to having children grow emotional maturity is to make them understand how to control their feelings, which is the base for interpersonal interactions. The latter helps them learn empathy for others.

The third is to help them learn to communicate their desires and emotions without needing to strike.

This ability set would prove more important to the joy of your child's existence than academic achievement, financial performance, or any of our other traditional acts. In reality, emotional intelligence — defined as the ability to control one's own emotions and to connect well with others — will be a key factor in his or her subsequent academic and career performance in your child's existence, perhaps more essential than IQ. And, how is it that you make your kid develop social skills?

Empathize and Sympathize

Children who get a lot of support from adults in their life for their own emotions are the first to build support towards others, and studies have shown that empathy for others is the foundation of positive interpersonal relationships.

Stay close over playgroups.

Most kids strike when they feel distracted through social encounters because they really do not know what to do about it. If you are there, you may ask, "Yeah, Ryan was taking your bucket is that all right with you? Doesn't it? You might say: 'My bowl! "When the kid understands when you're backing up, hitting isn't likely to become a routine.

Do not push kids to partake.

Unfortunately, it prevents exchanging skills growth! Children ought to feel comfortable in their possession before sharing. Alternatively, incorporate the taking turn's principle.

"It is the duty of Sophia to use the pot. Now it is your time. In addition, I am going to make you wait. "

Let the child determine how long it will take for his turn.

If children believe that adults can take a toy away after the adult's vague notion of "long enough" has gone, you are demonstrating picking, and typically, the kid is more possessive. If the kid is able to use the product as much as he wants, he will love it to the maximum and then give it up with a clear heart. If the same kid uses the same product every time, you should purchase a repeat item because either it is such a crowd-pleaser, or you can take different turns.

Help them wait for your kids.

If your kid is having a breakdown waiting for her turn, it is a sign that she has some huge emotions to get out and is taking advantage of the convenient chance. In an effort to shore up their delicate equilibrium, children sometimes get defensive about possession — just like adults!

Empathize: "Waiting is hard, you hope you could use the basket now" and help her up as she is weeping. You will be shocked to see that she actually will not really know about the doll she has been longing for after "showing" you those pent-up feelings and would happily pass on.

Think of compulsive picking.

Often when children snatch, they do not really think about the other person. Do not hesitate to enter, though. Instead, take notice. They are probably playing a game. Much of the way, when one of the kids is upset, you should not worry.

If one child is constantly grabbing, though, then you probably need to intervene. Children would also snatch whatever the other kid has, then drop the item and continue to the next one to replace their own miserable feelings. Such emotions require support.

So gather all your sympathy, place your hands on the disputed item and ask, "Would you like the truck? "In addition, look at the vehicle the kid is using. "Is that all right with you? "If that is — great. You do not need to be the arbiter of equity.

Assertiveness teaches.

If your child often allows other kids to take stuff from him and often appears sad, ask, "You do not want to give it up, do you? You might tell, 'I am really playing with this.' "Experiment with him acting this out at home and demonstrating it with teddy bears. You will need to be his "face" while he interacts with others before he learns the language skills.

Slow down. Make sure to reflect while talking to your toddler, then stop to allow him a chance to answer before jumping in. When your kid knows she has your full attention, Ecclestone suggests she is expected to communicate with you through noises, movements, and vocabulary.

Say something crazy

You will gain the attention of your child and provide an incentive for her to connect just by being dumb or doing anything unexpected. Seek to place her in a waterless pool, or leave her cereal bowl bare. She would have to convey that something is wrong with you, whether it is by movements, noises, or sentences. Then, speak to her about what you intend to do to get it changed

Rather than celebrating communication in the abstract, help her learn what is actually cool about it.

Research suggests that children do something most when we encourage sharing — but only while we are listening! They simply do it fewer when we are not, so our appreciation does not owe them much incentive to share beyond the moment of our focus. Instead, encourage her to make the decision of sharing in the future by making her see the impact of her choosing: "Look how delighted Michael is that he gets a turn with your car." If you follow the strategy of having children have a turn for however long, however, they wish, they gladly transferred the desired object to the other child at the end of their turn. They get to know how good it feels to send. So having children manage their turns is the perfect way of promoting cooperation and kindness.

Kids will get a chance to put away their most exclusive things before visitors come over if they do not want someone else to play with them. Using this practice as a way to demonstrate why the visiting child would obviously want to interact with Junior is other toys, even as Junior enjoys the toys at their homes with his peers.

Set the physical violence to reasonable limits.

"You should tell us how crazy you're without harming. Come; let's tell Henry how crazy you are because I'm going to comfort you." "You should yell NO and stamp your foot as hard as you want. You should yell, 'Mum! 'And I will still support.' Babies, like our arms and legs, are entitled to their emotions, which have a way to only exist in humans. Yet all people, including the small ones, are liable for their arms and legs and emotions about what they are doing. Our responsibility as parents should be to teach them safe methods of self-management without becoming harsh, which also makes the children more aggressively violent.

Giving the children language for their feelings is never too early.

Emotion marking is the first step of the brain's capacity to perceive it mentally, rather than physically.

"When you concentrate hard on your tower, it's so painful; then it falls like this. "The huge dog's bark is frightening, but you're protected on this side of the fence, and I'd never let it harm you. The exception to that is when kids are in the throes of a major emotion, where so many words will drive them out of their hearts and into their heads. Only tell your kid he's healthy at those moments, and save the phrases for later.

Remember that there is typically pain or anxiety behind the rage.

Recognizing such emotions is often more successful in transmitting wrath than merely marking the wrath, which just appears to intensify it. "I hear Jimmy is very angry with you. I wonder if you are sad because he needs to be interacting with someone else right now. "That's even more important when children say," I hate him! "Hate is not a feeling; it is a position.

"Right now, you're so upset at your brother that you sound like you're never going to figure out anything with him. That is what it means by the word hate. Even we feel that way when we are very, very mad, even at those we love. We are a team, and we are just trying to hash it out. Let us go and tell your brother that he hurt you by pushing you off the swing, and how angry that makes you feel. Continue incorporating the notion of understanding how people behave as early as possible.

Hold cool

Research suggests one of the most effective things parents can do to help children know how to control their feelings is to remain calm. During the turmoil of their tumultuous emotions, children need to perceive their parents as a "keeping environment "— a secure haven. If you will remain calm and soothe your girl, she can gradually learn to soothe herself, which is the initial phase in learning how to handle her emotions.

Keep in mind they are young

Only because James bites a playmate does not mean that he is going to be an ax-murderer. It's important not to encourage negative conduct against others, but that doesn't imply you're not giving understanding — and the confidence your child can gain. "Sometimes, even the children get angry at their peers. When you grow older, it will get better to know how to manage yourself as you feel angry, and you can sort through problems. "Children deserve to learn from parents because they are not evil people.

2.4 Ideal Montessori Learning Environment

The significance of a Prepared Maria Montessori's "prepared atmosphere" is the idea that the setting should be structured to promote the child's full autonomous thinking and discovery. There is a range of actions, as well as a lot of movement in the trained area. An instructor from Montessori represents the infant as the preparer and tactician of the world and is responsible for preserving the climate and order of the planned community. A structured atmosphere allows the growing child the freedom to thoroughly explore their abilities by tactile materials that are appropriate for growth. The materials vary from basic to complex and from real to theoretical, which conform to the age and skill of each boy.

Montessori classrooms are structured to deliver lessons, activities, and resources to suit the individual child's developmental needs and interests. It's necessary to remember that not every child is involved in any lesson possible. That's why children can pick the experiences they instinctively gravitate toward.

Many parents can ask what separates Montessori childcare from the regular daycare or preschool center. For example, as soon as you reach the typical childcare center, you'll find that it's most definitely busy, noisy, and messy. In the opposite extreme of the continuum, as soon as you step into a classroom in Montessori, you will find its calm, quiet, and organized. You may ask why the two childcare programs vary so far from each other. The distinction resides in something called the structured setting by Dr. Maria Montessori.

Montessori Classrooms

A Montessori classroom is typically a large, open-minded space with low shelves, various tables' sizes that comfortably seat one to four children and seats that are suitably designed in the classroom for the children (Figure 1.2). While not uncommon still, one of Dr. Montessori's inventions (Elkind, 1976) was creating furniture that was suitably made for the children who might need it. Practical Montessori classes often have communities of at least three years of age; all six years of primary education may be integrated with smaller schools.

The classroom at Montessori is organized in sections, typically separated by low shelving. -- the field has "materials," the Montessori word designating academic items, for research in a specific subject field (art, music, math, language, science, etc.). That contrasts sharply with traditional schooling, where learning is primarily extracted from texts. On the Montessori Elementary school, books are increasingly critical as instruments for learning, but even there, hands-on activities prevail. Dr. Montessori claimed that deep focus was necessary to help children achieve their true self, and that deep focus arises in children when interacting with their hands, and objects.

In providing a clean look, Montessori classrooms often contrast with other traditional schools. In a wardrobe, additional supplies are held out of reach and moved in and out of the school, when children appear to be eager for or no longer in need. Each material has its position on the shelf, and after usage, children are required to bring each element back neatly in its position, ready for another boy. Attention to the environment is strongly respected, with consideration for the interests of others. The focus is often expressed in how the classroom is organized by teachers. Materials are thoughtfully arranged both inside and around topic regions, and the structures make common sense. Children are not allocated seats but are free to travel about throughout the day at any tables they want to operate. They may even work on tiny rugs on the board. Children can choose for themselves, whether they want to work alone or in groups established by themselves, even when the instructor is giving a lesson. With very few exceptions, all lessons are given to individuals (most often at primary level, 3- to 6-year-old level) or small groups (most often at the elementary level, 6- to 12-year-old). When the children are ready for them, lessons are given; the instructor will write on the board or announce the expected lessons of the day early in the day so that the children can know what to expect. Care is taken that the purpose is not to exert power over the kids, but merely to warn them so that they can prepare their day appropriately.

Education at Montessori is structured to the heart. This often throws people back at the preschool stage. They reach a Montessori classroom, and it is very calm, unlike the preschools they usually see. Children operate individually or in communities in a peaceful way. And it organizes their jobs. They focus, carry out tasks in a sequence of actions that the instructor or other children have shown to them. Research shows that better child results are consistent with organized settings, but the level of order will make the parents feel insecure. The products on the shelf are intended to draw the attention of children and to teach lessons through repetitive usage. Much of the items are constructed of wood and are either organic or painted in chosen bright colors since they have been shown to draw children. Any content has a primary motive for being in the classroom; most even have many secondary reasons. Montessori instructors watch children at work, not offering assessments to determine competency, observing that children are utilizing the resources correctly. It is believed that proper usage would produce comprehension. Teachers revisit lessons where children seem to have misused a material and therefore do not derive from it the instruction that is meant to be imparted; new lessons are offered where children seem to have learned material and to be ready in a series for the next.

There are different methods of utilizing the items, which are demonstrated to the children in the classes, in accordance with each piece serving a primary function. With Metal Insets, which consists of standard geometric shapes made of metal, children are not supposed to make music; the materials break down essential practices into a sequence of structured moves that kids learn individually before putting them together to do the main activities. These measures also represent indirect planning; children are unsure of what the steps lead to, however, the instructor is conscientious, and methodically introduces the materials. A clear example of how Montessori learning continues is in writing and reading education.

What Is The Prepared Environment?

Throughout her book The Joy of Childhood, Dr. Montessori defined the goal of the prepared environment as follows: "The first aim of the prepared environment is to make the developing infant independent of the parent whenever appropriate." Thus, the prepared atmosphere is one of the central elements of the Montessori theory. The learning atmosphere and all that the child comes into touch with will promote independent thinking and discovery, according to Dr. Montessori.

Primary elements of Prepared Community

Independence —The right of choice is one of the critical goals in a Montessori-prepared setting. This is accomplished by allowing the child independence to experiment, free expression, free social contact, and free intervention from others.

Montessori believes in allowing our little one's more freedom to select their daily activities. During the meantime, we, as teachers, will be observing and advising them whenever possible. It enhances cognitive capacity (the awareness, reasoning, studying, and assessing process).

Framework and order — The theory behind this concept is to represent the framework and order of the cosmos so that the infant can internalize the meaning of its environment and thereby begin to make an understanding of the world around him.

Beauty — Making the atmosphere welcoming for learning is also essential. Therefore, the mood will be wonderfully and simplistically crafted in such a way as to invoke calm, tranquility, and harmony. The workspace will always be well controlled and uncluttered.

Culture and Truth — Dr. Montessori claimed that children would be motivated by religion. That is why teachers at Montessori often send the kids out into nature to use natural learning resources in the prepared setting. Such products are not synthetics or fabrics, but genuine timber, concrete, bamboo, structure, and glass. The tools should also be actual and child-size because the child can interact with the materials on its own without discomfort and without needing to rely on the adult for movement assistance.

Social atmosphere — The prepared community will promote social progress through the fostering of equality of contact. Montessori schools encourage the creation of a sense of dignity and empathy for others while rendering children more socially aware.

Academic Atmosphere — after all of the aforementioned ideas have been met, Montessori educators should be able to reach children in the educational setting that enhances the child's whole temperament and intelligence.

Creating an Ideal Montessori Environment at Home

Being autonomous involves being able to do something about yourself, being able to make your own decisions, and handle the effects of those decisions on your own. It merely implies 'not hanging from' anyone else or whatever. Dr. Maria Montessori witnessed small children struggling to become autonomous during their long lifespan. She believed the push toward independence that encourages young children is the same force that reinforces their growth. For this purpose, the classrooms at Montessori are designed so that children can choose their tasks individually. In these practices, children acquire not only necessary information but also how to take control of their own interests and their world on their own. Often, they know how to create relationships with each other. A Montessori classroom also referred to by Montessori educators as the 'world,' is specifically built such that a children's group can behave and communicate as individually as possible.

Montessori Activities for You And Your Child

Montessori-focused activities are interesting and unique, helping to stimulate independence and self-trust for your child. Here are a few basic and exploratory activities which you can try anytime. The Montessori curriculum teaches that student-led learning will encourage children to function at its autonomous level and speed. This, together with the instruction offered by devoted instructors, promotes cognitive, mental, social & physiological growth of your preschooler. No doubt a lot of parents love that style of learning!

If the pre-school of your child is already closed, or whether you only want to introduce the Montessori method at home, this is a perfect place to continue. These projects are only a Launchpad, enabling your child to try whatever areas and topics he or she is most anxious for. Follow her on. After all, she is the owner of the learning experience.

Water Play

It is a perfect opportunity to experience the surrounding world. Children learn essential lessons to float, fill, weigh, and sweep. There are several ways to integrate water related plays into your everyday life, which goes above the normal method of simply enjoying in the bath. Here mentioned are some ideas for you to begin with:

- Scrubbing: By using distinct scrub brushes, sponge like tools, and cleaning items, your child will learn about textures. They're willing to clean animals, walls, rocks, and even pinecones.
- Misting plants: Give them a watering that is child-sized, or have them go for the bigger version of it. We recommend you set the hose for gentle watering to prevent an unforeseen water fight.
- Bubbles: You can squirt soap inside a water-filled tub, pan, or cup. Let your kid blend it with a whisker, and watch the bubbles become bigger.
- Dishes: Your child is not too small to assist in simple cooking tasks. Set them up with a footstool or a tower standing at the bath. Start with plastic, metal, or wooden boards, tassels, and cups. It's cool if they only have fun with the dishes, and with the water — you can drop it all into the dish washing machine later.
- Measurement: Using cups to move water between jugs or bowls. Keep count of the number of cups a bucket or a tiny bowl needs to fill.

Food ingenuity

Indeed, little children will assist with food preparation. Only ensure it's enjoyable, imaginative, and play-oriented. Combat picky eaters? Okay, we've noticed that children are more inclined to choose to consume food when they help cook a meal. Although that may be suitable for every child, particularly young ones, it's worth trying! Below mention are a few things that you can try in your kitchen:

- Spread: Jam, butter, peanut whisk, jelly, or even hummus can be spread on crackers. Don't panic if something falls apart, that's an area of learning.

- Cutting: Let your children practice slicing softer fruits like melons using a butter knife.
- Peeling: Ask your child to attempt peeling an orange, and then hand it to stop.
- Squeezing: You can create the lemonade yourself. Have them by the side and push out the pieces. Having a mess is great!
- Dehydration: It is fun to see fruit move from normal to crisp the shrunken slices. Besides, using a dehydrator is safe for a little boy, as there is a different usage, unlike a danger in traditional stoves. (Yet it is also perfect for adult supervision.) Blending: let your kid choose items to place into the blender. For them, you should run it, but let them practice putting it in the cups.

Outdoor Exploration

Playing outdoors does not have to be restricted to sliding down slides, twirling, and playing tags (though these are also great activities). There are countless possibilities of allowing the children to invest some time outside.

- Gardening: having the kids interested in growing their own food helps to cultivate a wonderful interest in adulthood. Mark off one garden field as your own, letting them choose their own plants.
- Puddle play: That does not mean you cannot go outdoors just because it is rainy out. Get some fun rain boots and go leaping puddles!
- Treasure hunts: Create a list of items that they need to find — like a stone, a smooth rock, a yellow herb, etc.
- Outdoor art: drawing on leaves, creating pinecone handicrafts, putting flowers into a scrapbook, painting with mud – there are countless possibilities.
- Musical wall: Outside, you can hang a variety of things — pots and pans, old forks, tin cans, chimes, and even metal plates. Get some sticks, and begin to make music.
- Stick family: Locate and call a set of sticks. Find a place in your yard to build a house for them, with a mound of leaves for their nests, a

rock circle for them to cook, and some acorns for them to mumble on. Every day check on your stick mates.

Life Skills

A child learning his shirt buttoning is a life skill. The theory of Montessori interweaves realistic knowledge with freestyle games. That gives your child thumbs up on on being an adult that is efficient, positive, and independent. Always doing stuff as if lace up your shoes for them is good. However, if they can do anything on their own, let them. Only make sure you allow ample room to acquire new skills.

- Dressing: Begin by picking one object at a time and putting trousers on, for starters. Continue to focus on it and empower your child to do it alone. Then switch on to shirt putting. Definitely follow videos providing advice for the daily world.
- Washing up: Making sure General Grooming is included in the routine. You can also use a cloth to wash your preschooler's face, scrub his toes while in a bath, or use a shower brush to get all those trying to reach places like his back.
- Reusing: Your child will assist by rinsing recycled cans, throwing them in the bin, and even having you roll them out into the driveway. Talk to him about why reuse and recycle stuff is important.
- In an emergency: Kindergartners will begin knowing essential facts, such as their home number, address, and how to dial 911.

2.5 FAQs about Montessori

As a parent, it is very likely that you have many queries related to Montessori by this point. Hence, this part of the chapter is completely dedicated to all kinds of questions a parent can have regarding the Montessori Method.

Are the services recognized at Montessori?

The Montessori instructional approach is well established. The Montessori programs are based all over the world. In addition, many new childhood development and education textbooks are referring to Dr. Montessori's important contributions to the field of child education. Montessori applications are also recognized through different programs and societies. Of these societies, the most notable are the American Montessori Society and the American Montessori International. It is beneficial to be certified through one of these communities, as it provides parents with an assurance that, as Dr. Montessori intended, the Montessori syllabus be being professionally adhered to in all its facets. Bringing credentialed also guarantees that the proper materials are being provided and that the correct number of teachers have accomplished their Montessori training program.

Q. How are the children in a Montessori system disciplined?

Any Montessori system participants are surprised by how calm, friendly and well treated the kids are. Montessori programs are notorious for their children's self-discipline. What is especially noteworthy about this is that the approach does not require bullying, threats, or deception tactics. The kids do not consider their teachers as strict or evil. Energy or control methods are not required. What happens is that the children feel that they are fulfilling their needs. They want classrooms and coaches. They believe the instructor is responsible for them and is a source of support. The kid clearly wants to be taught how to fulfill his/her wants in a constructive way. Unacceptable behavior declines through this phase and eventually disappears. This makes the classroom an extremely pleasant place for both the teacher and the children. The secret to the cycle is:

- Development of an atmosphere able to fulfill the children's developmental requirements
- An instructor educated in optimistic, meaningful strategies to supporting kids

Q. The Montessori curriculum is geared to up till what age?

Montessori products are available and are meant for use for children up to the age of 12. There are a few middle and high schools in Montessori. Montessori, though, mostly produced resources directly during the years of elementary school. That was because she saw the need for specifically crafted products, especially for the younger kids, because the older kids should have the opportunity to benefit from widely accessible.

Q. Why do Montessorians use the term "work" to describe activities for children?

Dr. Montessori's profound appreciation for children is expressed in her philosophy of curiosity and discovery. She recognized that the students were in a self-construction cycle, constructing themselves constantly from inside. The specific classes, tools, and way of being in society (aka, "work") help the normal growth of the growing infant.

Q. What is the development of Montessori children, and are they good after leaving the Montessori environment?

There are no "classes" given in the school of Montessori. Evaluation is by portfolio, including the assessment, including record keeping of the instructor. The instructor closely observes any child's academic success, joy, development, and enjoyment of learning, and addresses it with the parents. Recent findings indicate that children from Montessori are well educated for their adult life – academically, psychologically, and emotionally. When exposed to a conventional school setting, they usually adapt well. In addition to doing highly on standardized exams, Montessori kids are graded above standard on factors such as following instructions, handing in on-time assignments, listening closely, utilizing practical knowledge, demonstrating maturity, posing challenging questions, displaying a passion for learning and adjusting to different circumstances.

Q. What about special kids?

The Montessori classes are built to support all children (those who are "gifted" and those with learning difficulties) at their own speed achieve their maximum potential. A classroom of children of different abilities is an environment where everybody learns from each other, and all participate. In comparison, multi-age grouping helps each child to reach its own rhythm in relation to peers, without feeling "fast" or "behind."

Q. What specialized qualifications do the instructors at Montessori have?

In addition to a bachelor's degree, teachers with Montessori certification have completed the course ranging from 200 to 600 hours of class and a year-long practical experience. The teaching includes concepts of infant growth and theory of Montessori as well as practical applications of Montessori tools in the classroom. There are training centers in Montessori in various places around the United States and around the world.

Q. What is the principle behind the Montessori approach to early childhood education?

Montessori is an instructional philosophy focused around the idea that learning will operate through, rather than against, the child's existence. Learning would also be focused on the child's empirical research and the subsequent perception of growth and learning processes.

Q. Are Montessori faith schools?

Some are, but the rest are not. Any Montessori schools work under the auspices of a church, temple, or diocese, much as most schools, but most are autonomous of any religious association.

Q. Are infants covered by the Montessori program?

Children under the age of two are extremely capable of learning about the environment around them. The Montessori Infants Program has been designed specifically to help the development needs and interests of young children. The most critical aspects that children acquire in the Montessori Baby Curriculum are activity control, good social skills, language learning, and basic conceptual principles that qualified them for the Toddler and Preschool Programme.

Q. How do teachers at Montessori meet the needs of so many different children?

Good instructors help the learners get to the stage that their hearts and minds are free, and they are ready to know. Students are not only inspired by having good grades in successful classrooms, as they are by a profound enjoyment of learning. As parents know the learning styles and temperaments of their own children, teachers, too, develop this sense of each child's uniqueness by spending several years with the students and their parents.

Q. Why do the classrooms at Montessori have mixed age groups?

Parents frequently wonder why Montessori classrooms divide children into two or three-year age ranges, while through their birth year, primary schools divide pupils. The main explanation for this is that mixed-age programs are promoting learning to mimic, a good sense of belonging, and empowering children to function within their growth level.

Q. How long will it take to for my child to settle in?

It takes a specific period for each child to move into a new childcare facility. Some kids decide on the same day when others can take more than a month. For children attending three or more days a week, they are expected to relax faster than children attending fewer days do.

Q. How do Montessori kids compare to the kids from other programs?

Children in a Montessori curriculum are frequently ahead in grade level by many years. They are generally involved in anything they like learning. They are usually polite, compassionate, collaborative, and respectful of their properties as well as others.

Chapter 3: Montessori & Child Psychology

Montessori products were systematically developed within the curriculum in an educational setting, with particular attention to the needs of children depending on the developmental period they were moving through and in the assumption that handling tangible artifacts helps to improve awareness and critical thought. Many of Montessori's views can be linked to psychological theories and child psychology. This chapter has elaborate explanations on child development from a psychological perspective.

3.1 Understanding Child Development

Reports and research suggest that children may profit from Montessori concepts emotionally and cognitively. A 2017 analysis compared Montessori students with regular schoolchildren between the ages of three and six reported that Montessori-educated students demonstrated "elevated outcomes" in many ways, including

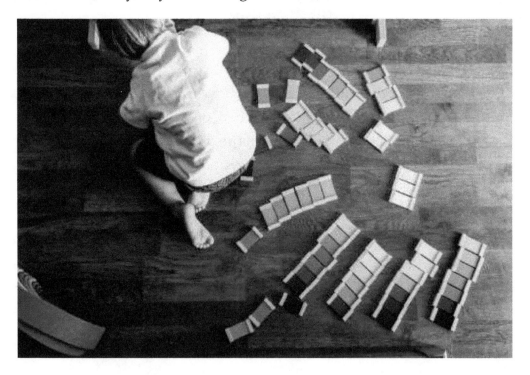

1. **Social Cognition**

Social cognition relates to the manner in which an individual collects and retains knowledge for later re-use. This research showed that the children of Montessori tended to grow social awareness quicker than their typical peers. In other words, across the three years, Montessori pupils displayed substantially higher rates of academic performance relative to their conventional school peers.

Nevertheless, one thing the researchers noticed was that it took some time for this to become clear. Children were originally monitored and found to be on equal learning standards in the mainstream and Montessori programs. However, the more the Montessori participants stayed in the curriculum, the higher the difference between the two classes of academic performance becomes.

2. Confidence in Learning Subjects

Researchers in the analysis observed that children participating in the Montessori program were more likely than their conventional classroom peers to display optimistic emotions towards school and learning events. That does not suggest they did not enjoy typical childhood things like playing football or watching TV. Nevertheless, in comparison to all other learning practices, Montessori kids were more likely to show an enthusiasm in literacy and other intellectual endeavors.

3. Mastery Orientation

This concept applies to the trust a child has in the abilities to answer and solve a problem, such as a puzzle. Children in the Montessori system were more inclined to choose difficult puzzles when they presented a variety of solutions, and they showed greater faith in their abilities to solve a challenging puzzle, too. The researchers then concluded and theorized that this might be in part due to Montessori's focus on intrinsic gratification as the primary incentive for a well-doing job, rather than the measurable incentive scheme that is sometimes found in a typical classroom setting.

Activities to Boost Toddler's Development

Check Out Textures

Toddlers are tactile learners that appreciate feeling, hearing, and experiencing the environment around them. Using a dark marker to draw alphabet letters and/or numbers on poster paper; then decorate your tot with textured things like sandpaper, shells, cotton balls, pasta, and pipe cleaners. Grabbing the letters allows children a chance to experience the way a letter is being shaped. For those little ones that begin to type, their fingertips will play with a letter form before finding a writing utensil. Say the letters and numbers out loud every day while your kid is brushing his fingertips through them. Earlier the practice is expanded by making a poster that spells out his first name. Your child will soon spot these letters on banners, advertisements, and posters.

Start Measuring Up

Learn how to weigh your child using daily objects. While a ruler is known as a popular measurement device, playing with months, seasons, or time of year to stimulate the learning method. Get your child lie on the lawn in the fall, and then line up apples next to her to determine how many "apples tall" she is at those ages. Or decide how many "Legos big" the sofa is in your house, or how many "wooden blocks long" the refrigerator is in. Figure out how many books your child would need to cover your room for extra fun. Just calculate when you lay down the numerous items, and your child will quickly calculate and weigh in many different ways!

Mark Your Home

Pick either one or two things in your house to be numbered, such as the refrigerator, windows, and furniture, and then change the branded products every few months. Allow stickers the same size and use a simple script, so that children can quickly distinguish them. Write, print, and cut off individual words; then use the blue painter tape to add them to artifacts (which enables quick removal). You may even add the terms on items on index cards and attach them. Labeling helps kids to realize that everything has a series of specific icons to write down and define. When your child is older and now ready to understand letters, show her the letter "lamp" starts with, and remind her to locate the mark that ends with "L." If she is still too young, pick out various letters, and expose her to the symbols. Strengthen the idea every day, and your child should be able to autonomously define the terms over time.

Sing Vocabulary Words

Build this ability by making humorous melodies with rhyming words and count to ten, or performing simple, popular songs like the Alphabet Song or "The Itsy Bitsy Spider." "In the pre-reader years, kids acquire an average of nine new words a day," tells children's author Eugie Foster in Pam Allyn's Writing Life / me for your Baby. "Parents have a greater chance of seeing that possible if they build environments for children that are like the nets of dream catchers, catching precious words and their vibrations," says Allyn, who is also LitWorld's Executive Director and founder.

Encourage automobile music, performing at home, and at bath time. If your child is undergoing daycare or pre-school, ask the instructor for favorite songs from the class and reinforce them at back when home. Teach grandma and babysitters songs such that this lighthearted practice includes all the significant people in your child's life. Your child will begin learning by song as she narrates letters, figures, weekdays, and sections of the body in melodic tunes.

Number Your Mornings

Build a calendar grid of 31 boxes on a piece of poster board, and then leave the room at the top to attach signs for each month. Write down the week's days through top and bottom 31 cards of numbers 1 to 31. Add Velcro to each card's back, then to each of the 31 poster cases. Hang the calendar at the stage of your child's eye and add a monthly sign on the first day of each month and the number 1 symbol on the correct day of the week. Challenge her the next day to locate the number 2 card, and work out the week's day. You can even aid in performing the Days of the Week album. Your kid will start to grasp the calendar and the numbering scheme. In addition, according to Allyn, "routines provide children with support in areas that adults sometimes overlook about."

Pin-Up Pictures

Place photos of friends and relatives in your child's space on a bulletin board to build word recognition and enhance recall. Write the names of individuals on sticky notes (include titles like "daughter," "dad," and "cousin") and mark them at the bottom of each photograph. Refer to the terms regularly, particularly at a family reunion. Delete any sticky notes from the photographs, as everybody is more comfortable with your child. Often, read books on brothers and sisters, or aunt and uncles, and encourage your child to describe every of the listed family members. As your child develops, expand the game by building a family tree that includes names and pictures—making this a continually evolving piece of work of art in your house.

Introduce Organization

Cultivates the helpful nature of your child by cultivating structure and organization in your household. Even if it can slow down tasks and chores, parents will accept the price. Connect your household operation to the mark by storing toys, clothing, plates, and kitchen products in different places. Render the cycle a guessing game when you placed items in their numbered bins and drawers.

Ask kids where other things go ("Where are your toys going? Where will your shoes be stored?") Alternatively, put forks in a sock drawer or play in the fridge and encourage kids to correct your "mistakes." They will love to reorganize for mum or dad, who does not seem to know where the cups go! According to the writers of Common Sense Discipline with Toddlers and Preschoolers, Bridge A. Barnes and Stephen M. York, "these exercises offer you a chance to start educating your small children about obligations, supporting others and becoming part of a team."

Plan a Scavenger Hunt

Children become natural explorers, and they want to explore. Scavenger hunts can be developed or conceived in preparation on the spot. Check the store for products that are one particular color (like purple) or search around the house for items in one form (like a circle). If your child wants to support, pick three things for her to select from when questioning, "Which object is pinkish? Which object is a triangle?" Extend the game on the Mark Your Household by organizing a scavenger hunt for various branded products, or encourage her to check the bookshelves for a particular letter, phrase, or number. You should always say you could not locate the carton of orange juice or a pair of shoes. Take your child on a pleasant quest to localize the house products.

Start to learn the area by pointing down the basic store, fire department, petrol station, and other important locations. Discuss the specifics of certain community staples when you visit each spot. It involves who goes there, the intent of your visit, and the things within you find. Then draw or print pictures of these locations and position them together with their information on index cards. Return to those "neighborhood" cards the next occasion you are out together with your boy. For example, if you drop by the dry cleaners, ask your child to find a corresponding "neighborhood" card and ask him a question: Purchase dry clothes or pick up washed clothes? Who works in there, a firefighter or a cleaner? Extend the area experience by organizing visits to a nearby fire department or a police station. Strengthen this practice by showing them the Sesame Street popularized the song "The People in Your Neighborhood."

Every toddler's parent knows that teaching them social skills is not straightforward. That is because even if babies want healthy, enjoyable experiences with others — their own anxieties and expectations get in the way.

They can't help wondering — is that child going to grab its toy? Will they bring the truck in front of the other? When the other kid is forced off the cycle and speeded off, can they get away with it?

In addition, the first move to having children grow emotional maturity is to make them understand how to control their feelings, which is the base for interpersonal interactions. The latter helps them learn empathy for others. The third is to help them learn to communicate their desires and emotions without needing to strike.

This ability set would prove more important to the joy of your child's existence than academic achievement, financial performance, or any of our other traditional acts. In reality, emotional intelligence — defined as the ability to control one's own emotions and to connect well with others — will be a key factor in his or her subsequent academic and career performance in your child's existence, perhaps more essential than IQ.

Work of Montessori, Itard & Seguin

Analysis of intellectual retardation and other developmental problems in children by Itard and Seguin Montessori led her to the research of two French doctors and psychologists, Jean-Marc Gaspard Itard (1774–1838), and Edouard Seguin (1812–1880).

The research of Itard and Seguin by Montessori has had a significant formative impact on the growth of her system of education.

Itard, an Otiatria nurse, has operated with adolescents who were deaf and hard of hearing. He was instrumental in converting the form of clinical assessment used by their medical doctors to infant assessment by the instructor.

His first notable case was his excellently publicized care of "Aveyron's wild kid," a feral man, seemingly abandoned or lost as an infant, who had been discovered living with animals in the mountains. The kid, around twelve years old, had no language, and had no functional skill. Itard had undertaken to educate the boy to teach him in real-life skills and voice. Although he had some modest improvements in training the boy, there were no encouraging findings in the experiment at Itard. A robust student of restricted skills, the boy defied much of Itard's attempts.

Itard's experience with the "wild guy," and his research with mentally disabled children prompted him to hypothesize that humans were going through unique, definitive, and essential periods of human development. Itard was not the first developmental thinker to emphasize the significance of social growth phases. The Roman rhetorician Quintilian (approx. AD 35–100), the Czech theologian and scholar John Amos Comenius (1592–1670), as well as the French intellectual Jean-Jacques Rousseau (1712–1778) all, had recognized the critical value of educational growth. Itard came to his theories through observational study of real children as opposed to those earlier educators who focused their ideas regarding creation on introspection or contemplation.

According to Itard, children encountered their developmental periods by participating in behaviors appropriate to the specific time and for which they were biologically and mentally trained. However, abnormal children, particularly those who were physically or mentally severely impaired, tended to miss the maximum potential of the developmental stage and were left with deficits that affected their further growth.15 He deduced that children needed to encounter the activities suitable to their developmental stage at the right time or bear the consequences of continuous and cumulative development.

Itard's research focused upon many significant themes: culture and human knowledge, and the extent to which human intellect is acquired or taught. There may be a distinction to the fictitious "noble warrior" of Rousseau, Emile, who learns mainly through simple sensory experiences, separated from civilization. Though Emile of Rousseau develops into a compassionate natural guy, itard's Introduction research was very different for the real wild child. Like the laissez-faire and permissive teacher of Emile, Itard was searching for unique forms to teach the boy. In coping with intelligence, Itard observed that knowledge, though a provided one, evolved at the right moment of growth by getting the correct experiences.

Itard's research had greatly influenced Montessori. A specialist such as Itard, Montessori has been qualified in clinical assessment. Readily embracing Itard's theories of scientific testing, she named his actions "the first behavioral psychology attempts." Seguin, a psychiatrist who had practiced psychiatry with Itard, consulted with psychologically ill children and implemented his techniques at the Hospice de Bicetre, a teaching school for children removed from Paris' insane asylum.

Seguin claimed that facilities for children with disabilities would become educational, rehabilitation centers, and that all scientific and pedagogical expertise could be used to address the state of impairment. He has continually emphasized the child's physiological assessment and evaluation as a method of diagnosis, care, and schooling. Seguin created a collection of academic apparatuses and tools to educate the senses and enhance the physical abilities of mentally disabled adolescents. Seguin introduced many methods that Montessori would incorporate in his research with these youngsters, such as basing teaching on developmental phases using didactic curriculum tools and preparing youngsters to practice functional tasks so they could gain a degree of independence. Seguin's groundbreaking special education initiatives became a spark that incited Montessori to dig further into schooling. Montessori derived two ideas from the research of Itard and Seguin: first, that intellectual disability demanded a different kind of education and not just medical care; second, that this specific kind of training was improved by the use of didactic resources and instruments. Nevertheless, the teacher's practices were moral in the education of mentally disabled children and indeed all children, in that it was essential to operate on the child's heart, which was a "kind of hidden key."

3.2 Child Psychologists & Montessori

The four aspects of Montessori teaching that were most out of line with the early 1900's ideas included Montessori's focus on mental or cognitive progress, physical input, the child's reactive growth stages, and the child's natural involvement in learning. Cognitive growth was also a key priority among educators. However, Freud's observations of the human being's mental and sexual growth, and his influence on his actions during his life, had a remarkable influence on the educational scene in America. For the first time, modern philosophers and educators have understood the child's instinctual urges and desires. Perhaps it was expected there could be an intense move away from academic learning and into an effort to interact with these recently identified trends explicitly in the classroom. Impressed by Freud's exploration of the mayhem that can push down repressed animosity and impulses, educators and parents developed a more permissive approach towards conduct that had not been accepted before. Even behavior that was physically destructive was sometimes accepted. It was thought that kicking dolls, hitting cement, tossing over blocks and toys, and smashing items to sort out their repressions was ideal for girls.

It is only lately that many parents have been conscious that their liberality and lack of control in this and other ways have contributed to children becoming undisciplined and depressed. Montessori felt that child behavior, which was physically abusive, was destructive. Far from helping the child feel better about himself, she noticed it left him more depressed than ever before. She did not tolerate such actions in the school, thinking that it was not part of true independence. In its place, she stressed the desire of the infant to explore himself and his willingness to react favorably to his surroundings through the excitement of learning and imaginative activity. She assumed a reduction of moral expectations or academic growth would contribute only to poorer schooling and culture.

If schooling is to be an assistance to society, it cannot be achieved by emptying the schools of intelligence, character, discipline, social peace, and, above all, independence.

Charles Darwin

Darwin's evolutionary philosophy, centered on natural selection, has left the early 1900s American culture with a conviction in xed knowledge. The importance Montessori put on early cognitive learning was completely out of line with the philosophy. Why worry about cognitive development if intelligence is a constant, not subject to modification of the signals? The accepted predetermined development theory was also a legacy of Darwinian influence. If the human embryo follows the development of the species in its formation, subsequent growth, including cognitive development, will well continue in predetermined stages, regardless of external inducements.

Arnold Gesell

Arnold Gesell is well known as the foremost literal depiction of these stages in the growth of the child. The resulting approach to child rearing has been one of "letting the child outgrow it" whenever unpleasant behavior. As one father told me, "Since he was two years old my son [now eighteen] has been going through 'a stage!' "Montessori claimed that the infant would have some factors in his life otherwise else he will not grow normally; so, however, when there are times of destructive behavior, that is because the infant is attempting to convince us that there is no great need for his. She noticed that this form of behavior vanished as the child started to concentrate on his job and gained self-confidence and self-acceptance by exploring himself and his skills. Both the trust of xed ability and the fixed growth hypothesis was given a deathblow in the 1940s as American psychologists started to shift their focus to the impact of early life factors on children's intellectual development. Freud's findings in the early 1900s had sparked curiosity in infancy and early childhood. However, the emphasis was on development, which was emotional, not intellectual. Following World War II, our emphasis on the cognitive development of the young child also began to our own.

It was reported that the children were suffering from extreme retardation in orphanages and schools. This happened despite the fact that outstanding physical treatment had been given well to the babies. Sixty percent of the two-year-old children did not sit alone in one such institution; eighty percent of those four-year-olds could not move. There was one clear finding regarding these institutions: these children provided little to no tactile stimuli. There was no vibration, next to no movement to watch, the walls were colorless. The lack of sensory stimuli in the premature environment apparently had an effect on these children's development.

Donald Hebb

Psychologists have also been conducting tests to explore the sensorial restriction consequences of certain environments. One of such psychologists was Donald Hebb, a man whose research and philosophy changed the direction of contemporary American psychology in a substantial way. Experimenting first with animals like rats and then gradually with dogs, Hebb found their adult problem-solving ability to vary considerably in the richness of their early environment. Hebb wrote his Behavior Organization, a novel theorizing on his experimental research, in 1949. This book provided Montessori's approach to early learning and environmental stimulation with the rest psycho-theoretical basis. Before a discovery that was made, it was commonly assumed that the brain should work via basic patterns or associations for stimulation response. Such relations were created for repeated interactions and comparisons to evolve and become lasting mental patterns. The functioning of the brain resembled a telephone switchboard. (It was on this commonly established principle of brain structure and function that Kilpatrick had based his criticism of the philosophy of transfer-of-learning and, thus, one of his key challenges to Montessori education.) This hypothesis of brain function did not sufficiently account for the Hebb effect, although some were ending in the laboratory in the light of early environmental influences. Hebb developed a much more critical theory of the neurological structure and brain processes that considered those phenomena. He argued that "cell assemblies" representing images or ideas are formed in early learning, and that these assemblies are joined into "phase sequences" in later learning, which facilitates thinking that, is more complex. Thus, later learning would depend on the wealth of the cell assemblies formed earlier.

Observation by Montessori of the child's spontaneous interest in learning was also supported by Hebb's theorizing. Any behavior was previously believed to be driven primarily by instinctual or homeostatic needs (the organism's need for a healthy physical and chemical state). If this were true, if no such motivation were present, the organisms would be quiescent. Physiologists, on the opposite, have recently identified that the central nervous system is continuously involved independent of external or endogenous stimuli. Hebb theorized that in addition to the already recognized motivation based on instinctual drives and homeostatic needs, there needed to be an intrinsic motivation for behavior. H did some of the critical research that would support this modern hypothesis. Harlow, F. In three different experiments, he observed that monkeys could and will learn to operate puzzles where no other incentive but the appearance of the puzzle itself has been ordered. Real learning had been demonstrated as once the puzzle had been mastered, it worked awfully and persistently. Harlow also showed that, rather than promoting, the usage of hunger-reducing incentives simply undermined incentive. He found that, as soon as they were finished, monkeys who had been rewarded with food for working their puzzles ignored them. On the other side, the unrewarded monkeys always continued investigating and exploiting the puzzle after it had been completed. Nearly fifty years ago, Montessori came to specific findings on the children's inner drive for learning through studying children specifically rather than animals in the laboratory. She had developed a classroom protocol based on this inner incentive, totally discarding the gold stars, special rights, qualifications, etc. that are now standard use as inducements to learning in classrooms today.

McVicker Hunt

Another visionary in the field of motivational learning is McVicker Hunt, who is particularly relevant to Montessori. He found that babies acquire habits of remembrance, and would attempt to repeat them after six months of age (crying to try the return of mother). The child often slowly becomes fascinated and may deliberately pursue the enjoyment of excitement within a known sense. "A major source of pleasure lies in finding something new within the context of the familiar." Novelty becomes a tool of motivation, then, if the old corresponds correctly to the new. The enticing novelty tends to be an ideal disparity in this partnership between the moment's input of knowledge and the details already accumulated in the cerebrum from experiences with specific circumstances. The child will be frustrated if there is too much excitement or incongruity; if it is too little, he will be bored.

Hunt called "the matching problem" the dilemma of finding the proper amount of each for any specific child at a given time.

Chapter 4: The Ultimate Parenting Guide

Becoming a new parent can be very exciting yet frightening at the same time. It can in fact get as scary as possible especially when it comes to the health of your newborn. As a new parent, it is essential that you realize you will make mistakes, but you will have to forgive yourself. Remember that, as a parent again, you are the primary caretaker of your child and that you will learn from your own experiences and take on responsibility rather than from others' take on parenthood. However, it is also completely normal to experience this roller coaster of emotions as there are plenty of ways to educate yourself about your little one. And, this chapter of the book has got you covered; starting from hypnobirthing to introducing you to baby sleep-training and feeding techniques and other effective parenting methods, it will provide you all the basics you need to become an expert parent.

4.1 The concept of Hypnobirthing

On its own, the word hypnosis implies "a treatment through which individual encounters proposed improvements in feeling, vision, thinking or actions." One specific marketed type of hypnosis is referred to as Hypnobirthing during the conception phase. Although this general concept has been around for decades, hypnotherapist Marie Mongan in the 1989 novel Hypnobirthing invented the precise word: A Celebration of Life. The theories are inspired by Dr. Jonathan Dye and Dr. Grantly Dick-Read, the pioneers of early "random conception."

Hypnobirthing, at its core, intends to help a woman deal with any apprehension or discomfort she might have around conception. It requires different methods of calming and self-hypnosis to help the body recover before and after conception and childbirth. Using breathing exercises and self-hypnosis, parents will support each other through a system that can help you conquer your worries and learn to disregard the painful birth myths that continue to spread and intimidate us during pregnancy.

The idea is that birth can happen faster and more painlessly once the mind and body are in a completely relaxed state because the body is not fighting the natural process. Hypnobirthing ideals seek to merge mindfulness and birth hypnosis, with the goal of eliminating any of the anxiety around childbirth and offering moms-to-be the encouragement and trust they need to make giving birth into a genuinely positive experience. Hypnobirthing provides moms-to-be with the courage to deal with discomfort, to aspire for an orderly birth (making reference to inducements), and to be comfortable if the delivery is not scheduled, for example, when an immediate C-section is required. Hypnobirthing's emphasis is on the relation and imagination of mind and body and looks at how self-hypnosis may help birth mums deal with the discomfort they feel in childbirth.

Relaxation is a term for the Hypnobirthing game. Yet how do you fall into a Zen-like condition amid all the theoretically turmoil of contractions? Well, several methods can be used, such as relaxing and levers.

Controlled respiration

The Hypnobirthing Midwife discusses two other methods of ventilation. You breathe heavily through the nose in the run, then through the nose back. Inhale into the four-count, and out to the seven counts.

The second is close in methodology. You adopt the same method of deep breathing, but lengthen the inhalation to the count of seven, and hold the exhalation to the count of seven. It will serve to stimulate your parasympathetic nervous system by relaxing in this manner, offering you some soothing vibes.

Concentrating on positive thinking and words

Concentrating on happy thoughts and expressions is another helpful tactic. You can use "surge" or "shock" for a more optimistic perspective instead of using the term "contraction" to explain the tightening throughout labor. Another way is replacing membrane "rupture" with the term "release."

Guided visualization

Other methods involve guided visualization, where you might imagine things like a flower opening to help calm the body, then use music then meditation to calm more. The aim is to give birth in a condition similar to daydreaming by utilizing such strategies. You may: be more conscious of what is happening to you and be able to come and go out of hypnosis when you please becoming more comfortable, holding the body out of the fight-or-flight state that may be triggered by the new atmosphere of a birth room to be more able to handle endorphin release pain and stress hormones By regulating pain and stress hormones, the body may let go and submit completely.

Related Hypnobirthing-like techniques are often called the Mongan Method. It is known to be the "first" form, which contains five classes that are 2 1/2 hours long, for a total of 12 hours. There are several accredited teachers in the Hypnobirthing worldwide. The key concept of this approach is that once the body is calm, extreme discomfort will not have to be included in the labor. Participants practice different methods of self-hypnosis and calming, including directed visualization and respiration.

Hypnobabies is another way of getting hypnosis during the cycle of conception. This is focused on the Painless Childbirth Program, which the master hypnotherapist Gerald Kein created. This technique has some key differences, although similar to Hypnobirthing. It depends on different approaches to deal relieve discomfort vs. purely calming strategies. Such methods include strategies such as hypnotic compounding (repetition) and even somnambulistic (sleepwalking) "professional school" hypnosis.

Hypnobirthing may:

- Reduce labor, along with confidence in the birthing cycle. In fact, birth hypnosis may help to shorten the first stage of labor. This stage requires both early and active labor where, when the cervix expands, contractions get longer, deeper, and closer together.
- Lessen the desire to interfere. A 2011 analysis of research found that Hypnobirthing could help promote natural birth, and people utilizing hypnosis may not need as much oxytocin augmentation. A

2015 report showed that just 17 percent of Hypnobirthing's Reliable Root moms had cesarean deliveries relative to a general 32 percent average in the United States.

- Manage discomfort normally. Hypnosis can also help if you are aiming for medium-free labor. Fourty six out of eighty-one participants (51 percent) did not use any pain medication in one 2013 study and reported their maximum pain level on a 10-scale as just 5.8.

- Offer them a feeling of power. Women have also indicated feeling more confident and in charge of the 2013 survey. As a result, they became less fearful of labor and conception.

- Good babies lead. Apgar ratings, which is the method for measuring babies in the minutes after conception, could be higher for babies raised utilizing Hypnobirthing.

- Help those women who have had trauma. In fact, Hypnobirthing may benefit birthers who have encountered distress around conception or who have a general apprehension of labor and childbirth.

If this is your first kid, and you are scared, excited, concerned, or just want any support to aid you through the birth process. Alternatively, whether this is your fourth baby and your previous births have not gone as planned and left you feeling nervous or depressed. Hypnobirthing applies to all! It can assist in any kind of birth, whether C-section, VBAC, home birth, college, at the car's back!

The course is intended to attend moms-to-be with their birth companion (husband, child, girlfriend, relative, family member). Your birth companion is the one you would like to be at your birth with you. If this is not approachable for you, even then you can still do the course on your own and still get a beautiful birth from Hypnobirthing.

Popular misconceptions about Hypnobirthing

- The hypnosis connected with hypnosis is a type of mind regulation or brainwashing.

- Hypnosis sends you to a deep state.
- A person who was hypnotized has no free thought.
- If you are hypnotized, you cannot do
- Regular activities and functions.
- When you are hypnotized, you do not realize what is going on around you.

Is it possible to hypnobirthing?

Hey. You are not going to be in a coma, or fall asleep, despite the name. You will be conscious of everything that is going on around you, and you will feel completely relaxed and in control. Do, however, remember that problems are not avoided by hypnobirthing.

How can I know about hypnobirthing?

Ask your midwife regarding lessons or seminars on hypnobirthing, since the NHS provides various courses around the world. These can not only help you but also help your family understand more about how hypnobirthing functions in more depth, what happens to your body through pregnancy, what your birth partner can do to support, and, among other items, what antenatal exercises you can do. In courses and seminars, such as extra audio content, you can typically get supplemental content for self-study.

If you are unable to join a course or choose to learn yourself, then you have other choices, such as CDs, DVDs, software, podcasts, and books explaining the methods of hypnobirthing.

When should I start training on hypnobirthing?

Following your 20-week check, the optimal time to book a course is, but it also depends on the quality of the courses in your field. Some NHS-run hypnobirthing courses, for example, can only begin from 28 weeks. Sessions generally last around two and a half hours a day, with four or five lessons over a month's duration.

If you are going to have your baby at a hospital, at a birth center, or at home, hypnobirthing will help you have a happier birth. The strategies you practice in hypnobirthing can only support to keep you feeling in charge, no matter how the labor progresses.

4.2 Baby Sleep-Training Techniques & No cry baby solution

Does your kid have to be rocked to bed by you — or getting up while it is still midnight looking for a breast, a drink, or a cuddle before going back to bed? If your little one is at least four months old, then it might be time to begin sleeping.

Because of that age, babies can — and should — fall asleep, or fall back to sleep by self-reassuring. If you are dreading sleep training (also known as sleep teaching), remember it is always done quicker than other parents expect, and it does not even have to require tons of crying.

When people add to sleep the word "Montessori," it always refers to the growth of freedom during sleep and bedtime. It is important to remember that Dr. Montessori rarely wrote about sleep and that there is no particular solution that all parent (or teachers) in the Montessori model identify with. The key idea is to focus on children being encouraged to obey their hormone sleep window to enable them to self-regulate themselves. Montessori sleep strategies may be useful for trouble sleepers and easy sleepers, as long as you select a system in which you are confident and which is a good match for the temperament of the infant.

Tips:

- Hold to it for a week or more.
- Do not expect everything to function in three days or shorter, some adjustments, and some kids need to adapt at least a couple of weeks.
- Do not allow sleep or penalty a result. Keep it nice. Lots of affection, cuddles, and routines and practices that are calming help make

bedtime simpler for children and parents. Ignore the kid as in all things in Montessori.

Floor Bed

The most commonly debated sleep system for Montessori is the floor bed, a crib- or kids-sized mattress positioned either directly on the floor or on a small bed frame. The principle behind this is that children can enter (or exit) their beds safely at any moment, which allows the bedroom to be completely child-safe. This is a perfect situation for some kids, and for some, it is just too much space. (In addition, there is nothing to suggest that if you decide to co-sleep, you cannot make your own bed a floor bed!)

Playing to Sleep

Another idea is "play to sleep" that encourages kids to have access to books and games at bedtime and offer them the right to choose when they are ready to sleep. There are also certain guidelines, so everything is special for each family.

Stimulation

An essential feature of Montessori-style bedrooms is that they do not believe in themselves over-stimulate. The rooms themselves will allow for peace and relaxation so children will indulge in hours of play inside them. Any items that would match the day may need to be withdrawn or changed during the night, such as stereos, shifting furniture to prevent injuries, etc. Montessori is compassionate and serves the infant above all others. When they show that they are willing, we motivate and teach children concepts and responsibilities. Many children require support more than others, so although it is the individual choice of each adult, the Montessori approach takes into consideration the children's wishes so preferences; children are not pressured to meet living arrangements or demands that they feel uncomfortable or disturbed by. That's not to suggest whether a kid gets a choice as to whether or not they're going to bed — they don't — but instead, whether a child feels uncomfortable going to sleep without a light on, with a parent present, etc., we understand that pressuring the child to adhere to our (well-intentioned, well-informed) bedtime arrangement may be counter-productive and doesn't appear as encouraging to the infant. It can help to think about it as eating: we do not let kids pick whether to feed or not, but we do not compel a kid to use a spoon that is not packed. We include the spoon as an option to display them, but we will not sit to watch a child not eat because they are not ready to use a spoon (or do not feel prepared to do so).

It is also necessary to insert some routine into sleep — as in any part of the day. Routine is comforting because they become more relaxed because secure relaxing into their bedtime as children can foresee just what will happen next.

Before Getting Started

It's important that even before you even think about "training" your baby to fall asleep on their own, make sure you follow a regular schedule and put them to bed each night at a consistent time (hint: usually better early, typically around 7 or 8 p.m.). It's a smart idea to try and put them down drowsy, then get up whenever you can, just to get them (and you) habituated to it, even if they fuss a little. Be sure they've been up for a decent period of time before bed (an over- or under-tired infant may have difficulty falling asleep), and set up a relaxing and regular bedtime routines, such as a meal, bath or relaxation accompanied by pajamas and stories or songs. To stop letting the kid equate the feeding with falling asleep, specific experts suggest feeding at the beginning of the day. Ideally, during your bedtime routine, your baby should not be beginning to nod off at some point. "You just want to make sure your kid is healthy for the night," says Montreal-based counselor Pamela Mitel man, who specializes in young adolescents and babies. Be conscious, too, of getting adequate exercise and relaxation to fill their daytime awake times, Garden says. "When they are awake, infants tend to be going in all manner of directions, not only sitting in a bouncy chair," she notes.

Here is how and when your baby should start sleep training to help everyone get a good night's sleep.

1) Sleep training no-cry-the fading method

For sleep training with no controlled weeping, the fading technique (a.k.a. gradual retreat) means just doing what you have done so far, and gradually minimizing the contact, you have with your child during bedtime.

The sleep guru and bestselling author of Kid Secrets this morning, Jo Tantrum, offers her top tip saying: "help your kid know how to sleep without a sleep aid" For example, if you usually put them down to sleep once they have gone to sleep, you'll put them down right before they fall asleep with the fading-it-out approach (FIO). If they wake up and cry, then take them back. If you rock them down to sleep, try to prevent doing this gradually. If they weep when you stop, rock them again a little bit, but keep trying to minimize that. Try to replace this with a dummy if your child sleeps on the boob, or get your partner to take the child to bed instead so that they stop affiliating breast time with bedtime. It is a method that is slow, but it can be achieved

2) Minimal contact sleep training method

This method is also known as the pick-up / put-down method and is a more gentle way of the sleeping train. That helps with the parent sitting with the baby until they fall asleep while attempting to lessen the touch, not holding the baby in your arms, for example. Place them in bed, pat them, shoot them, and try to get them back. If they scream, then again, you may pat and shush. If that does not work, then you can pick them up and put them down when they are quiet again.

They have to get used to putting themselves down. The entire idea is only taking up the kid for support then setting them down for the night. Try to keep the contact minimized. You will stop picking them up at some point, and just pat them until you can finally managed to lay them down at bedtime and let them sleep alone. We like that method, and so do babies. At first, it is tiring for the parent and might take much longer than any of the other methods, but it's guilt-free!

3) Sleep training Ferber technique

This system, developed by Dr. Richard Ferber, is also regarded as the technique of cry-out sleep training or the form of check-and-console.

If you have placed your baby in bed with their calming bedtime music or night-lights, you leave the house, and when they complain, you come back, touch them, and soothe them with phrases like "there, there," or "goodnight kid, go to sleep," or your choice terms, before you go. When they scream or complain, you go back in, massage and soothe them again; hopefully without picking them up and then leave again before they fall asleep. If they start crying, you should adhere to the same plan, adding one minute per time before coming back into the house.

The Ferber method's aim is to remind the kid that you are still there, but now its bedtime, so it is time to sleep. This technique is derived from a more severe variant of the Ferber System, and the somewhat divisive, the Extinction Approach, also known as the Cry it Out (CIO) form of sleep training. Marc Weissbluth developed this, so it means bringing the kid to bed, saying goodnight, and then leaving them there to sweat it out before they go to sleep. Many experts and parents highly criticize this method and consider it unnecessary, as there are many other ways of getting a child to sleep alone through the night. That said when they are at the end of their absolute wit, a lot of parents turn to this method as a last resort, with excellent results. If you can stomach it, getting your child to sleep alone through the night is a beneficial and quick way, often within a few days.

The aim of the CIO approach is to let baby stress and weep alone before she ends up sweating herself out and falling asleep alone. You may end up needing to let the baby cry it out at the beginning for 45 minutes to an hour until she goes to sleep, but it differs from baby to kid. Many parents who seek the technique of crying it out see their kids screaming fewer and less over the first three days until their weeping stops approximately anywhere between the fourth until seventh evenings. Eventually, infants will either whine or screech a few minutes of protest — or just fall asleep peacefully. Whereas it depends on your infant and the ease with the process to know whether to let the baby cry it out. Babies are usually able for production to sleep around 4 to 6 months of age. They will sleep through the night by around 5 to 6 months without needing to feed, making it a perfect time to test out the CIO system.

Note that your older baby may already have equipped you with feedings, cuddling as well as a return to your bed to react to her nocturnal cries. Around six months, infants are wise to the idea that screaming always contributes to being picked up, swayed, or eaten — a strong incentive to continue to do so. When that is the case, then baby and you may need any adjustments to the sleep routine. However, if they get the impression that you do not accept their actions, many will give up the game of weeping, typically within three or four days, often longer.

4) Form of sleep training chair

The chair system is a way to let your kid think you are there because it is always bedtime. A milder variant of the Ferber process, you are dressing the kid for bed and setting them down every night following the same procedure, taking a chair and staying next to them before they fall asleep. This strategy will take longer than other approaches as they will want your help if your kid sees you there, so you will have to stop. You should hug them every few minutes if they weep before they calm down. Try not to make eye contact, and if you see the baby scream and do not react, it would be rough for both of you. It is not fun watching a baby cry and doing nothing about it, and that is the same thing the child will ask. If you have perfected them falling asleep while seated next to them, the next step is to push the chair farther and farther forward, until you are totally out of the house.

5) The hybrid method of sleep training

No one size fits all. Some infants respond to dummies, while others do not. Some may like to be swaddled, while others may not. There is no right way, and every parent has to choose what is correct for them and their baby. There are no specific rules of a method for hybrid sleep training. It is just about working for the intuition. This hybrid method allows you to choose what is right for you. You may choose the relieve and comfort method for 20 minutes, then move on to the chair method for another 20 minutes, before proceeding to the Ferber method.

Remember that kids are going through phases, and even a big sleeper may have sleep regression, so, at certain times, you might have to go through sleep training all over again. If you want to make changes to your bedtime routine, gradually make them and lighten the baby into it. The key is consistency with whatever works for you.

Stand up, set down method. This strategy in sleep training includes you moving through the usual cycle of your baby's bedtime and placing her to bed drowsy yet wakeful. Wait a couple of minutes, when and where she starts screaming, to see how she slows down. Otherwise, go back to pick her up to soothe her. Place her back in the crib or bassinet, until she is quite enough.

Repeat until the kid falls asleep. Just be mindful that this form of sleep training will take a long time, which would demand a lot of discipline.

Tips

Sleep training tips the following sleep training suggestions can help make sure a smoother transition to dreamland: establish a bedtime routine no matter what method you are trying to use. Follow a coherent 30- to 45-minute children sleep routine to help your little one transition from awake to sleepy time. If she falls asleep in the breast or bottle, resume that feed in front of the shower or books, so you can put her to bed whilst she is waking.

Time to fix it. It is not the time to play with baby's sleep when his or her life has undergone a recent disturbance (a relocation, new nanny, ear infection, travel.). Wait before things stabilize until you try sleeping preparation.

Know when you have an exhausted kid. Watch for signs of sleep, such as yawning, eye scratching, or grumpiness, which can occur every night at around the same time. It is important to put your baby in bed when she is sleepy but not overtired, as overtired babies are more likely to sleep or wake up early. Place the kid up full. Sleep training is focused around getting the kid to fall asleep in her own — an experience she will not learn if you cradle her to sleep into your arms until she is moved to the crib.

Wait time for your reply. On the first groan, do not rush into the baby's room. In the night, babies make many noises, including weeping, and then fall back asleep. A nodding-off infant may wake up to any little noise or scream, or it can disrupt her attempts to soothe herself.

1. New Child? Support configure the "global clock" of your infant by introducing your kid to clear signs about the 24-hour day outside.

Like older adults, babies have sleep patterns or natural processes that commute every 24 hours, about once. You may think about such patterns as a clock that functions internally, there is a catch: no pre-programmed clock arrives. When babies are raised, their inner clocks are not aligned with the sunlight and darkness external 24-hour period. Babies need time to get in sync. Luckily, we do not have to sit passively to see that happen. We cannot, in reality, be inactive. Babies rely on us for help. Studies suggest that babies respond better when parents send them the correct "time-keepers" or external signals about the hour of the day. So reveal your baby to natural light and get your baby involved in your daytime activities' designed to stimulate the hustle and bustle. Guard the kid against sensitivity to artificial lights as evening comes. As I see below (see baby sleep tip # 2), light is a signal which tells the brain to postpone the onset of night sleep.

2. Use bulbs (or filters) that block the blue wavelengths when you need artificial lighting at night.

If you replaced both electric and artificial light sources at night, you and your baby would possibly consider sleeping easier. Yet complete blackouts are not a practical choice for most of us. When we decide to indulge in evening sports, what should we do, including reading? What do we do when we need a diaper change?

Happily, not all light wavelengths on the inner clock have the same effect. Yeah, white light (that is produced from both fluorescent and incandescent bulbs) has a detrimental impact on sleep habits, and the impact is highly important for small children.

However, one portion of white light — the blue part of the continuum — seems to be responsible for most of the problem. If we can obstruct that part of the light spectrum, the negative effects of nighttime light exposure could be minimized. A low watt, the amber bulb is capable of protecting your baby from blue wavelengths, yet providing you with enough light to perform infant care at night. Similarly, blue light filters can reduce the risk of sleep due to nighttime viewing of electronic screens.

3. Help your baby be settled: create a period of comfort, joy, and mental reassurance the hour leading up to bedtime. When we are anxious or irritated, none of us sleeps well, and babies are no different. So take action to ensure your kid feels protected, comfortable, content, and valued before bedtime. Try pursuing a schedule at bedtime (Mindell et al. 2015; Mindell et al. 2017).

Look for your own emotional state because of its contagious stress. Babies become more distressed with distress from their careers (Waters et al. 2014; Waters et al. 2017). In addition, if you sense negative feelings in your infant, combat them with reassurance and nothingness.

Studies at assessment say that this creates a difference. Parents who respond soothingly to the emotions of their children report fewer problems of infant sleep, and this is how it works regardless of the sleep arrangements in a family. If children share a bedroom with their parents or sleep elsewhere, when their parents are alert and attentive, they sleep better (Teti et al. 2010; Jian and Teti 2016).

4. Learn the art of stress busting — for your baby and for yourself. A baby who is very easily annoyed or becomes distressed is hard to soothe. This post on tension in babies in Parenting Research provides insights into what triggers babies. It also offers evidence-based advice to keep the babies happy and safe emotionally. However, what if you feel too stressed out for reassurance and calm project? Or far too depressed?

If it is, so you are not lonely. Caring for a baby can indeed be very worrying, troublesome, and even exhausting, especially when you yourself are sleep-deprived, coping with childbirth trauma or struggling with an excessively crying baby (see baby sleep tip # 10). If you are weak in your mental condition, check for postpartum depression and keep your psychological wellbeing a priority. Postpartum depression and postpartum stress are very normal, but many parents are still privately suffering. Discuss your choice with your psychiatrist.

5. If your kid does not seem to be asleep at bedtime, do not try to push it.

Getting bossy does not make children any sleepier, which makes them more hyperactive, if anything. In addition, you do not want to link the kid to a clash with bedtime.

6. Look out for those lengthy, late afternoon naps and seek to extend the last bit of waking until bedtime.

If your baby is not sleeping until late at night, the first rule is to guarantee that, your baby is not subject to bright lights until bedtime (baby sleep tip # 2). Next move? Test the duration of your baby's naps. For infants, naps do nice stuff, but infants are like us: late naps will set off the drowsiness they might normally have at bedtime (Nakagawa et al. 2016). Then see how you can prolong the period your kid spends up during the least productive portion of the day. When researchers tracked parents who used this advice, they found that babies were beginning to need less help sleeping at night (Skulldottir et al. 2005).

13. 13. Do not feel under pressure to burp or diaper your baby if your baby is waking up.

Something you would not want to do while your infant sleeps — or is about to doze off — is to jolt her up with unnecessary treatment. Could you wait, then? That seems probable.

Researchers find no proof of a new review of more than 70 children that burping has proven helpful to babies. It did not make them cry less, and indeed, it increased the chances of a baby spouting after being fed. (Kaur et al. 2015). In addition, an earlier finding shows that the feeling of a damp diaper does not activate babies (Zotter et al., 2007).

14.14. Get reasonable ideas regarding sleeping patterns for your kid?

What is the perfect time for bed? Your kid will sleep for how long? When does your baby start sleeping through the night for long intervals?

If you knew the answers to those issues, it would help you escape traps — and anger without use. For example, if your baby will not sleep the way you should like it to be, it is simple to believe that you are doing it wrong. New parents sometimes worry that if their young infants wake up multiple times at night, there is something developing awry. Night waking are always completely natural.

Parents may even make the error of scheduling the incorrect bedtime to seek to push their kids to fall asleep at a time when their inner clock is out of alignment. As noted in tip # 4 of baby sleep, the resulting conflict can create lasting problems with sleep.

In addition, parents are sometimes overly complacent about certain things — like a baby's nocturnal vampire-like schedule. If you believe that there is something you could not undo, it will become a promise that fulfills itself. You cannot use effective techniques, such as infant sleep advice on light signals. This helps to learn about the normal course of development of infant sleep and the wide range of variations that healthy babies can show.

Frequently Asked Questions about Sleep-Training

Can you sleep train for shorter sleep like naps?

The same overnight sleep management technique can be extended to naps. If you want to cry it out, or Ferber, bear in mind that a large part of the nap may be gone after 30 minutes of screaming. Moreover, you would want to put a cap on crying (say, 10 to 15 minutes) before you find some way to get your baby to sleep.

How long would it take for the sleep training?

Most infants are taught to sleep after three or four nights with strategies such as Ferber or cry it out (save a couple of minutes with fussing or wails before nodding off). Some methods of training — especially bedtime fading, the chair approach and pick up, put down — will possibly take longer, and for some babies, certain approaches will not function at all. Be faithful to the sleep-training approach you have selected to give it a chance to function for two complete weeks.

Is the teaching on sleep cruel?

Sleep has a negative reputation with those seeing raising an infant as an insensitive way to. Sleep is not about plunging a newborn into a crib and keeping it there until the morning after.

Of reality, most professionals warn against making a baby scream for longer than 15 minutes, and not all of the sleep strategies discussed above support that. There are plenty of other strategies to help the kid sleep through the night. Sleep training does not have to be associated with crying, it is not cruel, and it will help you and your baby tremendously.

Why train your child to sleep?

Even like we educate our kids to feed, drink, exercise, and talk – all the essential aspects of a human's everyday existence, so we have to educate them to sleep. Sleep is a big part of living. Even as adults, if we are disturbed by our nightly sleep and have trouble falling back to sleep, it could make us tired, grumpy, and disturbed during the day too. A safe sleep schedule is something that will always help a child well in their everyday lives as they develop. Sleep training can take some time to get the hang of and needs commitment, discipline, and energy, but in the end, it will be worth it.

How do I choose the right method for my baby and me?

One of the main aspects of sleep training is to find the strategy that works best for you. Ultimately, you are the only person who understands what your (and the baby's) ability to sob is. When a process for you does not look appropriate or seems too "intense," do not do it. Start with a gentle plan you are at ease with.

Keep in mind that you and your partner could have different levels of comfort and tolerance. Starting tiny is better then moving on to a less friendly approach if appropriate so you can know what you are happy with and what really won't fit for you and your family. In the end, the best method for you and your family will be the one you can change to suit your needs and comfort levels. There are several various sleep training approaches to pick from, although the most common strategies are described above as one or a combination of one of the five. You may find that one of these methods sounds like it is a perfect match for you, OR you may find aspects from every plan you like.

You may also have learned of the "sleep feeling" or the "sleep lady scramble," as opposed to a specific system, these are actually separate sleep training programs. Typically, though, they implement or function with the same principles that we discussed above.

The scale of sleep training approaches from gentler to less gentle when studying the numerous approaches of sleep training to assess which one is correct for you, note that growing kid and family is special. What one mom swears by, swears off another parent. If you use your instincts to choose, a system you and your baby know would be happy with, you will get the most benefit from sleep training.

How can I ensure successful sleep training?

Sleep planning for any family can look a bit different, based on which approach you want to adopt. To be effective, the numerous strategies need specific approaches from the parents. Tip to Melissa: take notice! Having a list of how your kid has done in the sleep training would be helpful when you are too exhausted to know how long they have been sleeping the night before.

Dream Feeding

Dream feeding: An evidence-based guide to help babies sleep more extended Dream feeding has been described as feeding a sleeping baby, as promoting the baby to sleep for longer. The word was often used to define any big meal that is scheduled to occur shortly before the parent falls asleep (delivered during sleep or waking time).

Are these effective measures? There is justification for believing that they might give you more quiet sleeping time. But dream feeds alone probably play only a modest role in the development of infant sleep. The most effective path to improving advanced sleep habits is to integrate dream feeds with other sleep-friendly activities.

Here is an outline of the subject — the meanings, the proof, the pros and cons, and the questions frequently asked.

What fuels dreams?

Tracey Hogg, who used the word for the very first time, describes dream feeding as feeding a young child while dreaming. In a very gentle way, hold your sleeping baby in a feeding position to accomplish this and try to enhance the rooting reflex by stroking the baby's mouth and offering your baby a breast or bottle. Several babies will eat without waking up in this way (Hogg and Blau, 2005).

Although some people make specific usage of the word "vision feed." For, e.g., Harvey Karp relates to intentionally waking a child as : "Vision feeding is when you wake up your kid to eat once more before you switch in for the night" (Karp, n.d.).

Others use the label "dream feed" to portray any effort to "tank up" your baby before you go to bed by yourself. It's not clear whether the kid is sleeping or alert. What is important is the meal arrives only before the parent rests. So with both these meanings, that's the basic denominator — the notion of having a kid to take in a large meal until you doze.

Newborns are quickly and often awoken by the empirical rationale for dream feeding, in part, because they are starving. If you start to sleep shortly after your baby has "boozed up," you may get some more time before your baby wakes up again.

In addition, every bit helps, particularly if you can sleep uninterrupted for a minimum of 4 hours. Our brains are built during the first few sleep stages of the night to target the most restorative period of sleep — NREM3, or intense, slow-wave sleep — And if only one part of your nightly sleep bout should be covered from interruptions, it would be the first 4-5 hours of sleep.

For many parents, it is impossible to achieve this ideal state in the days immediately after childbirth. If this is your case, you can take heart: When people are severely deprived of sleep — suffering from a significant NREM3 deficiency — their brains sometimes react by raising the duration of brief naps.

If you can take a couple of 30-minute naps throughout the day, you can get enough NREM3 to mitigate much of the sleep deprivation's harmful effects (Farout et al. 2015).

However, having your kid to sleep longer — enjoying at least one, 4-5 hour bout of sleep right at your bedtime — will make things simpler. It will offer you the ability to achieve the least and most significant amount of sleep you need to sustain your well-being. In addition, it may be an essential step for your baby to mature, nighttime sleep patterns.

However, will the feeding of dreams work? Will this contribute to more extended periods of baby sleep? Many parents that have tried it feel it works. Their babies sleep in longer, more centralized bouts as the weeks pass. Although we should, of course, allow it to happen anyway. Young infants grow more unified sleeping patterns at night when everything is going well. Below mentioned are the benefits dream feeding can provide you:

Synchronize Your Baby's Sleep with Your Own Sleep

One aim of a dream feed is to match up with your first period of sleep for your baby's more extended phase. Most babies get a longer period of rest, usually in the first half of the night, waking up only when moms calm down in a good stretch of sleep! If your newborn has one or even two night feeds, using a dream feed will get you a more extended period of rest.

Exception for a kid that eats more than one night: Without a dream feed: the child goes down for sleep at 7:00 pm and starts her long 5-hour period. You go to sleep at 10:00 pm, but at midnight, your infant is getting up for a snack. Only Two hours later, the night is cut short!

With a dream feed: Your baby will go down at 7:00 pm for bedtime. Shortly before you head to bed, you are getting a sleep feed at 10:00 pm. Your baby ends her long 5-hour period and wakes at 3:00 am. You have now reached 5 hours of the uninterrupted night!

For babies that sleep in even longer stretches of 8 or 9 hours, that may also mean that your baby sleeps straight to the morning: without a dream feed: your baby goes to bed around 7:00 pm and starts the long 8-hour cycle. At 10:00 pm, you go to bed, and your baby wakes you up at 3:00 am for a feeding. This early morning wake appears to be right in the center of the deepest sleep of a person! (You say that because it is tough to get up and it is much easier to get back to sleep later.) Fuel a dream: the kid goes to bed at 7 pm. Right before you head to bed, you are performing a vision feed at 10:00 pm. Your baby starts its long 8-hour stretch and makes it until 6:00 am. Now you will all wake up comfortable and ready for the day! You had a good night's sleep!

Tank Up Without the Sleep Alliance

One aim of a dream feeding is to start with night feedings with a decreased probability of developing a sleep relationship by night feed. This guarantees that your baby receives adequate calories, but when you start the dream feed as your baby sleeps, and not as a reaction to a call for action, it becomes less likely to become a sleeping crutch. The abdomen of your infant is tanked up, but it is not correlated with the process of falling asleep as he is still sleeping.

Maintain the Supply

A dream feed may be of special benefit to kids who sleep on their own early on in the night, or to moms who have returned to work. In both situations, the supply of mom's milk can take a drop, but you may sustain or even raise supply without needing to put in another pumping session by withdrawing milk from a dream-feed.

Eliminate the Guesswork

You have more power of what your baby eats because you are beginning the feeding process. No longer, go to bed worried over what the night is going to look like.

When does a fantasy feed come true?

The dream feed fits well with younger kids under the age of 6 months who are more prone to need a feeding scientifically. In older babies, the introduction of a dream feed appears to disturb the night. In older infants, whether following their lead or reducing excessive feedings is always more successful.

If you are using the dream feed to further balance the long duration of your baby's sleep with your own, you will want to feed your vision before you go to bed. This appears to work best from 10:00 am to 11:00 pm. If you do a dream feed to safeguard your supply or boost calorie intake, the feeding time is less important.

How do I feed on a dream?

It is pretty easy! If you're breastfeeding, just gently pick up your baby and bring it to the breast. Be sure to keep your stimulation low so that you won't wake your baby up completely.

You can pick up the baby or even prop up your baby right in the crib if you are bottle feeding. Never give a bottle to your baby while she lies down. It can contribute to tooth loss or ear infections (both of which will affect sleep — we don't need that!) When feeding is finished, just bring your baby back in her right sleeping place. There is typically no need to burp because your baby is so happy she is less likely to suck in food when eating. In addition, do not think about adjusting it until the baby's diaper is poopy or dripping.

What if I don't latch my baby on my nipple or the bottle?

The deepest sleep of your infant comes in the first half of the night, and at first, she increasingly is challenging to keep latched on. If your baby does not seem interested at first, you may need to transmit a bit of breastmilk by hand and place your baby's lips on your nipple. With formula and a bottle nipple, you can do the same. The scent and taste would possibly entice her to hold on. If your baby sleeps in the breast or bottle, you can use some tactile stimulation, such as rubbing the side of your baby's cheek or using compressions from the chest to increase your flow.

How can I tell that dream feed works?

Offer your baby over a week to calm down in the dream feed routine first. If you feel like you are getting more sleep, then it works for you! If it sounds off, then do not go for it! If dream feed contributes to a longer run, then it works.

For some babies, being even slightly roused during that deep sleep that occurs during the first part of the night can tangle with their rhythm of sleep. Here are few indications that dream feeds may not be perfect for your baby: your baby often wakes up a short period after the dream feed, and you do not have a good rest at night. Your baby wakes up more frequently than when you began to feed your baby during the dream feed and has a rough time resettling to sleep.

One of the dangers of a dream feed is giving the kid the meal period. Therefore, that means your baby can wake up hungry at that time if you do not do the dream feed. It is a smart thing to think accordingly about how you will wean away from the vision feed. It is like weaning your baby off other night feeds.

For younger babies who still need night feeding, push the dream feed over a few weeks later until it falls after midnight sometime. At this point, if she is hungry, you should let your baby wake naturally. You will also get a more extended period of sleep, and your kid will be able to wean this feed on her own. You should withdraw the dream feeding early for older babies who no longer require a meal so that she becomes less hungry and instead remove it entirely. If your baby seems to be hungry at this time, but you are still ready to drop it, you may need to reduce this feeding volume over time by reducing the length of time you're nursing for or the amount in the bottle. By slowly decreasing the amount you lower the risk, she will wake up with a hungry stomach.

Will I leave my baby swaddled to feed on the dream?

A: Most of the time, yes. Let us swaddle your son. You want to stimulate them only a little you can-only enough to feed them. Unsaddling could well wake them up.

What if my kid is too tired and is not going to eat while feeding on the dream?

Some babies are going to need a bit more excitement than some to get them awake up to eat, just make sure you don't rouse them too soon, or they're going to wake up entirely!

- Run a moist wipe or rag over his face
- Brush or tickle the bottom of his foot or jaw
- Place some milk on his lips

If those do not work, lay the baby back down. If you are still up, you can try again briefly a little later. If it is not functioning, so do not push it. "Never disturb a sleeping infant," as they claim. "You would never want to take the risk of making a cranky kid all night if you unintentionally got them up in mid-sleep. If you aim for a couple of nights without results, give it a few weeks' rest and come back to it.

When are you going to continue dream feeding? Is a vision feed too late to try?

Dream feeds work well in babies aged 3-9 months. They need to be fed regularly while your kid is an infant, as their little tummies will only accommodate too much. When they have achieved age around 3 and 4 months, they can continue traveling longer runs. If your baby still has not been able to sleep through the night after nine months of age, however, a dream feed will probably not help as much. Probably other associations of sleep at this age keep them from sleeping a longer stretch at night.

Once the dream feed is done, should I adjust my baby's diaper?

Just when you sense the need. You will learn better after a couple of nights of attempting a vision stream. Again, the idea is to get your baby stimulated as little as possible. They might be wakened by a diaper change, so avoid it if possible. However, if your infant wakes up an hour or two later due to a wet diaper, you may need to make a quick transition after the dream feed before turning them back down.

Bid farewell to Pacifiers

By implementing the Montessori method, pacifiers should not be used widely or will be phased out in the first year. When a small toddler often uses a pacifier, it should not be a complicated task to transition them out.

Even though the child is young, we can let them know we will make a change. The first move is to continue just sleeping with the pacifier. Once our kid wakes, we should place it out of reach in a box by the bed so our kid (or even the adult) will not be tempted to use it. Many days that our child asks for the pacifier, we should seek to understand why they have the urge to suck to fix the root cause. They may need something fun to do with their hands or a gadget to play with, maybe they are searching for a bond so we can give a cuddle, or maybe they need to settle down or ease their nervous system.

Here are a few suggestions that may help:

- sucking milk through a straw

- blowing bubbles

- hanging firmly on to a book or soft toy

- use a bottle through a straw

- blowing water across a straw to make bubbles

- a vigorous towel rubbing during a wash

- deep-pressure bear hugs

- kneading dough

- gripping bath toys

- a steady, hardback rub

We can then create a move for our kid to get rid of the pacifier at one common option is to offer this to a new baby buddy.

It normally takes the infant a couple of days to learn to fall asleep without it, after which they might require some – only enough – extra help. Be alert that no additional sleeping crutches are applied to the routine.

4.3 Understanding your toddler's brain development

The first few years of your baby are a path of learning when its mind expands; its body gets stronger as it learns to grasp the universe and its position inside it. Each and everything provides a learning point, and it is critical that he is introduced to as many development-potential experiences as possible throughout the early years.

Sensory Awareness

There is an old theory that kids know everything they do. Essentially, the same is claimed by Montessori. When we activate the senses of children in ways that allow them to identify and distinguish between the properties of different items, impulses are transmitted back and forth from the nervous system through the brain. The more that occurs, the better the brain neuropathy get, when the brain experiences substantial input that is necessary for proper functioning. Knowing how to think (assimilating, incorporating, and implementing knowledge) later in life relies on whether or not the brain has been "hardwired" correctly at an early age.

We have already identified how babies from the time of birth communicate with the environment through their senses. Montessori thought that we should expand on that by motivating babies and young children to center their attention on the real environment, investigating small differences in the properties of specified sets of items through increasing their senses – seeing, sound, contact, taste, and smell. Exercising the senses of children will significantly enhance their sensitivity through providing experiences that bring their focus to elements of daily life or by unique sensorial practices.

Brainpower boosting exercises to develop sensory awareness are particularly valuable in the years from birth to six, because this is when the nervous system develops.

Ways You Can Develop Sensory Awareness In Your Child

First, the overwhelming news. Your baby's brain is the one big organ that isn't completely developed before he or she is born; it's only 25 percent of the adult brain capacity. It's experiencing tremendous development in the first three years. His or her interactions in those early years continue to build the roots of the brain. In addition, the terrifying part is-what you do (or do not) as parents in these years will actually mold their brain. In addition, what is the better news? That is not complicated to do!

In daily life, we will do small tasks that will add up overnight and make our babies grow wise, socially well adjusted, and caring people. Many things on the list that come as a total surprise-especially their position in the growth of a child's brain.

React faithfully and lovingly

When listening regularly to the needs of your young kid, you do more than give them your affection. You are literally building a stable basis for their brains to develop. Yet still, we fall victim to misconceptions and uninformed suggestions, in spite of our best intentions.

Letting a child weep does not improve the lungs. It causes unnecessary pain. It does exploit him by not picking up a crying infant. It creates commitment and protection problems. Letting the little girl scream to sleep, not teach her to sleep. It encourages her not to confide in men. Any such early exposure allows the brain to wire. If its milk, warmth, and health needs are not fulfilled, the baby's brain is busy thinking about survival. Where is the time to study, learn, and grow?

Give them the power of your touch

'Because touch, more than any other sense, has such ready access to the brains of young babies, it offers perhaps the best and easiest opportunity to mold their emotional and mental well-being,' says Lise Eliot in What's Going In There – How the Brain and Mind Develops in the First Five Years of Life. Cuddling and hugging the infant as soon as we can is the best way to unlock the magic of touch. Not only in reaction to their cries but proactively as well. Yet there are tasks to perform, and homes to manage. Babywearing will assist with that.

You are holding the baby while you're bringing or 'holding' the infant in a sling or some other attachment on your back. Babywearing is shown to suppress screaming in children, allowing them to stay quiet and healthy overall. How is it going to grow the brain? "How do children do in their spare time if they waste less time moaning and fussing about? They are doing! Sling babies invest the most energy in a calm state of alertness. It may be considered a baby's optimum learning environment." says Dr. Sears. One established way we can give the kid major cognitive benefits is by offering him a regular massage.

Talk Loads, Talk Right

There is solid, irrefutable proof from years of study that is talking to your children or especially (who are under the age of 3) is directly related to their IQ and potential academic achievement. Speaking to your child, a great deal is the simplest and most powerful thing you can ever do for them. Day-to-day tasks and even chores give enough chances to chat.

Breastfeed

'The more kids breastfeed, the better they succeed in adulthood – large report,' says The Guardian, Breastfeed as much as your child needs, for as long as possible. Breastfeeding isn't always convenient, so should you encounter some issue, be sure to seek support. There is a range of community networks that are more than happy to assist, both online and offline. Know that breastfeeding is healthier than not breastfeeding at all, just for a brief period.

Talk aloud

To our children, we all realize the value of literacy. Any key points on reading to your child:

- Beginning reading to your kid is never too early – they may be in the nursery, a fetus, or a 6-month-old.
- Carry reading – do not be discouraged if they are just involved in chewing, tossing, or breaking the journal. It is normal; they are going to learn from it.
- Invest in a range of books – dining room, office, bathroom, fridge, baby bag, and car – and scatter them everywhere.
- Set an example – The more you know that you learn, and the more written content you have in the room, the more motivated you become to learn.
- Above all – equate reading with enjoyment. Never using it as a threat, nor force them to learn.

Let them on the run

Work shows close links between physical exercise and brain growth. Making sure your kid has at least 60 (even more) minutes of unorganized physical activity. Sometimes when a kid is upset or ready to throw a tantrum, it will transform the problem around and keep them going. Get crazy, force them to chase you or chase them, launch pillow battles, see who can leap to the highest, play horse-riding on the cushion, mimic animal motions-how frogs run, how rabbits hop, just go insane to get them to move! It will transfer their brain cells too!

Physical exercise includes tummy time for children and allowing them enough space to know how to turn over and crawl. Stop strapping babies in one place in rockers or prams or car seats, as far as practicable (except while driving).

Offer them novelty

'Studies consistently consider it necessary for intellectual growth to have play materials available. Toddlers with a wide variety of accessible playthings later tend to have stimulated mental growth, reports Kathy Hirch-Pasek and Roberta Michnik Golinkoff at the age of 3 and 4 in the novel 'Einstein Never Used Flashcards.' Luckily, we do not have to smash the bank to purchase a new gadget each. By utilizing household items, we should be imaginative; we should change their toys periodically so that only old toys are gazed at with fresh eyes. We may share mates' items or visit toy libraries.

Engage in Sensory Play

Sensory play involves games that allow children to use touch, scent, taste, visual, and hearing senses. The more you use your senses, the more you know. If you are a new mother, you might feel overwhelmed by all the lovely sensory experiences worthy of interest that some moms manage to set up. Fortunately for you, there are many daily household products and events that offer outstanding sensory play opportunities.

- Pool Fun – Bring them a bowl of water and fun to throw with two inside it. Bring them off to the ocean and love rolling in mud or sand

3. Experience Nutrition-Self-feeding is one of the child's greatest sensory opportunities. Let the kid experience and feel the texture of various foods.

- Closet Attack – Open the closet and take out garments in different materials. Play peekaboo with your woolen jumper, place in a tub your cotton dupatta and feel the silk scarf against his face.
- Hot and cold – Reach them with frost, and then a moist (not steam) teacup to tell them about cold and dry.

Encourage imaginative games, get help with chores

When your baby wants to feed a carrot on Teddy, or when your baby dresses up as a fairy and has a tea party, they're pretending to play. Pretend play helps to improve their vocabulary, language abilities, and social skills. Naturally, most children participate in imaginative play beginning about 12 months, and their play gets more complex as they mature. Often, we can support them along – by taking part in the action, introducing the 'show' for the younger kids, providing them with toys (doctor collection, kitchen set, etc.), taking turns playing with them.

When we get little children to support us with age-appropriate tasks, we encourage them to take part in another form of imaginative play, where they become adults. Using easy, day-to-day exercises to teach new ideas. Children who are not yet 3 do not need to study a classroom-type setting. The daily existence and artifacts provide ample opportunity to teach them simple concepts.

Encourage them to share stories

When a kid tells us a story, it brings all of her imagination into motion. 'The left brain will place things in order, use vocabulary and reasoning, to say a tale which makes sense. The right brain contributes to the body's feelings, raw emotions, and personal experiences, and we can see the whole image and interact with The Whole-Brain Kid, our experience' writes Dr. Daniel Siegel.

Modeling story-telling will build the groundwork for parents. Narrate previous kid incidents and envision potential 'lines.' As soon as they start talking, allow them to share their story, listen closely, address questions that will enable them to speak more. The best way is to spend a few minutes with your child every night passing the day.

Lay the framework for successful music

Listening to Mozart has a little long-lasting impact on the intellect of a boy. The theory was debunked. Yet playing a musical instrument remains linked to knowledge.

We can't teach babies to play an instrument, of course, but we can set the foundations for them to equate music with pleasure. Singing to them, singing rhymes while we sing, motivating them to sing along, will help them see music while enjoyable, and make them content. So maybe as they're a little older, we will expose them to different musical instruments and see what they're really loving playing.

Ensure sure they have the night.

'Sleep is the source of energy which keeps your brain alert and relaxed. Sleep recharges the brain's battery every night and at every nap.' says Good Sleep Patterns founder, Happy Boy, Marc Weissbluth, MD Young Baby Parents usually do their hardest to ensure their children sleep well. Or just lay it off! We can be sure we don't do anything that hampers their sleep unknowingly. Either allow them to have screen time up to 2 hours before bedtime, not providing enough productive daytime playtime, or prioritizing our routines over the sleeping timings of our kids.

Brain Development

From Birth to Age Three: An Overview of Early Brain Growth

First Trimester

In the first several weeks of pregnancy, brain development ends. Many of the brain's developmental features emerge throughout the embryonic stage (approximately the first eight weeks following fertilization); these constructs then begin to expand and mature throughout the fetal era (the rest of gestation).

The first primary process in brain growth is neural tube creation. Approximately two weeks after birth, the neural shield, a sheet of advanced embryo cells, starts to fold gradually over into itself, ultimately creating a tube-shaped framework. The tube closes slowly as the sides of the plate connect; normally, this cycle is accomplished four weeks after conception. The neural tube keeps evolving and finally becoming the brain and spinal cord.

The first neurons and synapses start to form in the spinal cord about seven weeks following conception. These early neuronal contacts enable the fetus to make the first movements, that can be sensed by ultrasound and MRI even if the mother can't feel them in most cases. Such gestures, in effect, provide sensory feedback to the brain that will accelerate its growth. More synchronized motions develop during the next few weeks.

The Second Trimester

Early in the second trimester, gyri and sulci begin to show on the surface of the brain; this cycle is nearly complete by the end of this trimester. The cerebral cortex increases in thickness and sophistication, and the development of synapse starts in this region. During the second trimester, Myelin begins to develop on the axons of individual neurons. This cycle persists through puberty-named myelination. Myelination makes for better information processing: for the brain to reach the same degree of output without myelination, the spinal cord will have to have a circumference of three yards.

The Third Trimester

The early weeks of the third trimester are a transitional time during which the cerebral cortex starts to fulfill specific roles formerly done by the more basic brain stem. Reflexes like fetal breathing, for example, and reactions to external stimuli, are more normal. The prefrontal cortex facilitates early learning that occurs during this time.

Year One

Newborn babies' impressive abilities demonstrate the magnitude of fetal brain growth. Newborns may recognize human images, which they favor to certain artifacts, and also distinguish between signs of joy and sorrow. A baby at birth acknowledges the voice of her parents and may remember the sounds of stories that her parents read to him or her while they were was still in the womb.

Throughout the first year, the brain begins to grow at a staggering pace. The cerebellum multiplies in volume, which seems to be consistent with the accelerated growth of motor skills happening during this time. When the cortex's perceptual fields expand, the formerly poor and restricted sight of the child grows into complete binocular vision.

The strength of recall in a child increases significantly at around three months; this correlates with substantial development in the hippocampus, the limbic system associated with memory processing. In the first year, the language loops in the frontal and temporal lobes are integrated, profoundly affected by the words a child learns. A baby at an English-speaking home can differentiate between the tones of a foreign language for the first few months. She lacks this capacity at the end of the first year: the vocabulary she learns at home has converted the brain to English.

Year Two

The most drastic developments this year include the vocabulary regions of the brain, which are forming more synapses and being increasingly integrated. Such improvements lead to the rapid increase in the language skills of children – also called the eruption in vocabulary – that usually happens during this era. The vocabulary of a infant even quadruples between the first and second birthdays.

There is a significant increase in myelination rate during the second year, which helps the brain conduct more complex tasks. Higher-order cognitive skills are increasing, such as self-awareness: a child is often more conscious of his thoughts and actions. He now wholly understands anytime he sees his image in a mirror that it is his own. Soon he can continue using his name as well as personal pronouns such as "I" and "me." **YEAR THREE**

Synaptic activity in the prefrontal cortex is expected to plateau in the third year, up to 200 percent of its adult point. The region is also continuing to develop and improve networks with other countries. As a consequence, they promote and combine dynamic cognitive skills. For starters, at this point, children are best prepared to understand current occurrences utilizing the context. They do have more exceptional executive ability and a clear perception of cause and effect. The first signals obtained by the brain have a huge impact.

Early brain growth is the foundation of human endurance and adaptability, but these attributes come at an expense. Since interactions have a high potential to impact brain growth during this time, children are especially susceptible to repeated negative influences. On the other side, these early years provide a window of development for parents, families, and communities: successful first encounters have an immense effect on the prospects for accomplishment, growth, and satisfaction for children.

4.4 Montessori Approach to Toilet Training and Feeding Toddlers

Toilet training is the method of training a young child to control the bowel and bladder and to use the bathroom to eliminate it. A child is known to be qualified as a toilet trained until he or she begins heading to the bathroom and is able to change the appropriate clothes to urinate or move the intestine. Toilet training is sometimes called potty training or toilet learning.

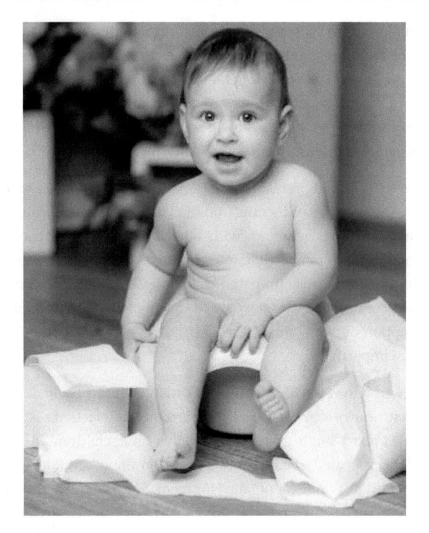

When is the child ready for toilet training?

Many parents are uncertain when and how to start toilet training or "potty training." Not all kids may be ready at the same age, and it's crucial to monitor your infant for indicators of preparation, including stopping operation for a couple of seconds or holding his or her diaper.

Watch for indications that your child might be able to start going for the potty instead of using force, such as:

- obey clear directions to recognize and use terms for using the potty
- create the relation between the desire to pee or poop

Your friend claims that by his second birthday, their little boy became diaper-free. On the other hand, your niece refused to perch at the potty till Montessori. What timeline is appropriate for the potty training? Or state it briefly: zero, neither both. Like for most developmental milestones, infants are equipped for one-of-a-kind routines — so having your child determine the tempo where to start potty training is important.

When your kid isn't equipped for potty training, so all the strongest bathroom methods would probably fall flat. And wait before you see the indicators of this surefire: What are the indicators that my child is about to be taught potty?

1. You change fewer damp diapers. Children pee too often before the age of about 20 months that asking them to regulate their bladders is definitely impractical. But an infant who stays dry at a stretch for an hour or two — and occasionally wakes up without wetness — is physically prepared for potty training.

2. The bowel movements of your infant are regular. If he's getting a BM in the morning, between meals, or right in front of the bed, a daily routine can enable you to know when to take out the potty — and therefore improve his odds of performance.

3. He transmits functions throughout the body. Any kids happily declare that a bowel movement is just about to happen ("I'm pooping right now!"). Some express by fewer vocal means — say, by moving back to a corner or creating a defensive grunt. Whatever the warning, once your kid indicates that he is mindful of the workings of his body, he's primed for the potty training.

4. He scoffs at messy diapers. At some stages, most babies go through a (fleeting) period where they are opposed to personal messes — they're bugged with errant crumbs and dirty paws, and yeah, they're ready to remove their soiled nappies as fast as possible. This is a perfect chance to set start the potty-training cycle, as your kid dislikes the stinky diapers as much as you do for the first time.

5. He will perform quick undressing. The potty will not be of any help as nature calls unless your kid can easily yank off his jeans and pull-ups or socks. Likewise, girls should be able to flash their skirts up.

6. He knows lingo in the toilet. Whether you prefer child-friendly jargon such as "poop" and "pee" or formal terminology such as "defecate" and "urinate," your child will be ready for potty training if he understands and can use the words of the family for bathroom functions and any related body parts.

Montessori Parents Toilet Training

What makes Montessori toilet training different is that it follows the child's development, and respects every child. It is slow, and at the speed of the infant. If your child/toddler attends a Montessori school, ask whether they have any childrearing or toilet learning handouts or if they operate any seminars or information sessions on the topic. It is better to read up on the subject wherever possible when your child is still in infancy.

Indirect Toilet Preparations

From birth, practice changing your child's diaper to give plenty of indirect kind of preparation as soon as it is wet (this can sometimes mean as often as every hour). From the beginning, the usage of cloth diapers allows tremendously to gain understanding, as they instinctively feel warm. This positive input makes the infant equate the desire to urinate to the outcome of relaxing her muscles. Thereby toilet training takes place slowly, over time. When the child is going to pull up and stand, let her rise when you are adjusting her and chat about what you are doing, include the child where you can. She will see what is going on and take an interest along that direction. Unless you have not already done so, as your infant begins to rise and walk, shift the diaper to the toilet. This helps them build the right connections between action and location.

The critical time for initiating toilet knowledge is between twelve and eighteen months when to start the toilet. Depending on the child, it will start eventually. Look for signs of readiness:

- Interest in cycles (bib is now going into the hamper, the hamper is going into the basement, into the machine, etc. Child watches with interest and even goes along).
- Baby runs.
- You note an infant is rubbing her / his genitals.
- For other hours during the day, the infant begins experiencing bowel movements.

Often a kid displays neither of these symptoms but gets excited as soon as you start directing her attention to the toilet, and we also suggest starting before 18 months.

Toilet Performance Tools

You could buy 30 pairs of thick underpants to get going. Gerber training pants that come three in a pack for around five bucks are suggested. They are the most absorbent but robust and the least costly. The leg holes must be wide enough for performance, and the underwear loses enough so it can be pulled up and down on the child's part without any additional effort. (Gerber training pants, size two, are suggested for an infant aged between 12 and 18 months. As the child reaches 18 months, or when she's large for her age, size three would be expected.)

Place a slice of rubberized flannel in the back of the car and purchase a couple of sheets for the bunk. Make sure you have plenty of pairs of pull-on pants for your boy because he will need to change sometimes. Include plenty of sheets, and you can rotate them regularly. Pick up delicate rugs.

Find "Nature's Gift" at a pet shop to clean rugs or the floor easily and efficiently, if desired. The item eliminates not only the mark but also the scent, which is suitable for good rugs and can be kept easily on the rug.

Place tiny potty chairs, a range if appropriate, and allow the child to sit on them, encouraging them when they do. Place a potty in each toilet with a small bucket to the left, and a clean underwear basket to the right. Under the three things, a folded towel or bath mat provides a non-slip base, and an image organizes.

The first three points are the most relevant as you continue the toilet, as they have to do with attracting your child's focus to this aspect of our everyday lives: let her see you and other family members seated on the toilet as soon as you can. Bring your kid to the bathroom every half hour or so in the beginning and allow her to stay on it whilst seated on the adult bathroom (as would be normal for just a moment). Doing that makes your kid how to use the toilet by the process, so that is even more than telling your infant, "Do you need to go to the bathroom?" That generally guarantees a "No!" except though they need to go!

It is really necessary that your child will quickly move into dry underwear after wetting it. We want her to be used to feeling dry, and to react to wetness right away. Your kid should wear only her panties from the waist down in the early years, and it's easy to use the potty chair to adjust, so it doesn't take long. Timing is crucial as bowel movements go into the toilets! If you note that your child has a bowel movement every day in the same period, make it a normal activity to go together to the bathroom and sit on the toilets. When your child's pacing is erratic, observe him closely and then send him to the bathroom because he goes in his underpants, and you can help him adjust, see the BM go into the bathroom, and push it downwards.

Start your effort to convince him to relax and hang out on the toilet anytime you know there could be a bowel movement coming his way-you might always read books together and pass the time if it happens. Start attempting to get the kid interested in the dressing and undressing. When the kid starts urinating in her bathroom, remind her that you place the pee in the wider toilet and flush. And work closely to remedy her, taking particular attention to making her learn to properly put her dry panties on. And work closely to remedy her, taking particular attention to making her learn to properly put her dry panties on. It helps to have a potty in whatever space he works in the early days so that he can see it and get to it in time. He can only wear pants that are simple to pull up and down himself, and when appropriate during this point, maybe naked or in underwear from the waist down.

When you commence this point, throw out all the diapers. Your kid needs to be set up to excel and have our trust that he will then easily be able to use the bathroom at any moment. A ton of kids sleeps too hard to get up to use the bathroom before they are older. Depending on your kid, her maturity, and the point you have reached in toileting, there are various ways to do that.

Carry a potty chair with you (to use at your destination) during the early phases of the bathroom training as you push your kid out of the vehicle. Place it in the house bathroom you are visiting, even though it is just a brief stay. It may create the bathroom schedule after entering the house and arrival at destinations.

Bring the kid to public bathrooms sometimes when out and about, when leaving home and returning. We suggest that you make it a routine and claim, "We're just sitting on the toilet for a moment before we head out and come home." (Just allow them to stop for a minute whether they stand up or don't urinate, just disregard it and carry on. Hopefully, they'll want to take advantage of the opportunity.) For special occasions or plane trips, we advise you not to bring your kid back in a slide, but instead to place a Nikki slide cover around her panties. With this diaper cover made of lightweight, durable cotton, you should also test for wetness so that the training time is not disrupted. For some public circumstances, this is a good "freedom net" to you. Always have a couple of jeans and underwear changes in the house, so you can run back to the car for a fast change as soon as your child gets dirty and then start shopping.

Tips To Continue Potty Training Once Your Kid Is Eager For Potty Training Success-

- Wear. All that gets in the way is overalls or tricky buttons. Get used to dressing your infant in the right potty training clothes (pants that pull up and down without any easy-to-hike fiddling or dresses).

- Choose a potty chair on the extreme. Some infants prefer a potty seat to their own, and others prefer a separate one. Decide what suits the little one best. If you purchase a seat connected to the toilet, search for a comfortable match — for weeks, a loose seat will spook a child back into diapers.

- Switch on Pull-ups. Pull-ups are a great intermediate level because they encourage you to start practicing in a not-so-convenient position without fear of an injury. Plus, they slide up like underpants, but they can be torn off instead of pushed to his bottom. The drawback is they sweep away moisture like a cloth, and the wetness that can slow down the cycle won't disturb your child. So turn to reusable training pants as you continue to get any accomplishments.

- Look out for signals. You may see them before your toddler at this age. Note whether the little one is straining or fidgeting, then run to the bathroom for a try. There are occasions that you might want to delay starting toilet training, such as: while traveling after a sibling's conception, transferring from the crib to the bed, that your child is unwell (especially if diarrhea is under consideration)

How long does toilet training take?

It's no easy job to train a child to use the potty. It always takes around 3 and 6 months, but for certain kids, it will take more or less time. The cycle appears to take longer if you proceed too early. So remaining dry at night will take months or even years or learn.

Potty Styles

The two main potty choices are a single, adults-sized potty chair with a bowl that can be drained into the toilet with an adults-sized cover that can be put on top of a toilet seat that can help the kids feel better and not scared to fall in. When you want to do so, have a walking stub so that your child can easily touch the seat and be comfortable when making a bowel motion.

Typically it is safer for boys to train to use the bathroom sitting down first before having to pee standing up. A potty chair could be a safer choice for boys who feel uncomfortable — or nervous — regarding standing on a stool to pee in the toilet. With any toilet in your house, you may want to have a potty or seat training. In emergencies, you may also want to have a potty in the trunk of your vehicle. Make sure to take a potty seat with you while driving long distances and rest every 1-2 hours. Then locating a toilet will take too long.

About Training Pants, effective training pants are a helpful move between diapers and undergarments. Since nighttime control of the kids' bladder and bowel sometimes lags behind their daytime regulation, certain parents enjoy using nighttime training pants. Some want their children to wear trousers for exercise while they're out and about. If the training pants remain dry for a couple of days, children will make the transition to wearing underwear.

But some people assume that disposable training undies may make kids believe it's okay to use them like diapers, slowing down the cycle of toilet-teaching. Ask your doctor if the use of disposable training pants as an intermediate phase will help your boy.

Tips for Toilet Training

- You should educate your little one by talking about the method well when your kid is able to use the potty: using phrases to demonstrate the usage of the bathroom ("pee," "poop," and "potty").
- Teach your child to let you know when a dirty or soiled diaper is in.
- Identify habits ("Are you going to poop?"), so your child can know how to understand the need to vomit and pee.
- Get your child to practice sitting on a potty chair. Your child could sit on it at first, wearing trousers or a diaper. Your child can go naked-bottomed when they're ready.
- If you have now made sure that, your child is ready to start studying how to use the potty, these suggestions will help: set aside some time to focus on potty training.
- Do not have your child sit against his or her will at the toilet.

- Show your child how to sit on the toilet and describe what you are doing (because you are helping your child learn). You may even get your kid sitting on the potty seat and observing as you (or a sibling) are using the bathroom.
- Set up a schedule. You may want to continue, for example, by making your child sit on the toilet after arising with a dry diaper, or 45 minutes to an hour after consuming loads of liquids. Only place your child on the potty a couple of times a day for a few minutes, then let your child get up if he or she desires.
- Make your child stay on the toilet for 15 to 30 minutes between meals to take advantage of the normal inclination of the body to get a bowel movement between feeding (the gastro-colic reflex is called this). Many children do have a time of day where they appear to get a bowel movement.
- If you see obvious indicators of needing to go to the toilet, such as crossed hands, grunting, or squatting, remind your child to sit on the seat.
- Empty a movement of the intestine (poop) from the diaper of your infant into the bathroom and warn your infant that poop is going into the bowl.
- Stop hard to pull off clothing, such as overalls and tops that clip onto the groin. Children doing potty training ought to be allowed to undress.
- Offer little incentives to your kid, such as badges or reading time, if your child goes in the potty. Hold a map to monitor milestones. If your little one appears to understand bathroom use, let him or her pick out some fresh pairs of big-kid panties to wear.
- Ensure that all guardians – including babysitters, mothers, and childcare staff – adopt the same schedule and use the same terms for body parts and bathroom activities. Let us exactly how to do the toilet training and remind us to follow the same methods so that the child would not be upset.

All efforts to use the bathroom are celebrated, even though nothing occurs. And note there would be injuries. It is necessary not to discipline children with potty-training or express frustration while wetting or soiling themselves or the room. Tell your dad, instead, that it was an accident, and give your help. Ensure your infant is well on the road to use the potty like a big boy.

Problems with Potty Training

A few kids get to use the potty, then never reflect back. Nonetheless, things happen for everyone. Young children sometimes train in stalls and in spurts. Often they also fail or lack their newly learned skills — such as using the bathroom.

As a mom, when your potty-trained infant has an incident, it's normal to feel disappointed, and even angry. Know that regression is simply, in certain situations, a positive emotional reaction to emotions that your child is also not able to convey. And staying calm and taking action to help your kid get back on track is the best option for managing a potty training setback.

What's the gap between the potty training events and the collapse of potty training?

Potty training mistakes arise as the kid tries to use the bathroom first — after all, it is a learning process. Regression, however, occurs when a previously potty trained kid unexpectedly has accidents and/or tries to go back to wearing diapers. The positive news: In most regression situations, the child will catch up only a couple of days or weeks from where she left off.

Popular sources of potty-training relapse. The trick to getting potty training back on track is coping with the sources of injuries, so be on the alert for specific reasons, which could include: lack of preparedness. If the timing is not correct, even all the strongest methods in toilet training do not avoid setbacks. Some children display signs of preparation for potty training between 20 and 30 months, but others may demonstrate these symptoms earlier or later.

Struggle. Every new scenario, such as a new parent, a new sitter, a new daycare, adjustments in the daily schedule of your child, or a family dispute can be upsetting enough to cause a decline in potty exercise.

Feeling sleepy or slow may prevent your baby from going to the potty in order to use it. Pressure on kin. It is possible that moving a child who is not ready or comfortable in using the bathroom would go backfire. During the potty training cycle, it's essential to be polite, compassionate, motivating, and calming. Letting your child set the tempo, too, is important. Length. Whether your kid is busy playing or engaging in some task, she might not feel the need to go to the potty until it's too late, or she might want to postpone going only because she doesn't want to interrupt what she's doing. Excitation. Just becoming excited may cause an accident for the tots who are fresh to the bathroom — they can fail to go or miss the impulse, culminating in an accident. Can't talk. Your child does not have the capacity to convey any apprehension or insecurity over using the bathroom or the actual pain that it might trigger, so that may lead her to want and escape the potty.

Importance of Potty Training

Because infants do not have the opportunity to educate themselves on how to clean themselves in a hygienic environment, potty training is still something any parent will undertake as part of their child's education, whether they reside in a tribal community or a developing country. The age of potty training varies from birth to preschool, but the benefits are the same, regardless of when you start or where you live.

American Culture specifies that individuals with a diaper will not be removed until early childhood. Therefore, training children to remove in a toilet is important, so that we will not annoy our peers. Even from other parents, this societal pressure comes when a parent considers when using a diaper is no longer acceptable for a child. When the social strain starts, however, it depends largely on what society you live in. In certain societies, potty training begins in infancy, and peers would consider a child in diapers at one or two years of age as socially unacceptable. In the United States, diapers are deemed socially unacceptable only before an infant reaches around four years old.

Self-Esteem and the smallest of children will sense the social burden to use a bathroom. As per pediatrician Jill M. Lekovic in the book "Diaper-Free Before 3," even preschoolers feel the pressure from society to be trained in the potty.

Lekovic claims that potty-trained kindergarteners are more confident than non-potty-trained preschoolers and that being potty-trained for the bathroom allows them "an incredible amount of faith in the environment of preschool socialization." Potty training tends to offer a kid a good self-image and power over her own body.

Good bathroom and potty training have a range of wellbeing advantages. Several research, including the 2002 report "Effects of a questionnaire evaluating the impact of various toilet training approaches on the attainment of bladder regulation" published in the "British Journal of Urology," and research published in the "Journal of Pediatric Urology" in 2009 indicates that subsequent toilet training is correlated with an elevated likelihood of urinary and intestinal disorders, such as urinary tract.

Child Psychology and Toilet Training

Did you know that even back in the 1920s and 1930s, little kids were forced into draconian and abusive measures to provide rigorous toilet training?

According to Gwen Dewar, author of the essay "The Psychology of Toilet Training: What Evidence Tells Us about Timing," in 1935, the U.S. Department of Instruction suggested the usage of soap sticks injection into the rectum at all hours to impose rigid regularity of bowel movement. Others also levied severe penalties on incidents concerning bathroom instruction. Dewar said such brutal practices were widespread shortly after the Second World War, where the scientific profession protested about their harmful impact on infants. Let's take a deeper look into the social effects of potty training to fully grasp this.

Potty Training And Erikson's Psychosocial Development Theory

Erik Erikson, inventor of the eight-step Psychosocial Development Theory, emphasized the significance of effective potty training in the second growth period called Control vs. Guilt and Skepticism. According to Erikson, when an adult grows up, there are many phases of psychosocial growth that need to be commenced successfully. Failure at any point to resolve the war will contribute to psychological distress and social misdemeanors.

He said in his hypothesis that when an infant hits 18 months to 3 years of age, they undergo an emotional conflict for sovereignty. If you have contact with kids, you realize that these kids like to tell "No" a lot and want to determine for themselves what food to consume or what clothes to wear. This is because they feel a sense of "control" over their kin. Through managing stuff themselves, they build a perceptual illusion of sovereignty. With respect to potty training that often remains true. If a child is taught effectively through these years, they will establish a sense of sovereignty that will ultimately lead them to "should" virtue. If the child does not do this, though, it may contribute to a psychiatric breakdown of guilt and doubt. Erikson theorized that failure at this point gives rise to certain negative effects on the psychological and social functioning of a child, particularly the following:

- The child may have low self-esteem.
- The child becomes overly reliant on others.
- They would challenge each other in accomplishing various activities.
- They are likely to grow up with a lot of insecurities.
- Sometimes, they'd condemn their own skills.

It takes us to another matter. How can we claim a kid has had a good potty training?

Successful Vs. Unsuccessful Potty Training

The position of parents, is very important in potty training an infant. Parents will encourage freedom for the child without resulting in a lack of self-esteem for the child. So a delicate balance should be kept in order to be effective in getting our child to learn his toilet routine. How do we continue to do this?

Let the infant demonstrate its readiness to be taught in the bathroom. We can verbalize a need to go to the bathroom or use the toilet. Forcing them to do so even if they do not feel the desire can result in psychological distress. Let your child have enough time in the toilet. Let them learn their routine themselves. Too much interaction and rigid habits will just discourage your boy.

Show not relaxation but gratitude. When your little one has been good, compliment them with stuff like "Great work! "And" You have made it correctly! "Instead of verbalizing gratification such as 'Finally, you did it' or 'Finally, it's over.' Encouraging the kid would make them more comfortable about their self-control and motivate them to do something again, whilst the other will offer the pessimistic notion that you're sick of waiting or that you only want to finish it up. Don't mention anything bad. Any definitions are, "You've never grown," or "You're always getting things wrong." Telling your kid of their failed potty training or making someone know about it can impact their sense of self-worth.

Evite the kid getting scolded for injuries. Your child has yet to learn its own bathroom routine, and accidents can occur. Scolding them will contribute to deterrence. Try rephrasing the sentences as something like, "I hope you should do something different this time" or "I'm sure you'll be able to make this error again."

Tips for managing potty training failures

Picking up pee puddles is especially stressful because you figured you'd already hit this landmark of progress. But have confidence. It's only a process, and your little one gets beyond it. These tips may help:

- Be relaxed. After an incident, your child can get frustrated, so be careful. ("You've had an incident, so that's all right. Tons of kids have incidents; maybe you're going to make it to the potty on time this time.")
- Never scold, threaten, or blame your kid for experiencing a failure.
- Potty Training Ideas for Boys and Girls
- Continue to play Fun Play Baby Playing, Walking, Leaping, and Kicking

Note that the method varies with all ages. Although most children are taught potty by around three years, all children grow at various levels, and some will require more time. So be confident that your child is old enough and shows signs of preparation.

Shooting problems

Does your child appear exhausted or stressed out? Worried? Discuss potential reasons for a setback with your kids. ("Are you worried about moving to our new home?" or "Has your new brother been changed at home?") And attempt to help her express her thoughts about what is troubling her. Then, you should provide reassurance to help create confidence. ("It's normal to feel scared of your new daycare, but those feelings are going to go away.") Go back to the starters of potty training. Be clear on when to use the potty and how. Suggest regular breaks in the bathroom at key times, like first thing in the morning, after meals and snacks, before a car ride and before bed, but try not to nag. Try utilizing (or re-activating) a stickered incentidve program.

Boost the likelihood of your child succeeding. Hold the potty in a convenient spot, and dress your kid in easy-to-use, easy-to-go bottoms. Look for training pants. Training pants will make potty training less inconvenient if you're on the early side, and help teach wetness sensitivity with adorable icons that disappear as they get wet. If your kid is in potty training later, you might choose to continue with pull-ups when incidents become uncomfortable (such as while you're away from home), only using regular pants during training sessions at home.

Offer appreciation for every move along the way. Play the "big baby" angle to help inspire your kids. When she effectively uses the potty, emphasis on constructive encouragement, and enthusiastic support. If you have ruled out any potential factors and the regression of your child continues for more than a month, she may just not be able. Under any scenario, offer a little break to the potty training. Only get back on track as soon as your child begins to display indicators of anticipation because discipline is vital to progress.

What to contact the doctor regarding the worsening in potty training or injuries?

Injuries is part of the cycle of potty training, but repeated incidents for an extended time may be a sign that there could be a medical problem that requires care. Test with your pediatrician whether your kid has either of these symptoms: persistent wetness Wetness after laughing A weak urinary stream Frequent urination or defecation Recurrent constipation Blood in the pee or stool Your pediatrician may help diagnose either physical or non-physical complications that your kid might have, as well as offer advice for treatment, behavioral changes.

Feeding Toddlers

For the young, fruits and vegetables make perfect snacks. They are filled with vitamins and nutrients, as well as valuable concentrations of minerals and trace minerals. They do happen to be small in calories, calcium, and fat, both of which are essential components to help the growth and development of your toddler. Fruits and vegetables will star at all meals and are an excellent addition at snack time, so by incorporating them along with other nutritious snack items, you are improving the diet's energy and nutrient content.

Here are a few, fast and simple ideas for baby snacks that include vegetables and fruits.

Fruit With Cheese Frais

As with all dairy products, cheese Frais is an excellent source of muscle and bone density protein. Fromage frais is also filled with B vitamins, required to release electricity. While the tiny pots of fruity cheese frais are always sugar-laden, serving fruit slices alongside simple cheese Frais is an excellent choice for a healthy snack. Fruit, peach, banana, mango, and melon strips all fit just fine for dipping. The smoother quality of cheese Frais renders this dip less sticky than regular yogurt.

Fruit With Cheese Cubes

Cheese is known to be high in calcium and phosphorus, which are both critical for bone growth. Apple bits, grape pieces, raisins, or even celery sticks come perfectly paired for a snack with the milk. Cream cheese pineapple as a coating cream cheese is lower in salt than strong cheeses like Cheddar but also a decent choice for calcium bone building. Top cut mini bagels, crackers, or toasted crumpets containing soft cheese and pineapple slices. Canned pineapple is a much more versatile choice than fresh pineapple, but only make sure that the rings or pieces are well-drained because the juice will get soggy the bread or crackers. For a cold, yummy snack or dessert during warmer weather, pulse light berries that are frozen with a blender, and stir through natural or Greek yogurt. The effect is identical to ice cream even without having all the sugar in it.

Freezing the mashed banana is another good ice cream option; you can also put it in lolly molds. If you don't have time to prepare, choose your hummus with frozen chickpeas, tahini, garlic, and lemon extract than store-bought hummus is always the right choice for your little one. If your tot continues to follow a vegan or vegetarian diet, then hummus adds additional protein, calcium, and iron as well. Naturally, pepper and carrot sticks are good, while cucumber and celery sticks are often ordinary when infants are growing teeth.

So now you know, there's no need for boring infant snacks. You could sustain your little one's diet varied with a range of sweet and tangy options to choose from and will provide them with nutrients they need for growth and development.

4.5 Effective Parenting Methods that actually work & Advice for New Mothers

You've gone through labor, labor, and childbirth, and now you're excited to go home and continue your baby's life. But, once back, you can feel like you have no idea what you are doing. These strategies will make even the most stressed first-time parents feel assured that they can take charge of a child within no time.

Having Aid After the Birth

Remember seeking assistance that may be quite hectic and stressful at this period. Speak to the professionals around you when inside the facility. Many clinics have diet experts or lactation counselors who will help you get breastfeeding or bottle-feeding going. Nurses are also an excellent tool for teaching you how to carry, burp, feed, and look after your infant.

You may choose to employ an infant nurse, postpartum doula, or a conscientious community adolescent to support you for a brief period after conception for in-house assistance. Your doctor or hospital may be able to help you locate in-house support records, and can refer you to home health agencies. Relatives and acquaintances are usually keen to support. Also, if you differ with specific issues, do not doubt their expertise. Yet do not feel bad for putting limits on travelers if you do not feel up to receiving guests or have any issues.

Handling a New Born

If you have not been around newborns for a long time, their fragility can be overwhelming. Here are a few tips you should remember: Wash your hands before touching your infant (or using a hand sanitizer). Newborns do not yet have a good immune response, and they are at risk of being sick. Ensure sure everybody who touches your kid has their hands washed.

Help to the head and neck of your infant. Cradle your back while holding your infant, and keep your head while bringing the infant upright or while lying down your baby. Never shake your baby, in practice, or out of rage. Shaking of the brain will cause damage and even death. Should not do so by tossing if you intend to wake your child — either tickle your baby's foot or softly blow on an ear. Always sure, the infant is safely secured to the backpack, car seat, or stroller. Stop some operation, which may be too rough or bouncy. Note that the infant is not equipped for physical activity, including getting knee-jiggled or tossed into the air.

Bonding

Supportive Bonding, perhaps one of the most pleasurable aspects of childcare, happens in the first hours and days after conception during the critical period when parents create a meaningful link with their baby. Physical closeness can encourage emotional bonding.

For children, attachment leads to their emotional growth, which in other ways, such as physical growth, often influences their progress. Another way to conceive about connecting with your kid is by "falling in love." Children succeed in their life by finding a parent or other person who loves them unconditionally. Start bonding by cradling your infant and stroke him or her softly in various patterns. You and your wife should even take the chance to be "head-to-skin," either eating or cradling, hugging your baby to your own flesh.

Babies may respond to massage, especially premature babies and those with medical problems. Other forms of massage can improve bonding and assist with the growth and development of infants. Many books and videos address the treatment of children-ask the doctor for advice. Be cautious, though — babies are not as heavy as adults are, so gently massage your infant. Babies seem to enjoy expressive noises like talking, babbling, humming, and cooing. Your kid will definitely love to listen to music as well. Some effective methods to enhance the infant's ears are baby rattles and electronic mobiles. Consider humming, reciting poems and nursery rhymes, or speaking aloud as you swing or softly rock your infant in a chair if your little one is fussy. Some babies may be unusually sensitive to touch, light, or sound, and could easily startle and cry, sleep less than expected, or turn away their faces when someone speaks to them or sings to them. Hold noise and light rates low to moderate if this is the case for your infant.

Swaddling

Swaddling, which functions best throughout the first few weeks children, is another calming method that parents will practice the first time. Proper swaddling holds the limbs of a baby tight to the chest, thus allowing any leg mobility. Swaddling not only holds an infant safe but also appears to offer a feeling of protection and warmth to most newborns. Swaddling may also help to limit the reflex of astonishment that can wake a child. Here is how to swaddle a baby: Stretch the receiving sheet, one corner partially folded over.

- Lay the baby face-up on the blanket, over the folded corner with his head.
- Wrap the left corner over the baby's body, and tuck it under the baby's back, under the right arm.
- Take the bottom corner up around the foot of the infant and raise it over the ear, pulling back the cloth as it comes near to the nose. Make a careful note to curl up around the waist too closely. Hips and elbows should be twisted slightly and will turn down. Too tightly wrapping your baby may increase the chance of having hip dysplasia.
- Wrap the correct corner around the infant; tuck it on the left side of the baby's ass, leaving just the neck and head uncovered. Make sure you can move a hand between the blanket and the chest of your baby to ensure that your baby is not bundled too closely, which would make for easier breathing. However, make sure the blanket is not so loose it might become undone.

Babies should not be swaddled after two months. Few babies at this age can turn over while swaddling, which raises their risk of sudden infant death syndrome (SIDS).

Everything Regarding Diapering

You will actually know whether you are going to use a cloth or disposable diapers before you carry your baby home with you. Your little one can dirty diapers approximately ten times a day, or about 70 days a week, no matter what you have.

When diapering your baby, be sure that you have all the tools within reach such that you do not have to put your infant on the changing table unattended. You will need: a clean diaper fastener (if disposable presold diapers are used) diaper ointment diaper wipes (or a hot water cup and a clean washcloth or cotton balls) after each bowel movement, or if the diaper is sticky, put your baby on his or her back and remove the messy slip. Using the bath, cotton balls, and washcloth or the towels to clean the genital region of your baby gently. Take very cautiously when changing a boy's diaper, because access to the environment will cause him to urinate. To prevent urinary tract infection (UTI), clean her bottom from front to back while wiping a child. Apply ointment to avoid or treat a rash. Mind also to wash your hands properly following a diaper shift.

A diaper rash can be a problem specific to you. The rash is usually red, which bumpy and should go away with warm water, some diaper cream, and a little time without the diaper over a couple of days. Some rashes develop when the baby's skin becomes responsive, and the dirty or poopy diaper is irritated. Use these strategies to prevent or treat diaper rash: adjust the baby's diaper regularly, preferably during bowel movements as soon as possible. Wash the region carefully with gentle soap and water (wipes may be painful at times), and add a very dense coat of diaper rash or "barrier" cream. Zinc oxide creams are favored because they create a barrier to moisture.

If using cotton diapers, wash them with detergents clean of dyes and fragrances. For a portion of the day, let the kid go un-diapered. This offers the skin an excuse to shine out. Whether the diaper rash lasts for longer than three days or appears to grow worse, call the doctor — it could be related to a prescription-requiring fungal infection.

Bathing Fundamentals

You can give your kid a bubble bath until the umbilical cord falls off and the navel heals fully (1–4 weeks) the circumcision heals (1–2 weeks) The first year's bath is perfect two or three days a week. More regular bathing will dry up on the skin. Before bathing your infant, have these things ready: a nice, warm, gentle washcloth, unscented infant soap, and shampoo a nice brush to relax the baby's scalp towels or blankets to warm Bubble baths and a clean diaper.

At first, you might be nervous to manage a baby but after practicing all these above-mentioned tips, you can establish a routine in a few quick weeks and be nurturing like a pro.

Conclusion

Montessori put forward an enticing contrast to her time's restrictive schooling. She took the blueprint from the factory and flipped it over on her back. The philosophy embraced by Montessori was to help rather than threaten, to inspire imagination rather than rote learning, and to inquire for suggestions rather than give responses. She frequently promoted problem solving over rote thinking, initiative over consequences, freedom over control, practical thinking over theoretical learning and preference of satisfying assignments over seeking to appease others. This book is a complete guide for anyone wanting to explore the roots of Montessori, how it emerged, how popular it is today and what exactly are the benefits of sending your child to a Montessori. Each chapter in this book is focused on a different but equally important aspect. The first chapter has not only briefed about who Dr Maria Montessori was but has also covered details of her journey creating the Montessori method. Chapter 1 has also discussed the benefits of Montessori education and compared it with the traditional education today, making it clear how both the methods differ and which one can precisely be more beneficial for your child. The second chapter, as the title says, is focused on making the reader understand the Montessori method in depth. It has discussed the curriculum, lesson plans and a lot of questions that are frequently asked about it. In addition to that, it also has a section for those who confuse Montessori as a constructivist method of learning. Next, the third chapter is a brief chapter yet has everything you need to know when understanding child development from the Montessori method. In addition to that, it has also enlisted the works of different psychologists and how their ideologies matched with Dr. Montessori. The last chapter of the book is itself a complete guide for new parents. It has everything a new parents needs to know, from safe and pain-free methods like Hypnobirthing to baby sleep & feeding techniques for new mothers. It has an interesting part that explains the Montessori approach to toilet training and how it differs from everyday toilet training.

References

1. A Brief History of Montessori Education. Retrieved from: https://www.bluffviewmontessori.org/about/a-brief-history-of-montessori-education/

2. Six Fun Ways to Boost Your Toddler's Brain Development. Retrieved from: https://www.todaysparent.com/toddler/toddler-development/fun-ways-to-boost-your-toddlers-language-development/

3. Benefits of Hypnobirthing. Retrieved from: https://www.bmhypnobirthing.com/hypnobirthing

4. Why Choose A Montessori Education. Retrieved from: http://www.webstermontessori.org/why-choose-montessori

5. Independent Sleep and Gentle Parenting. Retrieved from: https://reachformontessori.com/2019/01/07/independent-sleep-and-gentle-parenting-sleep-training/

6. 19 Simple Ways to Boost Brain Power in Infants and Toddlers. Retrieved from: https://www.mylittlemoppet.com/19-simple-ways-to-boost-brain-power-in-infants-and-toddlers/

7. How to Potty Train A Toddler In A Week. Retrieved from: https://www.parenting.com/toddler/potty-training/how-to-potty-train/

8. Dream Feeding a Baby: Its Benefits and Drawbacks. Retrieved from: https://www.momjunction.com/articles/dream-feeding-a-baby_00462342/

9. Learning In the Baby for Preschool Years. Retrieved from: https://raisingchildren.net.au/babies/play-learning/learning-ideas/learning-baby-to-preschool

10. Constructivism and the Montessori Educational Method. Retrieved from: https://www.slideshare.net/tcovert/constructivism-and-the-montessori-educational-method

Montessori Toddler Disciplines

Positive Parents: The Baby-Led Weaning Guide to Positive Discipline for Your Kids with Baby Sleep, No-Cry Baby, Potty Trainings and First-Time Mom Method (Age 0-6)

By

CALEMA DUMONT

Table of contents

Introduction

Most of us have been to college, primary and high school, but we realize that completing tests or graduation alone will not ready us for adulthood. However, when properly applied, Montessori education prepares children for life, particularly for 21st century life, it lays a strong basis by having the child support himself.

Montessori is a theory and tradition of education that fosters intensive, soul-motivated growth for children and teens in all aspects of their life, with the aim of fostering the innate need of awareness, comprehension and reverence for each individual.

What is Schooling at Montessori? The child-focused method founded by Dr. Maria Montessori, an Italian educator, for teaching children has been changing classrooms across the globe for more than a century now.

You realize that something new is in the making as soon as you reach a classroom. The classes at Montessori are easily visible. You can see kids functioning individually and in communities, including with carefully designed learning materials; actively interested in their work; and mindful of themselves and their community.

Your infant grows more quickly throughout the first 3 years of existence than at any other period. Via impressions and interactions your child learns vast quantities of knowledge from the world during this process. These are the years that set the foundations for later learning — and the greater the base, the better the child will expand upon it.

Montessori Child & Toddler programs offer a curriculum which arises from the specific abilities and interests of each child. The teachers introduce new materials and activities based on daily observations, which pique curiosity and stimulate learning. Learning goals for your child at this age include developing language skills, concentration skills, solving problems, visual discrimination, and physical coordination.

The Montessori Approach fosters systematic, self-motivated progress in all aspects of their development cognitive, mental, social, and physical for children and teenagers.

Chapter 1: Historical Introduction to Montessori Discipline

Know how, more than 100 years ago, the establishment of the first Montessori school contributed to a global phenomenon.

1.1 History of discipline

Dr. Maria Montessori, the Italian Teacher, mathematician, And the physicist who also judged the foreign exhibition On the basis of empiric pedagogy and behavioral psychology, a childcare center in San Lorenzo was set up, a deprived district in Rome's inner-city. There, she'd meet Just a selection of the neediest, and historically unschooled, children in the city.

On January 6, 1907, she opened the doors, naming the center Casa dei Bambini — Italian as "Children's House"." Dr. Maria Montessori was eager to render the Casa a Safe House educational place for these young boys, who others felt couldn't Know – because she has done so. Although at first the kids were unruly, they quickly displayed tremendous interest in interacting with puzzles, knowing how to cook Feed and clean the house, and participating in meaningful learning opportunities. Dr. Montessori found that the children displayed relaxed, cooperative behavior, intervals of intense focus and a common sense of balance in gentle for their surroundings before long. She saw the kids learn information from their environment and educate themselves ultimately.

Using experimental insight and knowledge learned of her previous research with small kids, Dr. Maria Montessori built for them innovative learning resources, numerous of those are now in operation today in Montessori schools, and produced a classroom atmosphere which fosters the innate ability of the children to know.

News about the progress of the school quickly circulated across Italy. Dr. Montessori founded a second Casa dei Bambini on 7 April 1907, again in San Lorenzo's. And she founded a third Casa October 18, 1907, in Milan.

Montessori gain momentum

Dr Montessori's schools' performance ignited concern worldwide. Far from countries, dignitaries traveled to Rome to see, first hand, the "miracle babies" who displayed focus, commitment and Self-discipline naturally.

The groundbreaking Montessori approach has now begun to draw the interest of influential educators who are keen to understand. Dr Maria Montessori herself instructed others. Her classes attracted children from Australia and Chile. and 5 continents had Montessori schools in only a few years.

Dr. Montessori wrote her first novel, Il Scientific Metodo della Pedagogy application to all 'education nelle infantile Case of the Bambins, in 1909. This has been published into ten languages within 3 years. His first five thousand copies were sold in four days, briefly dubbed The Montessori Process.

By 1910, the Montessori Schools, which can be found in Western Europe, were established around the country. In the United States the Montessori First kindergarten began in 1911.

187 papers and books in 1914 on Montessori schooling was written in English. Research describes Dr. Maria Montessori as "an intellectual wonder-worker," in the highly popular McClure's Journal. In 1916 Dr. Maria Montessori starts to revolve focus to the schooling of elementary-age children. Half the teachings of Dr Montessori based almost on freshly developed elementary materials in the foreign training course that year. She released Elementary L'autoeducazionne nelle Scuole a year later; outlining her views on educating children aged 7 – 11. Early work by Dr. Montessori concentrated on teaching small children but she shifted her focus to puberty in the 1920s. She found that students require opportunities at current period of growth which facilitate them appreciate themselves, discover place them in the universe, and Blossom of International People.

Dr Maria Montessori suggested uptown institute in which adolescent adults-whom she named "Children of the Planet or Erdkinder,"-could function and survive in a supportive environment, participating in actual-globe tasks such as cultivating or selling their own homemade products. He claimed that by observing human interdependence, the respondent must have known how to manage community, and gain the skills required to face the problems of the planet in a constructive way.

Dr. Montessori has often incorporated calm schooling into her lessons over time, as a consequence of living through it two devastating world wars. Montessori schooling is an important aspect of curriculum for harmony and global justice.

Dr. Montessori travelled widely, lecturing and offering classes and promoting the opening of new colleges. In 1929 she formed the Montessori International Association with her friend, Mario, to insure that her theory and education Strategy would proceed as she planned.

In America the arrival of Montessori

The Montessori Phenomenon soon caught on in the West. In 1911 Montessori first school opened, in Scarborough, New York, prominent banker home. Others also proceeded in fast chain. Like the first Bambini Casa dei by Maria Montessori, which was meant for kids from impoverished, deprived backgrounds, they were appealing to kids from affluent, educated backgrounds seeking to provide their kids with the highest quality education. Prominent people have offered their encouragement, like Alexander Graham Bell and Thomas Edison.

In 1913, on a three-week lecture series, Maria Montessori traveled to the US, Where she encountered thousands of eager and enthusiastic followers. A banquet was held in DC Washington, for her. Four hundred guests participated, like Wilson, President Woodrow Wilson's aunt, as well as other dignitaries and foreign ministers.

Dr Maria lecture to an audience of thousand at Carnegie Hall in New York City, where she presented "moving images" taken back to her Rome school; a second lecture was organized in reaction to the demand.

Montessori said she considers the schools close to her principles in America, and deemed the journey to be an incredible success.

In 1915, Dr. Montessori came to the United State. To show her system at the International Panama San Francisco in Pacific Fair and to offer an international preparation course for aspiring Montessori instructors. A "Glass Montessori Lab" was installed at the exhibition which is a lab with 3 walls of panoramic glass screens. This innovative concept allowed spectators to watch the young student's class that operated with extreme attention and determination with amazement, almost indifferent to the people around them.

In 1915 it was the similar time; Dr Maria Montessori was an official visitor at the Education National Association's influential annual meeting in California Oakland. Above 15 thousands representatives from the education industry participated.

The popularity of the Classroom of mirror and the lengthy journey to California by Dr. Montessori ignited American involvement in schooling Montessori and its pioneering creator, helping to drive Montessori education worldwide. For both her attitude and her pedagogy, American newspapers and educational leaders welcomed his author. By 1916 there were over Montessori hundred schools functioning in the United States.

A derailed movement

In United state the Montessori Trend was dying out as soon as it grew. Language shortages, transportation restrictions of 1 World War, anti-immigrant rhetoric, and the disapproval of a little prominent educators all added to the refuse.

One such detractor was Kilpatrick William, a well regarded leader in the modern education society, a longtime classmate of Dewey John. In his essay, The Montessori Program Discussed, he criticized the Montessori approach. Kilpatrick, a prominent theorist in the early on twenty centuries, attacked the qualifications, viewpoints and general theory of Dr Montessori. He ignored her views about the instructor position, the appropriate size of the classroom, and the resources in the classroom. And, he opposed her understanding of the creation theory and also the sum of independence that kids have in a classroom of Montessori. Montessori's poor portrayal of Kilpatrick soon became well recognized and embraced around the US.

Through the twenties century, with the exception of the odd school or teacher, Montessori schooling in the US has almost entirely died away.

A school of glasses

The Classroom Glass in Montessori had large screens, allowing tourists to gaze inside at the going on. Many returned everyday in their wonderful room of class environment to see the laborious "miracle babies."

The innovation of the twentieth century was on dazzling show at the Panama Pacific International Exhibition in San Francisco for the best part of 1915. In 10 minutes flat, Model Ts turned out to be an actual Ford assembly line. The brand new transcontinental telephone network was connecting callers three thousand miles away. And, for four months of operating the show, in a glass-walled Montessori classroom, 30 small children attended kindergarten, offering an exclusive view of the modern educational paradigm that was quickly catching on with American educators and parents.

The "Glass Classroom" was hidden within the Education and Social Economy Palace, one of 11 huge display palaces at the 635-acre, expansive show. There were large windows on three of the room's doors, allowing tourists to see the goings-on inside.

The students had an equally fair vision of the audience, but they attended their research tirelessly and gave rise to admiring comments regarding their concentrating forces. The children aged from 2 1/2 to 6 years old, and were chosen from a selection of several thousand applicants. Under the urging of Dr. Maria Montessori, only children who had no previous school experience were considered for the program.

An ideal classroom

The presence of Dr Montessori may be seen in the classroom of the layout. She knew the enormous promotional importance of the well-attended exhibition, and was keen to make it fine. Billowing fabric provided the space with a ceiling which gave the room a cozy feel. Designer Louise Brigham, famed for her "box furniture," designed the blue, brown, and white furnishings — simple, recycled fabrics made into beautiful items for the house.

The space was packed with items in varying types, sizes, and colours, carefully placed on low shelves to encourage interaction and discovery. These learning resources helped the children to individually solve issues, feel good in them, thought analytically, and enjoy the happiness that comes from achievement.

The role of lead teacher — whom Dr. Montessori believed would be a reference rather than a source of authority — fell to Helen Parkhurst, a star student of Dr. Montessori, and a respected American instructor of her own. Later in New York City, Parkhurst founded the experimental Dalton School and created the renowned Dalton Laboratory Program for secondary education, both influenced by Montessori theory and practice.

If embodying Montessori education was a daunting assignment for the world's visitors, as Parkhurst later admitted, there is no doubt she acted on it.

Inspired observers

According to historical accounts, the classroom became quite well-liked with the fairmen day after day with many guests persistent in their beautiful classroom setting to observe the laborious "miracle children." The day of school was going from noon Nine AM, and the crowds increased as the lunchtime arrived. The spectators lined the Place and ahead of plates, transfix by the exquisite of the set of dining table with china, linens, and candles in the classroom; the show of impeccable table manners; and the sight of small children feeding themselves and washing up afterwards.

Spreading the Pedagogy

The public of American and political figures of the time accepted both the woman and Montessori pedagogy who founded it, as a consequence of the Glass Classroom and positive publishing in American newspapers and magazines.

The Montessori campaign has been an interesting moment. Nevertheless, following global developments and specific incidents in the life of Dr. Maria Montessori lead to a deterioration in the educational method over the subsequently numerous decades in the U.S. In the Ninety century Montessori saw a revival in the U.S. that continues today, with new practitioners and the formation of AMS.

The resurgence

The cultural atmosphere in the U.S. was shifting by the 1950s, including increasing dissatisfaction with mainstream US schooling. Among those exploring alternatives was Nancy McCormick Rambusch, a single, ambitious New York City teacher.

Having "occurred on" Maria Montessori's works, Rambusch was fascinated by the freshness of her thoughts. She traveled to Paris in 1953 to attend a congress in Montessori, and learn more. There, she encountered Mario Montessori, son of Maria, who urged her to introduce Montessori back to the United States. One event contributed to another and through ensuing Montessori learning by Rambusch and concerted attempts to encourage the

System in the U.S., Montessori education took off once again. In contrast to this the American Montessori Community was founded in 1960, perhaps as a consequence of Rambusch's actions.

Montessori today

Montessori curriculum has taken solid roots in the curriculum environment from its modest origins more than 100 years ago as a single schoolroom for a community of underprivileged children in Rome, Italy. Roughly 5,000 Montessori schools currently educate over a million children in the United States alone, from childhood to puberty. There are thousands of Montessori schools worldwide. The American Montessori Society thrives, as do the Montessori Foreign Organization and its affiliate communities worldwide. Many Montessori organizations often provide networking resources, teamwork and professional development. In particular, China is currently seeing enormous demand, and educational organizations are working as hard as they can to train the teachers and develop the schools required to fulfill that demand. We at AMS are working to improve the consistency of chosen services in particular, and are preparing in the coming years to provide further assistance.

In the U.S., there has been a growth of community-specific programming; for example, public and private schools providing tuition-free Montessori instruction, colleges with flexible service hours, and services operated year-round.

There are also multicultural, immersive-language and/or faith-based Montessori classrooms; and services expressly for children with developmental exceptionalities, such as those relating to dyslexia and language-processing disabilities.

Recognizing the many aspects of intergenerational partnerships and aligning Montessori theory with adult care requirements, several Montessori schools now include opportunities with social experiences that put together children and the elderly. Others build cross-cultural partnerships in distant countries with Montessori colleges, opening the doors for students to establish global links, and enhancing their awareness of peoples around the world. Most, if not most, Montessori schools incorporate community-based service learning programs in their curriculum.

Well-known celebrities were taught in the classrooms of Montessori. Among them are NBA MVP, Stephen Curry; the creators of Google, Larry Page and Sergey Brin; and Julia Boy, the late cook, journalist, and TV personality. These individuals listed their Montessori education experience as leading to their performance, raising Montessori's public awareness as a method that helps people from all sorts of fields reach their full potential.

Day One Academies, an effort initiated in 2018 to fund $1 billion for Montessori-inspired full-scholarship preschools for low-income families, has brought fresh exposure to the process. The man behind this initiative? Amazon Chief Jeff Bezos, is a Montessori graduate.

The evidence is clear: not only is Montessori here to live, it is growing at a rate that would have gladdened the heart of its creator, Dr. Maria Montessori — a woman who sought to re-imagine how we know, and understood the integrity and capacity of all men.

Yet her influence persists through the excellent work of Montessori-credentialed instructors yet related professional preparation services at AMS. We are unified by one common purpose: to make the world a better place with our babies, who will act as our future leaders, by humility and courtesy.

1.2 Comparison between Classical Pedagogy and Modern Pedagogy

Over the past decade, something has been said regarding the propensity of pedagogy, pursuing the example of science, to move beyond the strictly theoretical stage and focus its findings on the promising effects of the experiments. Physiological and experimental psychology, which has been structured into a modern discipline from Weber and Fechner to Wundt, appears expected to provide the current pedagogy with the simple training that the old theoretical psychology had for conceptual pedagogy.

Morphological anthropology applied to children's physical research is also a powerful factor in the current pedagogy's development. But despite all these features, Scientific Pedagogy has never been clearly developed nor described yet. It's something we're worried about, so it doesn't really happen. We may conclude that it has been, to date, the pure hypothesis or idea of a science that will arise from the mist and clouds that have overshadowed it, with the help of the constructive and experimental sciences that have revived the nineteenth-century thinking. That man, who through science advancement has created a modern universe, must be prepared and established through himself by a modern pedagogy. But I'm not going to attempt to comment more thoroughly about this here.

A few years ago, a renowned doctor founded a school of scientific pedagogy in Italy, the purpose of which was to train teachers to pursue the new trend that had begun to be felt within the world of pedagogy. This school had such much success for two or three years that teachers from all over Italy flocked to it and was equipped with a wonderful equipment of scientific material by the City of Milan. In reality, its origins were most favorable and liberal support was given in the hope that through the experiments carried out there, "the science of human creation" could be developed.

The excitement that greeted the school was largely due to the warm support given it by the renowned anthropologist Giuseppe Sergi, who spent more than 30 years actively working to spread the ideals of a new society focused on education among teachers in Italy. "Our everyday needs in the social world," Sergi said, "are imperative – the restoration of the educational methods; and whoever fights for this cause, fights for human regeneration." He sums up the lectures he funded in his pedagogical writings, which have been compiled by a book named 'Educazione Ed Istruzione' (Pensieri)*.

"For many years I have been struggling for an understanding of man's teaching and education, which proved to be the more reasonable and beneficial the more deeply I thought about it. My theory was that, in order to develop normal, logical practices, it was important that we make various, reliable and logical observations of man as an person, especially during infancy, which is the age at which the human being was raised. "Measuring the head, the height, etc. does not in fact suggest that we are setting up a pedagogical framework, but it does imply the direction we should follow to achieve such a method, and if we want to teach a person, we must have a simple and precise understanding of him."

Sergi's reputation was enough to persuade others that the art of educating him should grow naturally, despite such knowledge of the person. This, as is always the case, contributed to a clash of ideas among his disciples, emerging now from a simplistic understanding of the master's thoughts, now from a misunderstanding. The main problem was the misunderstanding between the pupil's scientific research and his schooling. And because the one was the path leading to the other, which would have evolved from it naturally and rationally, they instantly gave what in fact was pedagogical anthropology the name of Scientific Pedagogy. These new adherents bore the "Biographical Map" as their flag, claiming that triumph would be achieved if this engraving was firmly placed on the school's battlefield.

Therefore, the so-called School of Scientific Pedagogy advised teachers to take anthropometric samples, use esthesiometric devices, gather psychological evidence, and shape the army of new science students.

It can be mentioned that Italy proved herself to be on track in this campaign. Experiments have been produced in the elementary schools in France, England, and particularly in America, focused on an analysis of anthropology and psychological pedagogy, in the hope of discovering the restoration of the school in anthropometry and psychometry. During such attempts it was never the students who carried out the research; the tests were, in most instances, in the care of physicians who had greater pride in their unique science than in teaching. Typically, they have attempted to bring a reference to psychology or sociology through their studies, rather than trying to coordinate their research and findings into the development of the long-awaited Scientific Pedagogy. Just summarize the case quickly, sociology and psychology never dedicated themselves just the problem of teaching children in classrooms, nor did the professionally educated instructors really live up to true scientists' expectations.

The reality is that the school's functional development requires a true convergence in action and thinking of these contemporary tendencies; a convergence that would put science directly into the school's essential sector and at the same time lift teachers from the lower academic stage to which they are confined today. The University School of Pedagogy, established by Credaro in Italy, definitely operates against this eminently realistic ideal. This is this school's aim to lift Pedagogy from the lower role it has held as a secondary branch of philosophy to the prestige of a definite discipline, which, like medicine, should encompass a broad and varied area of comparative research.

Yet Pedagogical Hygiene, Pedagogical Anthropology, yet Clinical Psychology can most definitely be included in the divisions associated with it.

Indeed, Italy, the nation of Lombroso, De-Giovanni, and Sergi, should claim the prestige of pre-eminence in such a movement's organization. In addition, in Anthropology, these three scientists may be considered the pioneers of the current trend: the first leading the way in criminal anthropology, the second in medical anthropology, and the third in pedagogical anthropology. For the good fortune of science, all three of them were the acknowledged founders of their unique lines of thinking, and were so influential in the academic community that they not only made important and brave followers, but also primed the minds of the people to accept the intellectual revival they promoted.

Today, though, the issues that concern us in the field of education are the needs of mankind as a whole and of society, and we can consider only one country — the whole world — before these great powers. So in a cause with so immense significance, all those who have made some effort deserve with consideration for mankind in the modern world, even if it is merely an endeavor not crowned with achievement. In Italy, therefore, the schools of Scientific Pedagogy and the Anthropological Laboratories, which originated in the various cities through the actions of elementary teachers and scholarly inspectors, and which were abandoned almost before they were clearly formed, nevertheless have great importance because of the confidence that motivated them and because of the doors that they had opened.

It is unnecessary to claim that such efforts have been insufficient and have emerged from too mild an awareness of modern sciences already in the creation phase. Each great cause has its roots in repetitive defeats and incomplete attainment. When Assisi of St. Francis in a dream met his Lord, and got the order from the lips of Divine-"Francis, restore my House!"-he assumed that the teacher talked of the small house in which he kneels at the time. And he then set up for the job, bearing the stones from which he intended to repair the collapsed walls upon his shoulders. Only later did he become alert of the reality that his goal was to revive the Church Catholic in the courage of deprivation. But the Francis St. who brought the stones so naively, and the Powerful representative who directed the country so miraculously to a moral victory, are one of the same man in development of different stages. And we, who are working for one perfect finish, are part of one of the same self, and all who come with us will only achieve the aim if those people who believed were there and operated prior to them. And, similar to Francis St., we have hoped that we could restore it by taking the rough and desolate gravel of the laboratory research to the school's old and decaying buildings.

From the same confidence as Francis looked at the granite squares he had to bear on his hands, we looked at the supports provided by the mechanical and materialistic sciences.

So we have been drawn in a wrong and restricted way from that we must safe ourselves if we are to build real and live teaching methods for upcoming creation. Preparing teachers in the sciences of experimentation system is not a straightforward issue.

Although we have directed them in the minutest fashion imaginable in psychometry and anthropometry, we would still have produced devices whose utility would be most questionable. Indeed, if our teachers are to be invited to explore after this pattern, we will stay in the theory field forever. The previous educate instructors, trained in keeping with the concepts of philosophical theory, grasped the thoughts of other people deemed to be experts, and to speak about them shifted the muscles of expression, and to interpret their theories shifted the muscles of the mind. Instead, our science instructors are acquainted with those instruments and know how to shift the arm and hand muscles to operate certain instruments; in addition, they've had advanced experience consisting of a set of traditional assessments what they did research how to conduct in a sterile and mechanical manner. The disparity is not significant, since fundamental variations in outer practice alone cannot occur, but reside inside the central guy instead. We have not equipped new masters for all our beginning into logical practice, after all, we left them without all the gate of real science; we did not embrace them in the most worthy and informative phase of such research, the knowledge which makes better scientists.

And what's a scientist, really? Not, surely, he who understands how to control all the equipment in the physical research lab, or who handles the different reactive with deftness and safety in the chemist's laboratory or who knows how to prepare the samples for the microscope in biology. Surely it is always the case that in laboratory methodology an associate has a better agility than the leading scientist himself. We assign the word scientist to the sort of man who felt experiment as a way of leading him to seek out the sublime truth of creation, to raise a curtain from its mysterious secrets, and the one who, in this quest, felt a reverence for the wonders of nature emerging inside him, so intense as to destroy his own mind. The scientist is not the sharp machine manipulator, he is the believer of god, and he holds the visible marks of his faith, as does the adherent of any religious group. To this group of scientists belong to those who, ignoring the environment around them, same as the Trappists of the Medieval period, exist only in the laboratory, always negligent in case of food and clothes as they no longer speak about themselves; those who are blind by years about unwearied usage of the microscope; those who immunize themselves with tuberculosis germs in their intellectual ardor. This is the men's spirit of science to whom nature freely tells its secrets, with the glory of innovation crowning their labors.

Technology, we didn't want to make such essential teachers professional anthropologists, expert psychologists or experts in child hygiene; we simply tried to guide them to the area in experimental research, training them to handle specific Devices of the same level of competency. Therefore, in connection with his own specific area, the classroom, we want to guide the instructor, attempting to stimulate in him the analytical spirit the opens up door to wider and more opportunities for him. In further terms, we want to awaken a curiosity in natural phenomenon in the brain and core of the instructor to such a degree that, in devoted environment, he can appreciate the nervous and expectant mood of somebody that has anticipated and hopes a breakthrough from the research.

The apparatuses are like alphabet, so we must learn how to handle them if we have to understand nature; just as the novel, which includes the unveiling of an author's greatest feelings, uses the ways of writing outer words or symbols in the alphabet, so existence, by the process of the experiment, provides us an unlimited sequence of discoveries, revealing its mysteries for us.

Now the one, who has learned to spell all the terms in his spell-book mechanically, will be able to interpret the terms in one of the plays of Shakespeare in the same mechanical manner, if the print was plain enough. He who is exclusively introduced into the creation of the pure experimentation is similar to one who points out the basic sense of the terms in the spell-book; it's on such a basis that we abandon the instructors because we limit their training to methodology alone.

Instead, we will make them interpreters and adorers of the force of god. They must have been like him who, having learned to spell, one day finds himself capable to read the Shakespeare play, or Dante or Goethe, behind the written symbols. The gap is fantastic as can be shown, and the path is wide. However our first mistake was a good one. The kid who learns the spell-book provides the illusion that he understands how to read. In fact, he reads the signs above the doors of the shop, the names of newspapers and each and every word that comes in his mind. It would be quite normal if this boy were to be misled into believing, upon visiting a library, that he learned how to interpret the meaning of all the books he looked there. Yet he will quickly feel struggling to do so, like "knowing how to learn technically" is nothing, and he wants to return to school. Hence it's with the teachers that we thought by teaching them psychometry and anthropometry, to prepare for scientific pedagogy.

But let us set away, in the agreed meaning of the term, the challenge of training science masters. We won't even try to detail such a planning plan, because it will bring us into a conversation that has no position here. Let us assume instead that we have already set teachers for the observation of nature through lengthy and easygoing exercises, and that we must led them, for instance, to the point reached by those natural science students who rise up at night and back into the forests and fields so that they might wonder the awakening and early actions of some family of the insects they are interested in. Here we see the scientist who, although he might be drowsy and tired of walking, full of vigilance, who is unaware that he is dusty or wet, that the fog wets him, or that the sun burns him; but only intends not to reveal his presence in the lowest degree, so that the insects may, hour after hour, keep up gently those normal function which he desires to watch. Let's say these instructors have entered the point of view of the scientist who is half blind, already observing the random movements of a unique infusory animalcule through his microscope. To this science watcher, these animals appear to hold a dim wisdom in their way of avoiding one another and in their manner of picking their milk. Then, with an electric shock, he disturbs this stagnant existence, seeing how others stick themselves around the positive pole and others around the negative. Investigating more, he observes how others sprint into the sun with a luminous cue, whilst others travel away from it. He examines such and other phenomena; often keeping in mind the question: if fleeing or running towards the stimuli is of the same nature as avoiding one another or choosing food – that is, if these variations are the product of preference and are attributable to the dim awareness, rather than to actual desire or repulsion comparable to the magnet's. And let's say that this guy, considering it as four o'clock in the afternoon and not yet having lunch, is mindful, with a sense of delight that he was operating in his research laboratory instead in its own place, where they should have called him some hours before, interrupting his fascinating discovery so that he could sleep.

Let us suppose, I suggest, that the instructor has arrived at such an approach of curiosity in the study of usual phenomenon, independent of his academic experience. Quite good, but a planning like that is not sufficient. Indeed, the master is supposed not to observe insects or microbes, but to observe man in his specific task. One is not to create an embodiment analysis of many of his everyday physical activities as one examines any insects' family from the morning hour waking, watching their motions. In the waking of his academic existence the teacher is to research man.

The value in humanity of whom we wish of educate the instructor must be defined by the personal relationship that is to be found between the educator and the individual; a relationship that does not occur among the students of botany or zoology and the environment that he is learning. Man can't love the natural process or the insect he's studying without sacrificing some of his own. This self-denial appears like a giant renunciation of existence itself, almost pacifism, to one who sees it from the world's viewpoint.

To offer an understanding of this second type of preparing, that of the soul, let us seek to reach into the hearts and minds of those first believers of Christ Jesus when they heard Him talk of an Empire that is not of this universe, much greater than every earthly realm, no matter how royally created. In their simplicity they asked Him, "Lord, ask all of us that shall be strongest in the kingdom of god?" To which Christ, hugging the head of a small child who observed His face with reverent, curious eyes, replied, "Whoever shall become like one of these little ones shall be strongest in the empire of paradise." Now let us imagine a passionate one of those to which these words were spoken. He sets himself to study any appearance of this little boy with a blend of reverence and devotion, holy interest and a determination to achieve certain divine excellence. Just such an outsider put in a classroom full of little kids won't be the latest instructor we want to shape. But let us try to embed in the spirit the scientist's self-sacrificing soul with the reverent affection of Christ's disciple, and we shall prepare the teacher's spirit. As an instructor he must hear from the kid himself how to improve himself.

Consider the teacher's attitude in the light of yet another case. Imagine one of our botanists or zoologists trained in research and testing techniques; one who travelled in their natural area to examine "other fungi." This physicist made his discoveries in the open world and then, with the help of his microscope and many of his laboratory equipment, he carried out the subsequent study work as far as possible. Yes, he is a scientist who knows what it is to research nature, and who is acquainted with all the instruments that contemporary experimental science uses for this analysis.

So let us consider such a man assigned to a chair in science at any university because of the unique work he has completed, with the challenge before him of carrying out more original research work with hymenoptera. Let us presume that, as he arrives at his location, he is given a glass-covered case having a variety of lovely butterflies, supported by sticks, their outstretched wings immobile. The student would suggest that this is a child's play, not science research stuff, and that these experiments in the container are more fittingly a portion of the game played by the little boys, pursuing butterflies and capturing them in a trap. The entire laboratory scientist can do for such content as this.

The condition will be pretty much the same if we were to put an instructor, who is medically educated according to our definition of the word, in one of the public schools where the children are repressed in the free expression of their personalities until they become almost like dead beings. In such a classroom, the children are fastened to their location, the desk, like butterflies perched on pins, spreading the worthless wings of barren and pointless intelligence they gained. This is not enough, though, to train the intellectual spirit of our Masters. We will always get the school accessible for their study. The school will accept the child's open, natural expressions, if empirical pedagogy is to be born in the classroom. This is the main change.

No one may claim that such a theory occurs now in pedagogy and in education. It's clear that certain pedagogues, led by Rousseau, have provided expression to impracticable ideals and abstract expectations for the child's liberation, but educators remain practically ignorant regarding the true definition of independence. They also have the same definition of independence that animates a nation from oppression in the hour of revolt, or even the definition of civil liberty that is still limited, even if it is a higher notion.

"Human equality" still means another step of Jacob's ladder. That means a partial emancipation, the emancipation of a nation, a class, or a feeling.

Instead, the principle of independence which must motivate pedagogy is universal. The nineteenth century biological sciences explained this to us when they gave us the opportunity to research creation. Therefore, if the old pedagogy foresaw or implicitly articulated the idea of observing the student before schooling him and keeping him loose in his random embodiments, such an concept, infinite and scarcely stated, was made probable of realistic accomplishment only after the experimental sciences' intervention during the last century. This is not a case of sophistry or debate, it is appropriate for us to state our argument. He who will suggest that the idea of independence governs today's pedagogy will make us grin like a kid who would wish that they were alive and could float before the box of installed butterflies. The theory of slavery still pervades pedagogy and the same concept, thus, pervades the classroom. I just need to offer one evidence the standing desks and chairs. For example, here we have a striking proof of the errors of early materialistic scientific pedagogy which, with misguided zeal and energy, brought the barren stones of science to the reconstruction of the school's crumbling walls. At first the schools were fitted with the large, thin benches on which the kids clustered together. Then, research arrived, and the bench polished. Significant focus has been given in this journal to the anthropology's recent contributions.

The child's age and the duration of his limbs were weighed while putting the seat at the appropriate height. The space between the seat and the desk was measured with utmost consideration, such that the back of the infant was not to be deformed, and eventually the benches were divided and the breadth determined such precisely that the infant could scarcely balance on it, although it became difficult to expand without doing any sideways motions. This was achieved so he could be isolated from his neighbor. These desks are designed in such a manner that the infant is rendered clear with all its immobility. The avoidance of unethical actions in the schoolroom is one of the objectives achieved by this separation. What are we supposed to do regarding this prudence in a condition of culture where giving voice to the ideals of sex morality in schooling will be deemed scandalous; for fear that we could thereby contaminate innocence? And still, here we have technology that contributes itself to this irony that creates computers! Not just this; obliging technology goes still better, perfecting the benches in such a way as to encourage the child's immobility to the fullest degree practicable, or, if you prefer, to repress any child's expression. It is designed in such a way that, although the child is well positioned in his place, the desk and chair itself cause him to take on the role called hygienically comfortable.

The bench, the foot-rest, the desks are positioned such that the child is never able to stand at his job. Also adequate room is reserved for sitting in an upright role. It is in such a manner that desks and benches in the schoolroom have advanced toward excellence. Through cults of the so-called science pedagogy crafted a science desk model. Not a few nations were proud of their "country desk,"- and these different computers were licensed in the battle for competitiveness.

There is certainly something that underlies the design of such benches in theoretical terms.

Anthropology has been used in the estimation of the body and in the treatment of the age; biology, in the study of muscle movements; psychology, in the perversion of instincts; and, above all, grooming, in the attempt to avoid spine curvature. Such desks were also empirical, despite the anthropological research of the child in their creation. Like I said, we have here an indication of the practical application of science to the classrooms.

I assume that we will all be hit by this mentality of great shock before quite long. This would appear surprising that the desk's basic mistake was not to have been discovered sooner by the emphasis paid to the study of child health, anatomy and sociology, and by the general development in thinking. The wonder becomes greater as we realize that a trend toward the security of the infant has been growing in almost every nation over the past years.

I assume that it will not be many years until the public, trusting barely in the explanations of these science benches, would begin to contact with curious hands the impressive seats which were designed to prevent the curvature of the spine among our school children!

The creation of these experimental benches indicates that the pupils were exposed to a system that made it possible for them to become humpbacked, even if they were born solid and clear! The vertebral column, scientifically the most basic, essential and oldest component of the backbone, the most stable element of our body, because the backbone is the most solid part of the organism, the vertebral column that resisted and was powerful during the desperate struggles of the primal man when he battled the desert lion, when he defeated the brute, when he quarried the s.

It is incomprehensible that so-called science would have served in the school to refine an instrument of oppression without being enlightened by one ray from the wave of social emancipation that is rising and evolving all over the world. For the era of intellectual benches the era of redeeming the working masses from the yokes of unfair labor was also. The inclination towards social equality is most obvious, and is expressed on either side.

People's representatives make it their motto, the laboring masses echo the protests, science and revolutionary journals express the same protest, our newspapers are loaded. The underfed worker is not calling for a tonic, but for improved economic opportunities to prevent malnutrition. The miner, who is exposed to inguinal failure through the stooping posture held for several hours of the day, does not ask for abdominal assistance, but wants shortened hours and improved working conditions so that he can live a healthier life as other people.

So then we see the children of our schoolrooms operating in unhygienic circumstances during that same social period, so ill suited to human growth that even the skeleton is deformed, our reaction to this terrible discovery becomes an orthopedic table. It's almost like we're selling the abdominal belt to the miner, or arsenic to the worker underfed. A woman some time ago, thinking that I was in agreement with all of the technical advances surrounding the classroom, gave me a corset or brace for pupils with apparent pleasure. She had created this, and thought the bench's work should be done.

Surgery also provides other ways for managing the curvature of the spinal cord. I may consider orthopedic devices, restraints and a technique of hanging the infant regularly, by the head or neck, in such a manner that the body weight extends and thereby straightens the vertebral spine. At college, the desk-shaped orthopedic device is in great favor; today someone is recommending the brace – one step forward and it would be proposed that we offer the scholars a comprehensive course in the method of suspension!

Everything this is the conceptual result of a substance applied to the decadent school of the methods of research. Clearly, the logical way of battling the spinal curvature of the pupils is to adjust the nature of their jobs, so that they may no longer be compelled to stay in a dangerous place for too many hours a day. It is liberation of democracy that the school wants, and not a bench process.

Even if the stationary seat is useful to the child's health, it would also be a hazardous and unhygienic feature of the area, owing to the difficulties of properly cleaning the space while the seating cannot be relocated. The foot-rests, which cannot be replaced, gather the many little feet of dirt taken in everyday from the driveway. There is a general change in the issue of house furnishings today. They are made lightweight and easier so they can be shifted, dusted and even cleaned quickly. Yet the school may appear oblivious to the social environment's change.

It is our responsibility to worry of what will happen to the child's soul, which is doomed to develop in circumstances so unnatural that the very bones will become deformed. When we talk of the worker's salvation, it is often known that beneath the most obvious type of misery, such as the starvation of the flesh, or ruptures, there is the other wound under which the man's soul which is subjected to some sort of slavery will endure. It is at this deeper misunderstanding that we point when we claim the worker must be liberated by democracy. We know far too well that when the very blood of a man has been eaten or his intestines have been stripped away by his life, his spirit may have lain in darkness imprisoned, made indifferent, or, maybe, destroyed inside him. The slave's moral decay is, above all, the weight which inhibits humanity's progress — humanity struggling to grow and be kept back by this great burden. The pleas of salvation talk far louder for men's hearts than for their bodies.

We know just too well the teacher's sad show which has to spill such cut and dried evidence into the scholars' heads in the ordinary schoolroom. She considers it appropriate to punish her pupils into immobility and compel their focus in order to excel in this barren mission. Prizes and penalties are all-ready and efficient tools for the leader, who will compel those who are sentenced to be his listeners into a specified disposition of mind and body.

It is probable that abolishing official whippings and repetitive strikes is thought expedient nowadays, even as granting awards has been less ceremonious. Such modest changes are just another science-approved tool, and provided to the decadent school group. These rewards and penalties are the bench of the mind, the tool of bondage to the spirit, if I might be given the word. Such are not introduced here, though, to reduce deformities but to cause them. The reward and retribution are rewards for artificial or coerced action, and so we should definitely not think of the child's normal growth in conjunction with it. Until hopping into the saddle the jockey gives his horse a slice of candy, the coachman beats his horse so that he can respond to the signals provided by the reins; and yet none of these runs so superbly as the plains' free horse.

And here, in the case of schooling, is he expected to put the yoke on him?

Real, we're suggesting the man in culture is a normal guy yoked to community. But if we take a thorough glance at the spiritual development of humanity, we will see that little by little the yokes are made lighter, that is, we can see that existence, or creation, is gradually progressing towards victory. The slave's yokes belong to the servant's, and the servant's yokes to the laborers.

Both aspects of slavery begin to collapse and vanish little by little, including in the woman's sexual slavery. Civilization history is a tale of colonization and emancipation. We should wonder what stage in society we are in and if, in fact, we require the benefit in rewards and punishments to succeed. When we have already progressed past this stage, instead introducing such an educational method will be dragging the younger generation down to a lower standard, not moving them through their true patrimony of development. Throughout the partnership between the government and the vast number of people serving in its administrative offices, anything quite close to this state of the school remains in culture. Such clerks work for the greater national benefit day after day, but they do not expect or see any tangible compensation for the value of their efforts. This is, they don't know that by their everyday activities the state carries out its big enterprise, and that their job supports the whole country. The immediate benefit for them is transfer, as for the child in school moving to a higher class is. The man who loses sight of his work's very big target is like a kid put under his real status in a class: like a slave, he is deceived by something that is his privilege. His honor as an individual is limited to the limitations of a machine's integrity, which must be oiled if it is to be kept going, because it loses the instinct of existence within itself. All these little things, including the need for gifts or medals, are just external stimulation, lightening the bleak, desolate road he is traveling in for the moment.

In the same way we are awarding school kids gifts. And the fear of failing to gain advancement keeps the clerk from running away, tying him to his monotonous job, just as the fear of not moving to the next class pushes the pupil to his journal. The superior's reproof is in some respect close to teacher's scolding. The correction of poorly done clerical work is equal to the bad mark imposed upon the deficient composition of the scholar by the teacher. The quasi-perfect relation.

Yet if the administrative divisions are not carried out in a manner that might appear acceptable to the glory of a nation; if cheating takes a position so easily; it is the consequence of having extinguished the true grandeur of man in the employee's eyes, and having limited his view to those low, immediate facts which he has come to consider as rewards and punishments. The nation stands because the rectitude of the overwhelming percentage of its workers is such that they reject reward and penalty abuse and pursue an unavoidable line of integrity. Just as life triumphs over any source of misery and death in the social world and continue to new conquests, so the spirit to liberation conquers all challenges, from victory to victory. It is this unique and fundamental force of existence that drives the universe forward, a power sometimes latent inside the mind.

But whoever does a really human job, whoever does something very wonderful and triumphant, is never driven to his mission by those trifling distractions named by the name of "prizes," nor by the fear of those trivial ills that we term "punishments." Even in a battle a great army of giants would fight without motivation beyond the urge to earn advancement, epaulets, or awards, or by fear of winning.

If true courage inside an army has fallen, rewards and penalties will only complete the job of destruction, putting about greed and cowardice. All human successes, all human achievements, rest upon the inner power. A young man will therefore become a fantastic doctor if he is motivated by a curiosity in his work that allows medicine his true vocation. But if he operates in the expectation of an estate, or a good marriage, or if he is truly motivated by some material benefit, he would never become a real master or a fantastic doctor, and because of his work, the universe will never make one move forward. He who wants this stimulation was much easier never to become a practitioner. Everyone has a specific inclination, a special vocation, maybe modest but definitely useful. The scheme of prizes that draw a person away from this vocation, that make him choose a wrong course, may be a futile one for him, and may be compelled to pursue it, can alter, diminish, and even annihilate a human being's natural behavior.

We still reiterate that the universe is going ahead, so we will encourage people to make changes. But change emerges from the fresh developments that are created, and these, unexpected, are not awarded with prizes: they always bring the person to martyrdom, instead. God forbid poetry has to be born out of the need to be installed in the Capitol!

Such a dream just has to reach into the poet's heart and the inspiration can vanish. The poem will emerge from the poet's mind, while he doesn't care of either himself or the money. Even if he earns the laurel, he'll sense the envy of an award like this. The real reward resides in the discovery of his own victorious inner power through the poem.

However, there is an intrinsic reward for man; when, for instance, the orator sees his listeners' faces shifting with the feelings he has aroused, he feels something so profound that it can only be contrasted with the deep pleasure in which one learns out he is valued. Touching and winning souls is our pleasure, because that is the only reward that will offer us true rewards.

Often we are granted a moment when we imagine being among the world's best people. These are moments of joy granted to man, so that he may live in harmony with his life. It can be accomplished by passion or by a son's gift, a magnificent finding, or the publishing of a book; at some stage we realize that there is no man beyond us. When, in such a moment, someone of power steps out to send us an award or a trophy, he is the essential killer of our true reward-"And who are you? "Our disappeared ego would scream," Who are you that tells me that I am not the first of men? Who is so high above me that he may send me a trophy?

As with penalties, the average man's soul grows better by development, and retribution is often a means of coercion, as generally believed. That carry outcomes in certain lesser natures that rise in bad, but there are very rare and they do not influence societal development. The criminal code seeks to discipline us if we become immoral under the boundaries specified by the rules. But we are not pure by fear of the laws; if we don't loot, if we don't murder, it's because we love goodwill, because the normal pattern of our lives takes us ahead, taking us ever further and more certainly away from the risk of low and evil actions. Without getting through the legal or philosophical dimensions of the issue, we should confidently conclude whether the perpetrator has experienced the intimidating weight of the penal code over him until he transgresses the statute, because he understands the nature of a penalty. He's ignored it, or he's been tricked into the felony, deluding himself with the possibility of escaping the penalty of the statute. But a conflict between guilt and retribution has arisen inside his subconscious. Whether or not it is successful in hindering violence, this penal code is certainly designed for a very small class of people; namely, offenders. The overwhelming majority of people remain truthful, irrespective of the law's challenges.

The true punishment of normal man is the lack of knowledge of the individual strength and grandeur which are the roots of his inner existence.

In the fullness of achievement such retribution also comes upon men. A man we should consider as crowned with happiness and wealth can suffer from this sort of punishment. Man all too much does not recognize the real penalty that affects him. And it is here that schooling will be of benefit. They keep the pupils in school today, restricted to body and soul, the desk – and content rewards and penalties by such devices. Through all of this, our goal is to limit them to the practice of immobility and silence, – to take them, – where? Too much for no definitive goal. Children's schooling also requires pouring the analytical substance of school activities, into their brains. And also in the official education department such services have been collected and their usage is enforced by statute on the instructor and the boy.

Oh, we should cover our heads in embarrassment and with our hands hide our guilty faces before such thick and willful disregard for the existence which is rising inside these girls! Sergi always says: "Today an immediate need forces itself on society: the restoration of schools and teaching systems, and he who battles for this purpose, battles for human regeneration.

1.3 Modern Pedagogical Approach and Science

Pedagogy is characterized merely as the teaching process, and exercise. Which includes?

- Teaching types?
- Teaching philosophy
- Teaching appraisal

As people think about teaching pedagogy, they'll be talking to how teachers present the instructional material to a community.

When an instructor prepares a lesson they will find different forms of presenting the material. This would be created on the basis of their own teaching interests, their knowledge, and the sense in which they work.

How will setting shift the attitude to pedagogy?

Differences in the pupils' age and the material being presented can influence the pedagogical practices that an instructor wants to use.

To addition to their expertise with certain age ranges, instructors can utilize studies from several various learning backgrounds to support their decision taking. An instructor at EYFS, for example, can respond to cognitive science studies and their understanding with adult-directed play performance.

The justifications behind the decisions should become the principles of pedagogy and over time each instructor can establish their own pedagogical principles.

What do the pedagogical methods mean?

The diverse methods to pedagogy may be grouped into four categories: behaviorism, constructivism, social constructivism and liberationism.

1. Behaviorism

Behaviorist pedagogy incorporates behavioral science to guide its method. A pedagogical response to behaviorism will suggest that learning is based on students. It will promote the usage of lessons focused on clear teaching, and lecture.

What does a pedagogical solution to behaviorism feel like in a classroom?

Behaviorism philosophy in a school environment originated from psychologists conducting pedagogical work. Behaviourist pedagogy is the philosophy of the instructor becoming the primary source of power, and guiding the class.

You might tend to see a combination of lecturing, modeling and presentation, rote instruction, and choral imitation in a classroom utilizing a behaviorist pedagogical method. Both these tasks are both 'seen' and organized, and are directed by the instructor. However, the change can occur when the student is the focus of the practice and show their learning throughout the course of the lesson. Behaviorism is often considered a conventional form of instruction. As is well recognized, behavioral philosophy as a therapeutic method was developed in the 1920s. It has been seen for a long time in school. Schools in the 18th and 19th centuries focus on a functional method (although functional science has not yet existed).

2. Constructivism

Constructivism is a philosophy people develop from their interactions and by thought. Constructivist pedagogy puts the infant at the forefront of instruction, often referred to as 'invisible pedagogy.' A constructivist method may include group research, learning focused on questioning, which might follow a Montessori or Steiner style.

And what does a pedagogical solution to constructivism feel like in a classroom?

Constructivism is rooted in Piaget's pedagogical work. Piaget spoke thoroughly about 'schemas,' a notion that learners are able to know, so teachers ought to create exercises that promote learning. Younger kids actively think it out, while older kids discuss conceptual and theoretical thoughts. A lesson may involve individualization, a relaxed speed, secret results, the expert's hat, and fewer speak by students. Any of this pedagogy's adopters will often stress getting outdoors and interacting with nature. Constructivism is often commonly characterized as a radical form of teaching.

3. Social constructivism

The philosophy of constructivism (social constructionism) was developed in the second half of the 20th century. There is a dual presence of social truth. It has factual interpretations, on the one hand, whereas it has subjective definitions, on the other. Each individual creates around himself a social truth. Language is an essential medium of social truth. An individual creates an area of information and understanding for himself through language and communication. The social and psychological building structures of community by human behavior and operation are taken into account. Pedagogy of social constructivism may be seen as a combination of two priorities: instructor directed, and student oriented. Lev Vygotsky, cognitive scientist, founded social constructivism, drawing on Piaget's research, but protested against Piaget's theories that learning should only happen in its social sense, and maintained that learning was a joint mechanism between student and instructor. What does an introduction to social constructivism appear like in a lesson?

The instructor will use community work features, but use smaller group sizes and limit the option of subjects. The instructor can may use teaching, interviewing, and a combination of person, pair, and whole-class instruction by instructor. In schooling, social constructivism is related to the socialization of the individual in community, the development of socialization skills in any individual and the instruction of learners in self-structuring. The method is related both to the development of the learning environment and to the creation of information. The principle is generally revised by usage of constructive and creative education training approaches (brainstorming, case studies, community instruction, etc.). We stress that the series of the emergence of hypotheses does not, in theory, contradict the previous series but complements it as if it was constructed on the former, fracturing the former and partly modifying its application. The new analytical theory of research, the concept of inclusion and complementation, illustrates this interpretation. Like at colleges, we use these patterns in the creation of the learning method at university. Note that social constructivism represents the environmental method to pedagogy.

Siemens and Downes suggested a different course for the evolving philosophy in conjunction with the creation of communication networks and new ways to use them in teaching. Information is obtained by engaging with the network group. Of example, such an information acquisition process may, on the one side, be indicative of an already trained child or an individual who can objectively assess, examine, pick and build knowledge. That is, it has certain awareness base. Around the same period, high school students themselves show an integrated comprehension of information and abilities — across networks. Therefore, we expect that this principle would slowly be infiltrated into lower-level groups (even initial). Networks have become popular among high school pupils and adolescents, and their networking abilities are far more established than those of educators.

The quality of the curriculum in Kazakhstan, which has the Soviet teaching roots, was based on encyclopedias, formalism, copyism (in Russian-eczemplyaric) and other theories. They are listed in the didactics textbook. The transition from behavioralism to cognitive and constructivism is known in Western education theory. The move to the domination of constructivist ideologies calls for the successful introduction of novel methods of teaching. Changes in fact explicitly determine the need for learning to step away from encyclopedia and cognitivism.

In schooling, learning results have moved from information, knowledge and skills to skills training. As awareness is continuously developed, abilities grow in a complex way. Skills are difficult to build in a single lesson, so we can address "learning techniques" that have been applied for some time. The learning technique combines strategies and concepts, growth path, techniques and training styles. Training approaches depend on performance — predicted educational outcomes. Strategies for involved, creative, project-oriented and interactive learning will incorporate building and connectivism principles

4. liberationism

The Brazilian educator Paulo Freire founded liberationism as a vital pedagogy. Freire was the Department of Education's Head, and established a training method that he could teach illiterate people to read in only 45 days. Freire concentrated on overcoming the two literacy barriers: deprivation and hunger. Freire was eventually arrested following a military takeover. When published, he wrote a book entitled 'Pedagogy of the Marginalized' in which Freire spoke about the dehumanization of school students and advocated for solidarity and unification. A liberationist philosophy is one that positions the student voice at the core, and brings a democracy in the classroom. Esteem is put on making the instructor as a learner, and on letting the class explore topics. What should seem in a lesson to be a social constructivist approach?

The instructor may use literature references that include non-standard constructions, such as hip-hop, or graffiti. Students will assume the teacher's position and settle on the subject of the lesson. The instructor will provide the students with room and ability to demonstrate their progress, and that may take the form of a presentation, voice, or dance.

The twentieth century pedagogy

The twentieth century introduced major improvements in instructional approaches and didactics. Twentieth-century pedagogy varies from twenty-first-century pedagogy. Since the beginning of the twenty-first century, the growth of national and world education has changed a great deal. The most visible trend today is the internetisation of culture and the introduction into information of new technology. The term internet, socially interactive, and generation Z is related to the new generation of schoolboys. Awareness is the process from information learning by comprehension, from the monolog of the instructor to visual experience, or conversation in classroom.

New technology alters our attitude, modes of communicating, way of thought, emotions, and sources of control over people, cognitive skills and social behavior. As Myamesheva says "The high-tech world-machines, video games, mobile phones, and Internet search engines-reshape the human brain,"

The most noticeable pattern lies behind the fundamental shifts in didactics and pedagogy. Pedagogy in domestic science has been redefined from the "study of reading, teaching, and studying" to the "technology of culture." The topic of the pedagogy of the twentieth century was "knowledge" (in Kazakh — tarbie, in Russian — vospitanie, in German — Bildung). "Upbringing in the specific pedagogical context is a purposeful effect of culture to train the younger generation for adulthood, according to scientist. In the limited pedagogical context, growing up is a purposeful effect on the creation of unique personal values. ". The topic of the pedagogy of the twenty-first century – the "reading" concept – has broadened the spectrum of interpretation and comprehension. It incorporated integrity and personal-oriented strategies.

This is how the post-Soviet trends in the Silova, Yakavets experiments to change schooling are expanded. There are several commonalities between countries in terms of the "post-socialist education reform bundle," "a series of policy changes symbolizing the acceptance of Western educational principles and involving such 'traveling initiatives' as student-centered learning, the implementation of curriculum requirements, decentralization of school finance and governance, higher school privatization, standard. This definition agrees with the Russian researcher Romanenchuk's assessment that "the growth of the 'westernization' of the (transfer of the Western style of education to Kazakh soil) is completely embodied in the 2004 philosophy of education." On the one hand, we should comply with these evaluations, and on the other, the strong trend of the restoration of Kazakh schools and the ethno-pedagogical roots of education need to be taken into consideration. Six reasons for modernizing education are identified by Kazakhstan scientist Akhmetova: standard of education, globalization and internationalization, politization and the development of an information society, new teaching technology, marketing and financing. Kazakhstan is a young, autonomous state that has just turned 25. Kazakhstani education reforms in the early twenty-first century were thus aimed at creating a regional education structure as an element of democracy. Actually Kazakhstan holds leading roles on the post-Soviet space trends of educational reforms.

Simple didactics

New pedagogy from the "technology of education" has become a "method of schooling and upbringing." Twentieth-century concept of "schooling" has been changed and extended. Didactics was known as a philosophy of learning since the days of Jan Amos Komensky. Education was known in Soviet didactics as a "learning result," "the method and consequence of mastering the framework of scientific information and cognitive ability ..." That is, schooling has a meaning of receiving an academic degree or a university diploma.

In current books on pedagogy, for example by Bordovskaya and Rean, schooling is more generally understood: (1) as a method and product of learning, (2) as a good for community, as community has spent more than eight centuries constructing a complicated educational system; (3) the importance of the citizen, as modern man spends more than fifteen years of his existence on schooling and occupation; (4) a witness of social institution;

Education theories recognize the relationship not just of the pupil and the teacher (the micro-level of relationship) but also of the connection between the state and the education system, the social classes of pupils and teachers, parents and pupils, parents and colleges, schools and public institutions, schools and faiths, schools and cultural, social growth. This is the macro-influence degree that schooling has on employment in culture and community. That is why didactic ideas and challenges are viewed not only from the point of view of the teachers and students internal relationships, but as an instructional and at the same time social climate, subject to creativity and intervention, complex transition. Therefore, we plan the development of psychological, communicative competences, life skills at the same time, shaping topic competences.

Environmental education strategy

In the 1970s–1980s of the twentieth century in the URSSR the teaching method started to be clarified from the viewpoint of the action framework to national pedagogical textbooks. The teaching and learning cycle includes: priorities and expectations, material, strategies, teaching resources, modes of learning and outcomes. When designing the class, we build these components. This idea is related to the L. Vygotsky's school experience hypothesis, L early learning hypothesis. Zankov, V. Davydov, I. Lerner, M. Skatkin and Z. Kalmykova.

The environmental approach to learning has been widely used since the 21st century. According to Manuilov, it is everything in which the topic resides that we identify the functional setting, shaping his way of life, which mediates his growth and averages his character.

The Italian physicist Rizolatti found mirror neurons in the 1990's of the twentieth century. Mirror neurons are brain cells which are both activated while conducting a certain action and when another individual witnesses the success of this activity. These neurons have been consistently identified in primates, are reported to be present in humans, and certain animals. Such neurons perform a crucial function in adaptation, empathy, adaptation and language learning processes.

Human activity is not so clear according to the principle of social learning by the Albert Bandura. Piaget and others assumed that when they grew up, skills and attitudes were created. Therefore certain continuity is implicit in behavior, as we are conditioned to assume. A. Bandura believes human nature isn't that reliable. It depends on the conditions, really. Human behaviour is defined more by an individual's current circumstance and its perception than by the level of his growth, character traits or styles of personality. From the principle of social learning by A. Bandura, one can infer that teaching is figurative, abstract, and may ultimately be carried out situationally.

Knowledge and resources are essential categories in the attitude towards the climate. There's a fluid sharing of ideas, experience and energy between the instructor and the student during the class. In our view here is embodied the foundation of the synergetic method of pedagogy. According to Mukazhanova's theory of self-cognition, the essence of "joy" is known as the sharing of energy between individuals, such as mother and her infant. Positive attitudes in research and profession, the positive energy produced by the instructor, set the spiritual environment to be especially positive. Ironically, one should transform back here to the past of the Plato Academy. As you know, the term "platonic love" derives from "spiritual contact between instructor and pupil." Thus, in didactics, it is best to use more emerging, positively inspiring approaches and instructional tools that can create a successful learning climate. The advisor is made the infant growth facilitator. Hence art-pedagogic, innovative training approaches are advised.

In fact, all details and constructive energies must be saturated to the environment. If he is a major personality to the pupil, the instructor himself plays a huge part.

This research trend of pedagogy related to the social climate and human socialization has culminated in a modern academic science — social pedagogy. This addresses other socializing mechanisms — printing, copying, naming. The upbringing hypothesis explores coping mechanisms, coping actions and the idea of a lifestyle due to the growth of psychology.

The age of internet

In modern school, we note major developments in information technology and in the implementation of digital into the educational setting. Global scientists — teachers, sociologists, futurists, too — speak about a new wave about pupils, i.e., 21st century schoolchildren. This century is the "Next," the Z century, the new revolution and the social media age (developing L. Hietajärvi, K. Lonka). Let us reflect on the fact that "the learning space extends beyond the classroom" Now that we have decided earlier with students, during the clarification and during group research we will use the internet video tools to encourage students to use laptops and tablets while they are planning a community solution.

The new generation is named by Hietajärvi and others 'socially and digitally engaged' and it is written that 'digital and social technologies are interconnected structures of technology, Internet and social networks the providing a continuous and deep online engagement with knowledge, people and artifacts;'

According to the research carried out by Soldatova and Zotova, there are changes in digital generation memory, thinking and attention. "The distribution of nearly all knowledge from an early age affects the function of mnemonic systems at every moment. Second, it is not the quality of any knowledge source in the net that is recalled, but the direction of that knowledge and the path to it, more specifically. The average concentration time compared to the 10-15 years ago reduced ten times. A new phenomenon is the thought of a clip. It is based on the processing of graphic images by fragments rather than "logical and text associations"

Teachers vary diametrically from conservators (leaving all aside, schoolchildren continue to be educated as they have been in the preceding century), to the desire for a complete overhaul of the schooling system. Our stance is built upon the ambivalence theory, the convergence between practice and creativity, the need to critically explore the phenomena between electronic and graphic culture, and the study of visual culture's effect on the identity of a schoolboy. Online innovations transform the way we work, interact, perceive, hear, impact on people, cognitive social behavior and skills.

School students and children have more short-term memory; modern forms of knowledge-building and capacity growth of long-term memory are also required. Educators are mindful of the question of the cogent reasoning of school children. It is important to consider the "superficial" and "serious" path to information acquisition. 'Knowing the term by heart, not knowing the definition, comprehension - is regarded as a superficial approach, and a thorough and objective evaluation, analysis of the subject as a profound approach.' 'Superficial studying is a superficial approach; it requires replicating experience, instructor instruction, passive epistemology, dual perception, and absorption of information. Deep method, transformation of information, automated learning, successful epistemology, relative views and approaches to information-building will contribute to deeper learning stages. Such challenges confronted the instructor and his professional practices with different criteria. Teachers ought to be more interested in studying new information and emerging technology. Moreover, new work in the field of psychology of cognition and thinking through the active usage of e-learning is required. Practical teachings of digital and ICT tools students, computer literacy teaching, the incorporation of these courses in teacher instructional programs are now important.

Education breakthrough

"The proportion of pupils to knowledge holders was around ten in medieval schools, according to Volov; with the advent of the pedagogical method, Ya. A. Comensky, pupil count to instructor is hundreds (I to 100); new creative technology raises the education development element by tens of thousands (I to 100,000) The research method "pedagogical invention" continues to establish advances in education and helps to create, introduce and disseminate inventions in the teaching environment. We are offering a range of its requirements.

Innovation is the nature, processes, approaches, technology and modern material of the phenomena. The launch of a previous one, the addition of older ones (Latin in-in, nove-new)."The creative method is a dynamic operation in creating and designing instructional materials and planning a new one," according to Taubaeva and Laktionova.

Innovative teaching methods are teaching methods which include new ways of communicating between teacher-student, teacher-student and some innovation in practical action during the phase of teaching the content. There are two specific kinds of "modern": "purely modern"-first formed, is at the correct stage of experimentation, a new truth; "new" with an old mix, more specifically, consisting of an old sheet, a new one, etc. We are proposing a further form of learning innovation (technology, system and techniques): total innovation (absolutely new technology); modernized innovation (significantly enhanced technology), amended innovation (slightly enhanced technology), innovation, technology brought into new territories (such as RK teaching, credit technology for Kazakhstan).

Innovative training: (1) anticipatory, expected development; (2) accessible to future; (3) constant uncertainty, in many words, the non-equilibrium of the method, in particular the individual himself; (4) emphasis on identity, its evolution; (5) the mandatory existence of the elements of creativity;

According to science, any concept in pedagogy unites: conviction that human ability has little to do with it; the pedagogical method seeks to conquer the truth in the system; the relaxation of nonlinear thinking; it is based on the hedonic theory, which is the enjoyment of learning, the happiness of accomplishment, and the pedagogy of performance. The teacher's smartphone role-playing area – the instructor advises and learns from the pupil concurrently.

Firstly, creative learning technique itself is focused on a specific approach. It is named student-centered learning in Western literature. Second, it summarizes synergistic, systematic, competence-oriented, dialogical and productive, economic, material, technical, environmental and other approaches. Third, the rules and values of the invention cycle can be defined in education and the framework for the teacher's creative community. The creative instructional approach is expressed in the instruction manual.

In 2010 UNESCO proposed the following educational approaches for the 21st century: literacy, communication, principles instruction, curiosity literacy, effective evaluation, potential troubleshooting, research beyond classrooms and the solution of group problems.

The intensive usage of teachers of creative instructional approaches is now a requirement. The greater the teacher's instructional techniques and approaches, the more engaging, complex it performs courses, inspire the cognitive practices of the pupil more, forms the practice of addressing non-standard issues, facilitates of-depth instruction and the gradual assimilation of modern technologies.

A strong instructor is constantly refining his instructional abilities, selecting and implementing new instructional approaches and technology.

To older-generation teachers graduating from colleges, specialized instruction ("About Training" in compliance with Republic of Kazakhstan legislation at least once every five years) is carried out.

Most schools in Kazakhstan are now undertaking changes and are consciously utilizing teachers' creative teaching methods. Next, we look at the instructor test findings about the usage of novel instructional approaches.

Six approaches for early childhood education in the 21st century

It is no secret that over the last ten years or so, the landscape of schooling has drastically shifted. Teachers around the country strive tirelessly to empower children with the resources required to excel in the environment of the 21st century. As well as giving students the versatility to adjust easily to new technology, teachers must promote learning environments which encourage critical thinking, innovation, problems solving, collaboration, teamwork, international awareness and social responsibility. The following six approaches are commonly utilized by early childhood teachers in schools to train children for the future.

1. Technology integrated

Youngsters of today were raised in the Internet era. Some are more technically advanced than the role given by the adults to educate them. To communicate with these students, teachers need to learn to talk their language and become conscious of the technologies that come so easily to young people. Integrating technology involves tapping into the needs of students and improving their technological abilities, all while providing learning experiences that are enriching. Like every new technology, several instructors, keen to keep up with the latest trend, are merely going through the integration motions. If they want to excel in it, however, they need more than the movements – they need a clear knowledge of the relevant resources, as well as practical contemplation about how to utilize them to boost learning. Furthermore, the increased accessibility which accompanies this technology makes it imperative that teachers emphasize the importance of Internet protection.

2. Cooperative mechanisms to understand

Instruction based on the instructor has had its day. Successful teachers use a student-centered methodology gradually. Cooperative learning fuels classroom participation by promoting cooperation within the students themselves. Rather than selecting one pupil at a time, the instructor encourages children to address learning content with buddies or in classes, thus increasing engagement rates. The students are as hard working as the instructors. Not a one-man display any more, instead the position of the instructor is that of a facilitator. This in effect contributes to higher accomplishment, though at the same time encouraging team bonding and class equality. Kagan Cooperative Learning has established over 200 realistic, easy-to-implement instructional techniques, or "structures," which turn classrooms into vibrant scenes of both action and engaging discussion. Cooperative Learning Materials by Laura Candler includes a number of instructor task sheets and backline trainers, which are helpful for communication during cooperative learning.

3. Instruction differentiate

Teachers should adapt learning environments in the classroom to distinguish between the specific needs of the students. There are three primary types of learning: visual, additive, and kinesthetic. Cognitive learning styles in children identify the features of these learners as well as the forms of behaviors in which they excel better, with the exception that it is only learning styles that are defined, that are distinguishable from cognitive styles (holistic, logical, field-dependent, etc). Teachers may often differentiate themselves by matching tasks to skill standards, providing suitable training or extension opportunities if required. Another perfect way to distinguish is to encourage the children to choose experiences based on areas of interest. It is an important motivator for children to make decisions. Working in community classes is one of the most successful methods of addressing the demands of varied learners in large-scale class environments. Differentiation Central includes informative material, as well as a brief video of Carol Ann Tomlinson, instructor, journalist, and writer, sharing her insights and views on differentiating classrooms.

4. Setting goal

The engagement of children in the cycle of establishing targets is an ideal way to enable them to take control over their learning. In the early stage, the target will be defined very simply and simplistically, such as regular two-way meetings with children regarding their success in particular fields. Teachers can find it easy to accomplish targets by utilizing guides, anchor maps and related resources. Free Printable Activity Maps offers early learners with specific graphics templates. Teaching and Tapas share the goals of a curriculum primarily planned for reading and writing. K-5 Math Education Tools display a set of quantitative target maps. In addition, helping children meet their objectives relies for teachers to include clear guidance and room for self-reflection.

5. Teaching cross-curriculum

In comparison to conventional teaching of single topics, studying several topics at the same time will allow students to expand their comprehension and skills. Of example, this technique tells the instructor more. Math, scientific or social sciences material of reading or writing may be conveniently combined. However, integrating both topics at once is more difficult. Here are some of the major simultaneous learning methods. Project-based learning requires children performing a project that ends in some form of tangible outcome. Problem-based curriculum requires instructors to assist children in creating real-world approaches. Children produce their own questions according to their curiosities or preferences in surveying-based research, which they then explore. Such approaches perform very good, as teachers don't only suggest what they will learn to pupils, but rather inspire children to investigate and uncover knowledge in a more engaging manner, where all subjects come together to play.

6. Assessment to know

Learning Evaluation, or Formative Evaluation, is a tool utilized by teachers to gather data and help them tailor teaching and match the needs of the students. Summative appraisals do not often give a good view of what a pupil understands. Often, it's already too late by the time data is processed! The instructor is already moved on to the next task, leaving behind several students who have not yet completely mastered the previous material. Teachers should track how the children think while they instruct, use questions, probing techniques, class conversations, exit cards, lesson records, peer reviews, self-assessments, and slate research, and other approaches, to avoid this issue. Teachers may measure the success of people, classes, or the whole class and change the process by encouraging or questioning students when appropriate.

Chapter 2: Effective parent-child communication

Communication is the transfer of knowledge from one human to another. Communication may be audible, for instance, one person talking to another or it may be nonverbal, for instance, a scowl on an individual's face that is sure to let someone think he's upset. Good or negative contact may be efficient or inefficient.

It's really critical that parents are willing to interact with their children freely and effectively. Open, efficient contact not only helps the children but any family member. When there is good contact, interactions between parents and their children are significantly enhanced. Generally speaking, if contact between parents and their children is nice, then even their relationships are nice.

By staring at their mother, the children know how to interact. If parents interact freely and easily, their children are more likely to interact. Strong communication skills can support children across their entire lives. Children start developing opinions and perceptions about themselves dependent on how they interact with their parents. When parents interact with their children successfully they display love for them. Children also start thinking like their parents are listening and recognizing them, which is a boost to self-esteem. On the other side, inadequate or hostile contact between parents and children may cause children to believe they are unimportant, unheard of, or confused. These kids can even come to see their parents as unhelpful and distrustful.

Parents who interact with their children consistently are more likely to have children that are able to do as they're asked. These children learn what to expect from their parents and they are more likely to live up to those standards because children realize what is expected of them. They are therefore more likely to feel comfortable in their family role, and are thus more inclined to be cooperative.

2.1 Ways of connecting with infants favorably

Start meaningful contact when the children are small. Both will be secure enough to do so until parents and their children can talk. Since their kids are still small, parents will start setting the foundation for free, efficient communication.

Parents may do that by being open to their kids when they have concerns or just want to chat. In addition, parents who offer compassion, empathy and acceptance to their children help build an environment for effective communication. Kids who feel cherished and welcomed by their parents are more apt to speak up with their parents and express their opinions, emotions and concerns. Often it's simpler for parents to sound appropriate to their kids than seeing it in reality. Parents ought to convince their kids they value them and support them. Adults will do this orally as well as nonverbally.

Verbally, parents will let their children realize from what they're doing they support them. Parents will seek to give their children encouraging messages. For example, when a kid gathers up his toys when they're done with them, parents should let him or her know they love it by saying things like, "I like it when you pick up your toys without being asked." Parents can be cautious when communicating to their children about what they're doing and how they're speaking. All that parents tell their kids gives a hint about how they feel about them. For instance, if a parent says anything like "Don't disturb me now. I'm occupied," their kids can end up feeling that their needs and desires are not important. Parents should convey nonverbally to their children that they support them by movements, facial expressions and other nonverbal actions. Parents should seek to avoid activities such as shouting and they should not pay attention to their babies. These activities are impeding successful contact.

Work makes it perfect: parents ought to know how to demonstrate appreciation when picking up their kids.

Communicate on level with your family

When parents interact with their children, it is essential that they both verbally and physically fall to the level of their children. Verbally, parents will try to use age-appropriate words so their children will grasp quickly. This can be achieved with younger ones, use clear terms. For starters, small children are far more inclined to follow a message such as "Do not hit your sister," as opposed to "Hitting your sister is not appropriate." Parents should strive to recognize what their children are capable of understanding and should seek not to act in ways that their children are not capable of understanding.

Parents, for example, do not literally stand above their kids while chatting or engaging with them. However, they will seek to fall to the stage of their kids by reducing themselves, either by standing, lying, stooping, etc. That would make eye contact much harder to sustain, because while parents are eye-to-eye, children are much less likely to be threatened.

Learn how to really listen

Hearing is an ability that has to be learned and mastered. Listening is an integral aspect of efficient contact. When parents listen to their kids they show them they are interested and they care what their kids have to say. Below are few important measures to becoming a successful listener;

1. Create and maintain eye contact

Parents who do so demonstrate their kids they are engaged and active in doing so. Kids may get the reverse idea-which their parents are not involved in what they think-if the eye contact is limited.

2. Removes obstacles

Parents will give them their undivided attention while children are showing a willingness to speak. They were expected to set down what they were doing, meet their kids and show them their indivisible focus. Of example, if parents start reading the paper or watching television as their children attempt to interact with them, they may get the impression that their parents are not interested in what they have to say, or that what they have to say is not relevant. If children show a need to chat at a time the parent cannot, parents should arrange a time later to talk to their children.

3. Speak with the mouth closed

Parents will strive to limit the interruptions when their kids speak. They can give motivation without interruption, for example by a smile or a touch. Interruptions also interrupt the line of thinking of the speaker, and this can be quite stressful.

4. Let the kids think they're noticed

When children have stopped communicating parents will prove them that they heard just in slightly different terms, by restating what was said. Of starters, "Boy, it sounds like you've had a pretty nice day in pre-school." That's not just trying to help kids think their parents cared. It would also offer a chance to explain whether the parents misunderstand the idea their kids are attempting to get across.

Keep up short communications

The younger students, the easier it is for them to sit during lengthy speeches. One clear guideline for parents is to talk for no longer than 30 seconds with small children, then invite them to elaborate about what has been said. The aim is for parents to pass on details at a time when ensuring that their children pay attention to what is being discussed at frequent intervals, and knowing it. Fathers will let their kids know whether plenty would suffice. Parents are eager to search for signs that kids have had plenty. Such clues involve fidgeting, loss of eye contact, distractibility, and so on. Parents need to know when to interact with their kids, but they do need to know when to ease off.

Tell the correct questions

Many queries help improve discussions and others can stop dead discussions in their tracks. In their discussions with their children parents will continue to pose open-ended questions. These queries also involve a thorough answer to keep a discussion moving. Open-ended questions that start with the terms "what," "when," "whom," or "how" are also quite helpful for opening up children. Parents will seek not to ask questions which just involve a yes or no response.

While asking the right questions will lead to a dialogue, parents need to be cautious not to pose too many questions when talking to their children. When this occurs, discussions will easily become interrogations, and kids become far less likely to speak up.

While engaging with them, communicate your own thoughts and ideas

To be successful in contact it must be a two-way path. Mothers not only need to be responsive to their children and respond to them for good communication; they do need to be ready to express their own opinions and emotions with their children.

Parents will teach their children many lessons by sharing their thoughts and emotions, for example, morality and principles. However, parents must be vigilant to do so in a non-judgmental way while voicing their thoughts and feelings. The more parents open up to their children, the more their children should open up to them, seems reasonable.

Provide daily family gatherings or chat periods

The daily scheduled opportunity to chat is one really important bonding method for families with older children. This can be achieved in a variety of different ways. First of all, the family gathering is in there. For e.g., family reunions may be held once a week and/or if there is anything the family wants to talk. Families will use family gathering time to work out daily life information, such as tasks, curfews and bedtime. Family gathering time can often be used to address complaints and resolve problems.

These moments should also be used to address the good things that have arisen in the past week. What is crucial is that each member of the family is allowed opportunities to talk and be understood by other members of the family. Regularly arranged occasions for speech and talking should not be as structured as the family reunion. For starters, families may use the dinner hour as a time to catch up with each other every night. Or, parents should set aside time to play games of conversation, such as taking up different subjects of debate and offering everyone in the family an opportunity to share their beliefs. What is crucial is that the families set aside time to connect with each other at regular intervals.

When you do not know anything, confess it

When children pose questions their parents are unable to respond, they will realize they do not learn. Parents should view these occasions as examples of learning.

Parents will show their kids how to find the knowledge they're searching for, for example, by sending them to the school, utilizing the internet, etc. It's much easier for parents to remind their kids that they're human and so don't know anything about it than thinking up some solution that may not be real.

Seek to full clarification

Children will strive to give them as much detail as they can while addressing their children's concerns, particularly though the subject is one child don't feel confident sharing. It is not to suggest the parents ought to go into considerable depth. It's only important that parents realize how much knowledge they need and then offer it to their babies. Families should consider the age-appropriate details they offer their children. Parents will allow their kids to pose questions too. This will help parents figure out just what details their kids are searching for. Not providing adequate facts will cause kids to draw assumptions that are not actually accurate.

Communicating through conflicts

For one point or another all the communities would have disagreements. While these disputes may be disturbing, they don't need to be too destructive. There are plenty of various strategies parents should do to move through disputes easily and at the same time maintain the contact channels accessible. Here are a couple tips.

- **Act one question at a time**

This is safer to seek to address one question at a time through disputes. Bringing up several separate things at once is not a smart strategy. That can be really frustrating for both kids and parents. When this occurs families will lose sight of the actual challenges easily.

- **Look for new solutions to problem solving**

Parents will strive to keep in mind when attempting to settle disputes that there is typically more than one approach to every issue. Parents and kids will work closely to identify approaches that fit both parties. Learning to be creative when it comes to problem solving is a perfect resource for youngsters. Parents will strive to be versatile enough to seek different approaches if one approach doesn't fit.

- **Be respectful**

Parents do not necessarily neglect the ordinary rules of politeness because they are concerned with their kids. Parents should handle their children with the same level of reverence they should give any other adult through disputes, or at any other time. Children, too, are people and they deserve fair care. Many parents suggest something to their children during the middle of a dispute or conflict that they will never inform any person or a near friend. Parents will make an attempt to prevent this.

- **Use "I" message**

Parents should always try to state issues in terms of how they feel when discussing conflicts with their children. For e.g., parents should do something like "I feel irritated when you don't pick up your clothing." By utilizing "I" texts, parents inform their kids how their behaviour makes them feel, instead of criticizing and/or shaming them. "I" signals are successful as children are much less inclined to fight or protest against what the adult feels like. Specifying things in terms of "I" messages is far less of a threat to children than they are accusing and/or blaming. "I" signals often teach children how to take control over their own acts.

Parents who show their emotions in such a way always encourage their kids to do likewise.

How to Avoid Negative Communication

Unfortunately, often parents don't realize how much they use derogatory modes of contact with their babies. As a consequence these parents might be growing in their children the seeds of distrust and poor self-esteem.

That is why it is particularly crucial for parents to become conscious of and fix any inappropriate ways of contact with their children that they may use. Here is a compilation of controversial news cases. Parents will go over the list to find all of those seemingly common problematic contact habits. The parents will then continue making adjustments after finding trouble areas.

Examples of Negative Communications Parents should be avoided

- **Nagging and offering lessons**

Nagging is saying that which has been stated before. Reading is providing more knowledge than is required without not listen to certain thoughts or opinions. Parents can prevent nagging and lecturing by remaining concise about their interactions with their kids. Parents can always bear in mind that there's no reason to mention anything again after they have asked their kids something. Families should have a punishment rather than nagging (for starters, time-out) when their kids don't do what they've been asked to do, instead of nagging. Nagging and lecturing lead kids to avoid learning or become resentful or aggressive.

- **Interrupting**

When kids chat, parents will allow them the chance to finish what they're saying before they speak.

This is the courtesy that is that. Children who believe like their parents can't get a word in edgewise can stop speaking with them entirely.

- **To criticize**

Parents should resist criticism of the emotions, feelings, opinions, and/or actions of their own family. Children frequently interpret critiques of this type as overt threats, and the effect may be decreased self-esteem. Parents will condemn actions as appropriate, or what kids have accomplished, not the children themselves.

- **To focus on the past**

After settling an issue or dispute, parents should seek not to discuss it again. Kids will be given a blank sheet to start from. Parents who regularly bring up previous errors committed by their children encourage their children to keep grudges over lengthy stretches of time. Children ought to realize that after a dispute has been resolved it stays resolved.

- **Trying to monitor the children by utilizing culpability**

This includes attempting to make kids feel bad about their emotions, feelings and/or behavior. Parents who use shame to manipulate their kids will do significant harm to their relationship with their kids.

- **Uses sarcasm**

Parents use sarcasm as they utter something that they don't intend, and suggest the reverse of what they think by their voice language. An example is a parent saying things like, "Oh, you aren't elegant" as it falls. Children get hurtled by utilizing sarcasm. Sarcasm is never a useful tool for parents who strive to communicate effectively with their kids.

- **Asking the kids how to fix the issues**

It occurs as parents step in to instruct their kids how to handle something instead of having them get more insight into problem-solving strategies.

Parents who tell their kids how to fix their issues may cause kids to believe they have no power of their own lives. Such kids can end up thinking that they don't trust their parents. Or, they may hate being asked what to do, and therefore reject the guidance of their parents.

- **Putting down children**

Put-downs may arrive in several different forms, including naming names, ridiculating, criticizing, accusing, etc. Put-downs can hurt successful contact. Put-downs will destroy self-esteem for children.

Children who have their parents placed down frequently feel abandoned, unloved and insufficient.

- **Lie.**

No matter how enticing it is to make up a lie, parents cannot, for example, stop thinking about difficult subjects like sex.

Parents should strive to keep their children transparent and truthful. This will allow children to be transparent with their parents and to be frank. Children are really perceptive too. They are also really effective at detecting despite not being absolutely truthful with their peers. That can contribute to feelings of mistrust.

- **Denying love for babies**

Parents do not make fun of these emotions when children inform their parents how they feel. When a parent thinks his or her kid shouldn't be bad after missing a football game, for example, he or she shouldn't say so. Rather, parents can suggest something positive, for instance, "I know you always wanted to win. Sometimes it's hard to fail." That can be achieved for younger children using clear, descriptive phrases. Kids like their parents to be helping their emotions. Parents ought to demonstrate empathy towards their children when it comes to their emotions. Unable to do this will result in adolescents becoming misled by their community.

2.2 Helping children deal with their feeling

Much like people, kids encounter complicated emotions. They are upset, anxious, nervous, depressed, jealous, afraid, afraid, angry and ashamed.

Typically, however, small children don't have the language to speak about how they feel. Rather they express their emotions differently. Children will communicate their emotions by facial gestures, their faces, their actions and their playing. They can often express their emotions in emotional, improper, or troublesome ways.

From the moment children are born, they begin to learn the emotional abilities that they need to identify, express and manage their feelings. They know how to do this through their social experiences and connections in their lives with significant people including friends, grandparents and cares. Being a parent ensures that you have a very significant position to perform and help children appreciate their emotions and behaviors. Kids ought to be taught how to interact respectfully and constructively with their emotions.

Strategies

Parents should help their children identify their feelings, and communicate them. The following techniques are some of the ways you can help your child communicate his or her emotions:

• Help your kids appreciate their emotions by first providing the names of the feelings and then allowing them to speak about how they feel. You might say to your child for example, "Daddy left on a holiday, you're sad. You said you needed your daddy. "Through developing a mark for your child's emotions, you allow your child to build a language to communicate about feelings.

• Offer children lots of ways to recognize emotions in and about themselves. For e.g., you might say to your kid, this is so much fun riding your bike. I can tell you are laughing. Will you sound happy? "Or you could point a problem out and encourage your child to talk of what anyone else would feel:" Joey knocked his head on the slide. How is Joey feeling? "

• Show the children how to react to different emotions, disagreements or issues.

Talk to the kids about their own thoughts. "Remember yesterday when the water wasn't going down drain in the bath? Mommy became so angry and do you know when I was crazy what my face looks like? Can you render that crazy face like that of Mommy? "Talk to your kids about various ways you approach similar emotions."When I get angry I take a deep breath, count to three, and then try to think of the right way to cope with my question."

• Encourage your child to recognize and communicate their feelings in ways that are appropriate to your family and friends. You could say to your brother, for example, "Grandfather often gets upset when things are not going well at work. What's He doing? He is still on the porch while he figures out what he needs to do about it. When you get upset, you should sit down and reflect.'

What are the Steps?

Explain the emotion, use terms that your child will comprehend quickly.

1. To better bring the point across, consider using pictures, texts, or images. "Look at the face of Little Red Riding Hood; when she sees the wolf in her grandma's house, she is so terrified!"What is happening?

2. Teach your child the different ways we should treat the emotions. Have your child come up with ways she should control her emotions. Speak of constructive ways to convey emotions, and not so good. There are plenty of techniques you can use to demonstrate different methods of communicating emotions appropriately:

- Using real-life illustrations, or actually instruct. For starters, "You're having a hard time getting your trike into the carport. You look irritated. What do you do? I hope you should ask for assistance and start again, or take a deep breath. What is it you like to do? "

- Show your child different forms of reacting to emotions by addressing specific circumstances that your child can remember or that sometimes happen. For examples, "You were angry yesterday because Joey wouldn't let you play with his truck. You were so furious you knocked him down. What do you do when you feel mad Joey won't let you take a turn? "

- The children's books should be used to think about emotions. For example, while reading a novel, ask your child "What is feeling (character in novel) right now? What do you know? Have feel like this? What do you do because that's how you feel? "• Keep things clear, use images or illustrations to help bring the point across, and also seek to link the lesson back to anything that occurs in the life of your kid.

- Educate your child with different techniques to use when expressing feelings that could be incorrectly conveyed (e.g., rage, disappointment, sadness).

- Talking techniques for your child may involve taking a deep breath when upset or irritated, allowing an adult to help settle a disagreement, requesting for a turn when others don't cooperate, requesting for a hug when depressed, and seeking a safe place to relax when distressed.

3. The first moment that he wants to speak about his emotions, compliment your kid instead of just responding. It's also necessary to let your kid realize just what she's doing well and how happy you are to speak about feelings with her. Everything we believe will still be OK to express. It's how we want to display and react to our feelings which take special effort.

4. Help your child to chat about feelings and practice her latest techniques to properly convey emotions any opportunity you can. For e.g., when you play a game, when you're traveling in the car or while you're having dinner, you might chat about emotions. There will be all sorts of stuff happening every day which will give you wonderful chances to chat about feelings. The more you teach your kid, the better your child understands.

Training makes it better

Below are some of the things you should use to help your kid appreciate his or her emotions.

- **Play Make Your Kid Face**

You start the game by saying, "I'm going to create a smile, by looking at my smile, and you determine what I mean." So, make a happy or sad face.

If your child conjectures the word feeling, respond by saying, "That's right! Will you know what makes me the feeling? "Take a picture of something easy that helps you feel this way (e.g.," Going to the park helps me smile." "I feel bad when it rains and we can't go to the park). Please note that this is not the time to discuss the adult circumstances linked to your emotions (e.g., "I feel sad when your daddy doesn't call me."). So advise your kid, "Your choice, you're making a face so I'm trying to infer what you're thinking." Don't be shocked if your kid selects the same emotion you've already shown; it's going to take time until your child will be imaginative about this activity. Ask your child to identify what makes him experience the feeling, and then you assume. Keep taking turns before your child tells you he doesn't want to play the game.

- **Share a story**

Write a novel that involves protagonists feeling various feelings (e.g., sad, joyful, scared, nervous, puzzled, etc.). Stop on a page where the phrase occurs on the character. Tell your kid "How do you suppose he feels?" How would he look like that? "See her profile, how do you tell she's?"Could other queries be "Have you ever thought? How makes that make you look like this? "Or" What comes next? "Or" What does he do? "Don't stop on one page for long, only start the conversation as soon as your child displays an interest.

- **Make a emotional book**

Creating a home crafted book is a fun activity to do with your kids. You only need ink, crayons or markers, and a stapler.

You can create a book about one emotion and fill the pages with items that make your child feel like that. A "Good Book," for example, might contain images that you and your child draw from items that make her good, photos taken from magazines that are taped to the covers, or photographs of friends and family members. One solution is to make the book be about a number of terms of feeling and do one page on each of those feelings (happy, crazy, shocked, scared, annoyed, and proud, etc.). For kids who have a lot to talk about their emotions, maybe you want them to tell you a sentence about what makes them sound like an emotion so that you can put the sentence on the paper. Your child will then cut an image from the book to add in or create a photo to go with the emotion. Alert, if you do it together this task is more likely to be fun to your child, but it will be challenging for your child to do it alone.

- **Play "Mirror, Mirror**

Play "Mirror, Mirror ... I see what?"With the boy. Play this game with your child using a hand mirror, or a mirror on the ground. Look into the mirror and ask, "Mirror, mirror, what am I seeing?"And face up to sentiment. Support by asking, "I see a sad mom staring at me." Turn to your child and tell, "Your choice." Make your child recall the word, "Mirror, what I see?" "With your kids, you might have to tell it.

So advise your child to make a smile and encourage him utter the next sentence "I see a smiling Patrick gazing at me." Don't be shocked if your kid will just choose the expression you've just demonstrated. Play the game until your child is losing interest.

Expressing Feelings

Children often express their feelings in inappropriate ways. If upset, your child may scream, or throw toys while mad. Here are a few different approaches you should show your child how to behave on feelings: ask for advice Fix things with words Say something, don't do it (say "I am crazy" instead of throwing toys) Tell a grown-up Take a deep breath Explain what you feel like Think about a better way to handle it Smile and start to Step away Ask for a hug.

Putting it altogether

This is up to parents to educate adolescents to consider their feelings and to cope with them appropriately. For the first time, they learn too many unique and thrilling items. This can be amazing! We will make careful that we still affirm the desires of our children and do not blame them for sharing their feelings. You may want to say that, "Tell me how you feel, but it isn't good to harm people and stuff while you feel (name feeling)." Teach them about their feelings, encourage them to discover alternative methods of coping with feelings, allow them lots of opportunities to use their new techniques, and please try to have a lot of constructive reinforcement while utilizing the new pressure.

2.3 Engaging cooperation

Cooperation is the capacity to align one's desires with others. Cooperation is also thought of as youth following what adults want. This is conformity. Real partnership requires a shared endeavor, a mutually satisfying contribution and recognition. In order for children to grow a cooperative attitude, we will encourage them to realize whether our demands and legislation are beneficial for everyone.

There are no simple ways to participate in cooperation; it is primarily a patience and continuity approach. There are also three A's to be practiced that will lead to stop cresting tensions and temperaments: pay attention; achieve an agreement; and allow time to accept it.

Look out for the sound.

Many sounds – anger, agitation, even hesitation – in the voice of the adolescent will quickly force a parent in a defensive way to compromise with him or her. When you're in reactive mode, go out. It is time to change the chat from reaction to response.

A reaction is a solely emotional occurrence. The answers are more constructive because you step back and take a break; evaluate your feeling and you're teen before offering a perspective or an opinion.

It's not about paying attention to the speech of your daughter; it's listening to your own too. Children are at times hypersensitive to the tone in their parent's voice. What can seem to be a stern sound for you is noticed by your adolescent yelling. When you hear yelling or talking, you avoid listening.

Are you afraid to repeat yourself, watching the sentences going in one ear and out the other? Seek to sit down with your child and make a to-do list together. What do you think that needs to be done? How do you think your child wants to be done?

Include it on the agenda if you have exciting activities, including going to the cinema. Good things on the agenda bring the drudgery out of the jobs. Together, the value of the products is decided. The list is your mutual understanding that places you in cooperation rather than in dispute.

Instead of calling for anything to be completed at once, commit to a timetable, from Friday afternoon to Sunday night. Let the young individual realize if they want to use this opportunity to accomplish their goals. They know what to do and where, which will help to avoid the whole nagging process. Parents have one of the greatest problems is to let go.

Ensure that the collection and time period are practical. You want your teen to handle the activities instead of getting distracted. When the kid is interested in determining what is in the plan and the time period, they can take control of it most frequently. If they will not follow as they have decided to do, they are therefore more willing to consider the implications.

Recognition of development

Always neglect your child's ability to reward and desire to perform more. Recognize what they've achieved along the way. If you judge their success and condemn their performance, begin with genuine positive statements and ease the criticism. Think of it like an internal bank account before you can borrow, you must make a deposit. Olympic athlete reports have found that one critique needs 13 constructive responses.

Having to collaborate is a vital skill in adulthood for your young person to develop and create confidence. Threats, sarcasm, blaming and branding are not sufficient enough to show our youngsters how to communicate.

Then enter the higher ground. We want to learn about the qualities that are great for our girls - their commitment, their sense of duty, their sense of fun and their openness to others' needs. As a mom, you are responsible for cultivating a positive interaction, strong communication skills and emotional management.

They don't often do it, of course, but that's all right, too. Both are parents fine. Youth do not need a perfect parent to see that a parent is trying to work constructively with them, a parent who helps them to collaborate rather than demeans them.

It is worth the effort to find ways to communicate with your kids, an effort which can push and make you feel good about it.

Birute Regime was the founder and co-facilitators of Iron Butterflies: Mothers and Daughters Negotiating Cycles of Transformations, a four-day program for mothers and their preteen children, "Transforming women themselves and the environment."

Are you afraid to repeat yourself, watching the sentences going in one ear and out the other? Seek to sit down with your child and make a to-do list together. What do you think that needs to be done? How do you think your child wants to be done?

Include it on the agenda if you have exciting activities, including going to the cinema. Good things on the agenda bring the drudgery out of the jobs. Together, the value of the products is decided. The list is your mutual understanding that places you in cooperation rather than in dispute.

Instead of calling for anything to be completed at once, commit to a timetable, from Friday afternoon to Sunday night. Let the young individual realize if they want to use this opportunity to accomplish their goals. They know what to do and where, which will help to avoid the whole nagging process. Parents have one of the greatest problems is to let go. Ensure that the collection and time period are practical. You want your teen to handle the activities instead of getting distracted. When the kid is interested in determining what is in the plan and the time period, they can take control of it most frequently. If they will not follow as they have decided to do, they are therefore more willing to consider the implications.

Tools for Collaboration with Children

Here we discuss tools for engaging cooperation in children;

1. **Be playful**

According to author, that won't always be a device since you typically can't be humorous while you try your utmost not to yell. Nonetheless, if you can use it, it is a really versatile and valuable device. It may involve transforming things into sports, creating amusing sounds, thinking about inanimate items and everything you might think about.

2. **Offer a choice**

It doesn't mean whether they should respond or not, but there are choices of listening. So offer them a preference between a rose shirt and the blue instead of picking their uniform. Or put it all and make interesting decisions. Jump on or race to the ride! The ultimate effect remains the same; children are seated and dressed in the vehicle, but they act as though they manipulate the results.

3. Put the child in charge

Let the child pick or inform you when it's time for a change, as much as possible! The book contains some more detailed examples of how to do this, but essentially allow your mind to rest, to establish certain borders or restrictions and to decide for itself. That's the end target correct after all? Getting children who are people and will know for themselves instead of just being asked what to do? ….

4. Give information

This is more about the unmoved truth. It is impossible to revolt against the truth. You don't know what to do specifically, so you understand what the possible implications will be if you didn't follow through, which will give you an incentive to change yourself. I often think it throws you off as a parent or instructor because the "law" isn't that you're a huge mean mom or daddy...

5. Say it with a word

KISS- Hold it Easy Silly, mind. The river is murky in so many terms. Whenever necessary, keep the instructions clear and emotionless. So instead of "pushing your chair" and all the emotions they have when they don't do what you want to do immediately, you just say chair and give them a chance to figure out what they want.

6. Describe what you see

Perhaps, the loss of empathy is the most significant aspect here. Emotions are wonderful in many respects, but when it comes to your kids, they can only end. You simply explain what you see in this device. Basically, if one term isn't appropriate. And you may tell "I see a chair in the walkway" when "chair" is not necessary.

7. Describe how you feel

Be vigilant of this because it's easy to hack it before you even know it. It is a helpful device, though, which helps children understand the language and logic behind those emotions and to teach them how they cope with them. Often, it is impossible for a kid to disagree with you as you explain how it makes you feel. And instead of "If you don't sit down, you'll collapse!"Try, emotionally pure, probably inaccurate and quickly disagreed with, 'I'm afraid that you are standing on the chair. I'm afraid you slip and strike the eye. "An extra advantage to this device ... helps create empathy.

8. Write a note

The method is perfect as you talk, it sounds like a parrot. And, for whatever purposes, the children are more open to words than voices ... even though they cannot read yet (although they will of course be of the era where they realize what words is).

9. Take action without insult

The device when anything else fails. The trick is to calmly use this tool, not as a forced penalty. Instead, that is the goal and you won't let it proceed for the health and moral well-being of everyone.

Tips and strategies for making children collaborate

- "Don't transform a decision into a threat"– You can consider both options ... plus anything else you're prepared to obey.
- "We acknowledge success before explaining what needs to be done"– we consider this a productive sandwich in education. By showing what has been accomplished right, you set them up to really desire to know what is next. That always encourages them to know like they have achieved everything good and they're not completely losing

that ... "Say the term I, stop the term you while voicing rage or disappointment."- It enables us to communicate with emotions and not just coercion and calling.

- "Display intense frustration sparingly, you will sound like an attack"- be mindful what" feeling "terms you use to keep your kid (or anybody really) from feeling attacked. That will just render the other individual defending and physically shut down.

Example of cooperation in child

The explanations below illustrate how cooperativeness evolves in the first three years of childhood.

- A 3-month-old wakes and continues screaming for milk. His mum, who's just placing the dish in his final bowl, says, "In one minute I'm going to be with you, darling. The baby calms a little and sucks on his toes. I know you are tired. This baby discovers that his needs are vital and will be fulfilled, even if he still has to wait on him.

- A 14-month-old happily loses socks and t-shirts from one tub of clothing in the other. His grandma says, "Thank you for helping me find the washroom. Why don't you come in the washing machine as I place it? I'm going to pick you up to press the button. This young boy learns that a part of being in a family works together to complete everyday tasks.

- Two 30-month-olds search in the sandbox for the same light red shovel. Each seizes, the other seizes. Tears accompany each other's assurances: "No!"The father of one child enters and gently separates the two and transfers a red shovel to one and a plastic bulldozer to the other. He shows them how to bulldoze a pile of dirt that the other person can throw into a bucket. Such children know how to settle disputes, deal with frustration and develop connections by working together.

Tips to Cooperate Your Children

Below are strategies to improve the child's incentives and cooperative skills.

Take breaks

Between 6 and 9 months, babies can start to interact back and forth. They learn to mimic as well. This is a wonderful way to promote turnaround when playing with your children. If you put a block in the container, allow it time to copy. Taking turns and pour items into the bin. When he grows older, tends to placing pieces in the puzzle or types in the sorter. When it's time to tidy up, take turns to place the things on the table. Such encounters give him the ability to enjoy the joy of doing it as a squad.

Explain the weaknesses and demands explanations

Many children at the age of three use and appreciate words well enough to clarify clearly. Identify how the rules benefit the entire family. "We support everyone to clean up. So we don't drop our toys and locate them again." "I finish easier when you help me put the laundry away, so we can play.

Take time to solve the problem

You should support the older two- and 3-year-olds discover answers to everyday dilemmas while also promoting teamwork. There are measures to help you teach your child problem solving skills:

- State the problem. "You want to draw on the board, but mama says no." "Where else you could draw?
- "Try a solution. Offer two choices that are either paper or cardboard box suitable to you. Set a cap whether she thinks she needs to draw on the refrigerator.
- "I should put the pencils away before we decide to draw a spot." Most young children need help to find acceptable ways to channel their wishes. "You can put on the refrigerator magnetic letters."

2.4 Alternatives to punishments

Spanking remains one of the most frequently discussed subjects on parenting. Although most pediatricians and parenting specialists will not advocate spanking, the overwhelming majority of parents worldwide agree that they cover their babies.

For certain parents, spanking will sound like the easiest and most successful method of improving the actions of a kid. And, in the short term, it always succeeds. Studies nevertheless suggest that corporal punishment has long-term implications for adolescents.

Below are eight approaches to control your kid by utilizing physical violence, if you're searching for an option to punishments.

1. Put your child out of time

Hitting children for misbehavior (particularly aggression) sends out a confusing message. The child would ask why hitting her is OK but not Okay for her to hit her friend.

Placing an infant in time-out would be a much safer alternative. If performed properly, time-out shows children how to settle themselves, which is a valuable trait in life. However in order to be successful on time-out, children need to have lots of meaningful time-in with their guardians. Then, the lack of focus would be unpleasant until they are separated from the scenario, and the frustration may motivate them to act differently in the future.

2. Put Privileges Back

While a spanking stings for a minute or two, it takes more to strip a right away. Taking away the screen, computer games, his dream gadget or an afternoon enjoyable experience and he'll have a chance not to make the error.

Keep it plain when you will enjoy the rights. Twenty-four hours is normally sufficient enough to encourage the kid to learn from his error. Then you might say, "You've missed television for the remainder of the day so tomorrow you will win it back by picking up your toys the first time I inquire."

3. Ignore minor abuse

No, selective indifference may be more successful than spanking. That does not mean that if your child is doing anything harmful or immoral you will turn the other way. But, behavior that seeks attention can be ignored. When your kid starts crying or moaning to get publicity, don't offer it to him. Look the other way, claim that you cannot hear him and don't speak. Then switch your focus to him when he asks politely or when he is acting. He should realize, over time, that respectful conduct is the only way to fulfill his needs.

4. Teach Different Skills

One of the big spanking issues is that it doesn't show the kid how to act properly. If he's having a temper tantrum, spanking your kid won't show him how to settle down the next time he gets angry.

Children profit from understanding how to fix challenges, control feelings and create choices. When parents develop these techniques it will dramatically mitigate issues with behavior. Using training that is built to instruct, not to punish.

5. Provide clear consequences

Logical outcomes are a perfect approach to support adolescents dealing with individual behavioral problems. Logical effects are linked directly to the abuse.

Of starters, if your child isn't enjoying his meal, don't let him have a snack in bedtime. And if he fails to pick his cars, do not make him play with them for the remainder of the day. Linking the result closely to the issue of actions lets children understand that their decisions have clear effects.

6. Enable Natural Implications

Natural outcomes allow the children to benefit from their own mistakes. For starters, if your child decides he won't wear a sweater, let him go out and get cold as long as that's healthy to do. If you believe your child can benefit from his own error, using natural consequences. Track the scenario to insure there is no possible risk your child may face.

7. Pay good behavior

Rather than spanking an infant for misbehavior, praise them for positive behavior. For starters, if your kid sometimes battles with his parents, set up a scheme of incentives to encourage him to get along with them better.

Providing an opportunity to conduct will easily turn misbehavior around. Rewards help children concentrate on what they ought to do to receive rewards, instead of stressing the negative actions they can prevent.

8. Praise positive behavior

Preventing behavioral issues by catching well on your kids. When he plays happily with his siblings for starters, point it out. Say, "You're doing such a nice job sharing and taking turns today." If there are several kids in the house, offer the most emphasis and encouragement to the kids who obey the guidelines and behave well. When the other kid starts to act so show him the encouragement and care.

2.5 Encouraging Autonomy

Autonomy in early childhood education includes letting kids realize they have power of themselves and the decisions they make.

Kids are just like The Little Machine That Could, confronted with challenging challenges they are motivated to excel alone with a single mind or objective at times and they are not prepared to let any mountain (or grown up) get in their way. That always appears to happen in front of 100 other customers in the midst of a busy grocery shop. However uncomfortable as such circumstances can appear the intention of understanding and demanding minor bits of adult sovereignty is characteristic of and anticipated of children.

Autonomy is an internal drive and is perfectly natural. Across all regions infants are witnessing accelerated growth and development between the ages of one and three. When their reasoning abilities improve, or their thought, they hear about cause and effect, playing with how their behaviors affect their life (i.e. what happens if I throw my cup on the floor)? They are improving their motor skills along with this cognitive growth and through their regulation over their bodies. If you pair this cognitive and motor growth with innate enthusiasm and high energy, you get a hungry toddler to influence the environment around you.

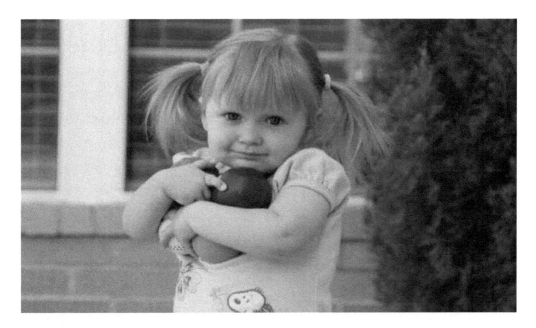

Build Autonomy Opportunities

You should build incentives to help your child thrive. If you realize that your child loves to have their own treats, place them on a shelf where your child can touch. Let your child practice brushing their teeth (and wash them before or after!). Offer them ways to exploit their behavior always helps. As irritating as a mom might be let them drop the blocks on the floor or take the books off the bookshelf. You will model supportive skills when they are finished by telling them to assist in packing them away.

Let them work

Toddlers are always on the move and this enthusiasm will also get them (or you) in trouble. Carrying out the child's duties will harness their motivation and therefore offer them feelings of freedom. You may ask your child to help move food from the shelf to the basket, bring packs into the building, fold the laundry, feed the dog or have them take the mail inside. Just when adults have a sense of pride after having finished a tough mission, as they work hard, you toddler should feel fulfilled and happy.

Offer choices

Everyone needs power, and too much of the life of a child is out of their grasp. Whenever you can give your kid a preference, not only can you give them control, but you also teach them the opportunity to make choices. No matter how tiny the job might be, if you can give your kid a choice go for it. If it's what they're going to have for lunch time, which novel to read or something to carry. There are definitely occasions where options are not at all suitable (like taking an adult's hand while crossing the street), so you should offer your child a restricted choice in any of those cases. If it's chilly outside and not appropriate for a short-sleeve jacket, take out two or three long-sleeve tops and let your child select.

Acknowledge their thoughts, mark them and accept them

Toddlers are quickly irritated as they struggle to accomplish a mission. They might scream, throw a tantrum, or show angry acts. This is also part of the normal training for toddlers. To help your child build strong social emotional communication skills, letting them identify certain feelings is crucial, but still showing them that a balanced display of feelings is fine. If your kid is upset that they can't take the cover off a cup you can console them "You're so unhappy because you couldn't keep your cover off." "You might tell" You're too mad when your kid pierces their foot and screams. You paddle your foot. It's okay to be upset. "Children often only need time to convey certain feelings. Help them realize in this situation that you are there to comfort them once they are happy. Giving your child the opportunity to exercise freedom and individuality helps build a feeling of control over their body mind and setting. It encourages autonomous and analytical thought, facilitates inherent encouragement and inspires confidence.

 Strategies to improve the autonomy of your child

Here we discuss following strategies to improve the autonomy of your child;

Trust is important

Autonomy implies so more than merely growing up. It always requires the courage to do such stuff and to be confident, to be willing to behave and to think for you. By being self-sufficient, and therefore similar to parents, the child gains self-esteem through the development of a secure and rich inner existence that helps deter him from forbearing and removing his dependency on others.

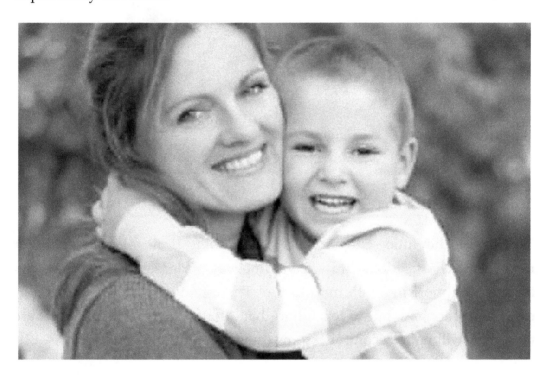

Through encouraging your child to gain his individuality, you indicate that you support him and are proud of his success; it also involves enabling him to express his independence whilst shielding him – though not overprotection. Parents sometimes do something with their children to support them, catch up, or because they're falsely persuaded that the job cannot be done by their child alone. How many times have you tied the shoelaces of your child or put his coat in the wardrobe, without telling your child to do so? The most frequent excuse parent's offer is that it is moving quicker! It definitely helps, but you don't inspire your kid to take an action by doing it yourself. In everything, you deter him from attempting to tackle small problems he most definitely will encounter.

His own little schedule

Giving every morning to your child little things, such as preparing his room, brushing his teeth, dressing, etc. Remind him whenever he continues to think about such things, but leave him alone.

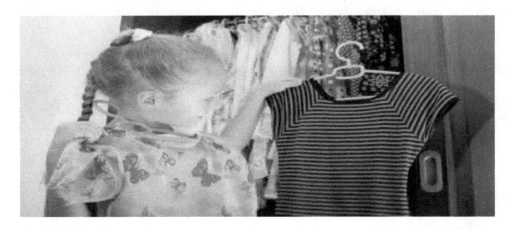

"You alone should do this!"

Seek to use this little sentence rather than doing it all for your kids. For moments such as: "Mom, draw me a dinosaur," "Please open my juice box for me," "Support me with my puzzle." The intention is not to leave your child to his hobbies, but to teach him that, though he understands you are near, he is willing to accomplish some things without your support.

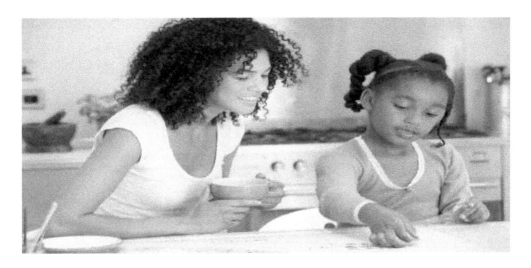

A wardrobe, a broom and a duster for him only

To motivate your child to take part in household tasks, plan your home so that he may give you a hand easier. Leave the kitchen cabinet at its height where the children's cups, utensils, bowls and dishes are placed. The child will help you set the table, clean the dishwasher, make treats, etc.

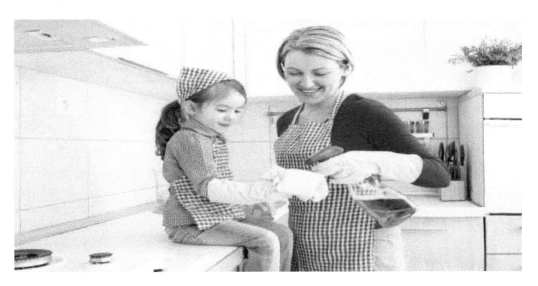

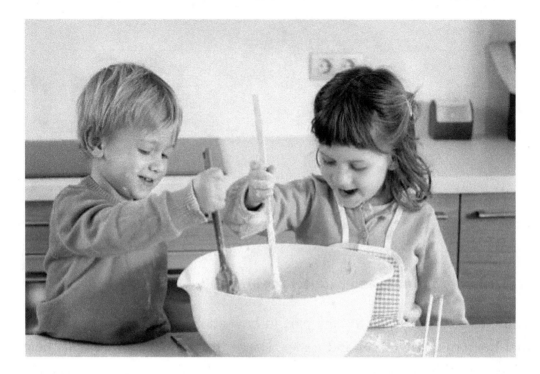

Relax

Are you overwhelmed about time constantly? Are you thinking with leaks and messes? Learn to remain patient and have your kid explore his or her own.

We love a contest! We need a fight!

Each day, seek to encourage your child to increase his ability to do something different and certainly be proud of his accomplishments! Will you need ideas? Ask him to drink a glass of milk without, for starters, dumping it out or joining his shoelaces by himself.

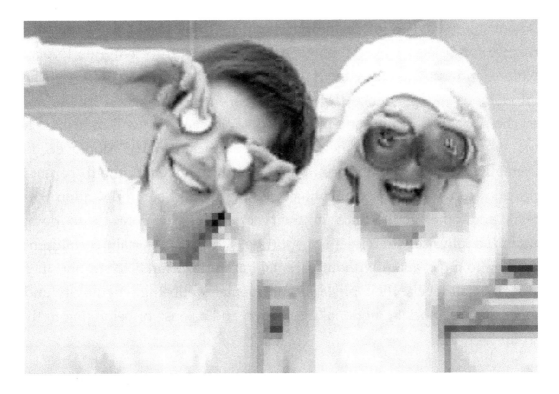

Encourage his feelings

Seek not to disturb the imaginative impulse of your kid or to regularly address his thoughts. If not, he may be hesitant to take initiative. Encourage your child to gamble nothing, do different activities or adjust tactics. You are his performance map. Failures also can be used as life experiences or fresh obstacles.

Learn to take accountability for your kids!

Although your child is small, that does not imply that he cannot be kept accountable for actual acts including feeding the cat, delivering the mail, coupon cutting in weekly flyers and so forth. Such acts will be viewed as jobs, but your child should perceive them as a blessing and a show of trust.

What research shows about Autonomy (The ability of parents to view infant autonomy as predictors of greater adult school independence?)

Childhood is important as habits of physical activity are formed that are likely to continue during adolescence and adulthood. The World Health

Organization advises that children perform mild to intensive physical exercise for at least 1 hour a day. The normal reason for children to play, explore and run about without adult control is physical exercise. This autonomous independence (IM) dimension encourages good fitness and psycho-social well-being for children and adolescents. IM will contribute to and support children with their everyday physical activity. Moreover, the alternative of playing and running around the area without parental guidance increases the social contact of children and communication with peers and other individuals in their community in contrast to doing organized physical exercise (e.g. sporting activities). Certainly children's freedom to travel about without parental interference tends to support their growth at all levels: their physical and mental wellbeing, cognitivity and, above all, their social-emotional interaction and a sense of belonging to the group.

According to study, the Independence of children is described as the opportunity to play in their world without accompaniment by the parent (e.g. go to school, go to local parks to play, meet buddies, go shopping, catch a coach). This versatility is an example of personal freedom. "Free autonomy is a critical feature of liberty per se," scientists claim. When children grow up, they get the license to cross the roads on their own, go to school independently, board busses and use bicycles. This expanded mobility has several physical-cognitive and psychosocial benefits. In comparison, children with more IM appear to avoid gaining endurance and are best suited for the environment of adults. Given these advantages, IM decreased in comparison with previous generations, especially in countries such as France, Portugal and Italy. The scientists have claimed that it is extremely impossible for children to play or travel on the highways, open fields, parks etc. in Western countries without strong adult oversight. Another practice that has significantly decreased children's IM is IM at home as less and less children go from home alone. In the United Kingdom, the number of children aged 7-8 years old attending school without oversight by parents was 80% in 1970, but just 10% in 1990. Throughout Germany and the United Kingdom, from 1990 to 2010, the number of primary school students supported by a parent on the ride from school. In a recent survey carried out in Germany by a professor, at least often about two thirds of elementary school children are accompanied to school by a parent. From 1991 to 2012, the number of children moving separately to school in Australia decreased from 61% to 32%. However, this IM to school is good for them. The study by scientists shows that 52 experiments were carried out, several of which centered on IM from and to school, and that IM to school has important positive ties to physical activity. We agree, however, that no study has extensively studied those children who go to or from school separately and those who exercise IM in both ways.

Previous research showed certain geographical, social and cultural shifts that influenced children's behavior: fewer opportunities for children to play in urban centers, less public room for them to play and socialize, less opportunity for them to walk about have been avoided. Therefore, less physical play involves the following reasons: fewer adolescents in community today, less households with babies, heightened worries regarding parenting and children's health, and middle-class homes that purchase more indoor cultural services. The researchers' analysis demonstrates the value of promoting outside play as they play games like 'disappearing' or 'getting away' and take up dangerous outside play, their physical activity and psychosocial wellbeing improve and monitored children become more sedentary. For the above-mentioned writers, the term 'danger' relates to a circumstance whereby a child may accept and evaluate a threat and agree on a course of action." The impression of parents that they assume that their children might experience a car accident and that the risk of "strangers" was also related to the limits on independence for their children.

Spending less time playing outside means adolescents becomes less free in today's generations. The definition of autonomy is characterized as a state of self-governance and often applies to three domains: mental, emotional and cognitive. Parents who view their children as more self-contained in cognitive, emotional and behavioral terms may also be more receptive to greater IM. In addition, the mindset of parents about the value of increasing their children's autonomy may be a significant predictor. The family definitely plays a crucial role in the children. According to the principle of self-determination, parents are principal socializes that promote the sovereignty of their children and are mindful that they require such sovereignty, taking their opinions into consideration and allowing the preference, mistakes and decision-making of their own issues. Mothers, in comparison, should behave by managing more and handling their children according to the standards of adults. The position of parents is therefore central to the growth of children's autonomy. This autonomy may be strengthened by actions, such as requiring greater IM for their children. Yet what does it rely on for parents to display one mindset or another?

Even if variables such as risk tolerance are related to children being given fewer IM, certain variables like the number of children and their place in the family or the ability of parents to give them more or less IM can be important. Such factors have, however, been less documented. The present research considered exploring in detail the function performed by the sociodemographic variables of certain children and parents and the variables linked to the parents' view of the infant in relation to enhanced MI of children. About their child-occupied parents, other research have shown that those not born first and those not just children love IM beforehand while their parents are watched. Older parents often require more IM for their babies, because they valued their independence more than later generations. The reality that all parents function influences the IM of children as well. More and more babies, whose school hours overlap with work hours of their parents and their parents go to school before going to work.

Different surveys have shown that IM has to do with parents who see their districts as providing a greater sense of identity, that is, their neighborhood has greater coherence, is stronger related and secure, and has schools in their proximity, since they are part of a smaller city. The study reveals how the ability of parents to raise children's IM is affected by social stability in the community. Parents are more likely to encourage their children to travel longer distances for spontaneous trips and outdoor play. The reasons that parents give to either promote or exclude IM from or to school for other leisure activities contribute to children's specific characteristics, such as their sense that they are adequately stable and respected their need to secure them or other older children in the family. One aspect that indicates that parents trust their children is to send them house keys.

Latest studies indicate the presence of multiple types of education IM and the significance of discriminating between children going to or from education alone (IM both ways) and those only going to or from school alone. Children exhibiting IM in both directions indicate more IM in their social activity and find that their home is easier and less stressful than others that only ride one route to school. These kids also regard their school trip as free, unlike the kids who do not use IM at home. In addition, each IM form has specific predictors. These results suggest that IM is correlated negatively with certain IM influences.

2.6 Freeing children from playing roles

Most scholars, early theories and clinicians agree that play is essential to the growth of the infant. That is the primary method of inspiring, taking choices, solving challenges, observing one's own rules, managing impulses, having friends and engaging with them, and loving.

One of the great psychologists and play advocates, Frobel, claims that play is the process of an outward expression of children's inner feelings. Where else can the kid express his inner thoughts more plainly than in free play? Throughout this way, we claim that the "reflection of free games is not just the most valuable gift we may offer them; it is also a profound opportunity for them to become potential professional adults physically, intellectually and emotionally."

Although the benefits of play in general and free play in particular are obvious, we note a "departure from it in favor of schooling" in the last half-century. According to the reports, anxiety, depression, helplessness and narcissism among infants, teens and young people increased drastically during that era. The American researcher Peter Gray still accepts these circumstances, who note that the deterioration in function has contributed to the rise of psychopathology in these days. It is not known whether lack of play is the primary cause of such issues, but definitely that is one of the key triggers. Play is observed in human interaction from the moment of conception where the infant works naturally or imitates. With aging, the game evolves, different versions and forms are added, guided more or less by adults, and its contents are fuller. Sadly, however, free play is reduced as time and meaning when the infant pursues an institutionalized method of education: children play openly for the first 6 years of their childhood.

We must first attempt to establish a theoretical delimitation of this style of action. In this word, thus, the following names have been established in early childhood literature: unstructured play /self-playing / realistic play / free play/ deliberate or self-initiated activity. In Romania's early education documents, the term free play is used. They would provide a set of meanings found in research at the regional and foreign rates, in order to describe the various valences of children's lives from the moment of conception to primary school age. Of accordance with the Early Childhood Education Guidelines for the 3-6 / 7-year-old, free playing is the style of activity that children perform in their childhood. Free play is the chosen, proposed, child-initiated play without the intervention of adults. He alone chooses the place he / she want, the toys and the type of play.

In Pedagogy Dictionary, researchers define free play as a "form of playing in which kids freely select their teammates, content as well as learning objectives. The work from playing to learning, where the authors support free play, is defined as a natural learning process that ensures that the individual, child or adult, has full meaning and profound learning." It is not a set plan, and adults are not guiding the operation. Children go from spatial and social education environments to arrange different activities with resources or rings, shouting, play-role, kites ... "In Imaginative Schools, renowned British instructor Ken Robinson describes free play as" the process by which children learn to make friends, resolve their worries, conquer their problems and in theory gain charge of them. It is also the primary way to learn and develop physical and mental skills in youngsters. Stuff children know in their own open play programs cannot be learned in certain forms.

Open play is one of the core practices of the pedagogy of Waldorf and Montessori focused on reverence for the rights of the infant. In the regular Waldorf kindergarten, free play lasts between 1.5-2 hours a day and is particularly necessary because the child's personality grows through it. The established environment is focused on peace, calm, but also movement and involvement. The educator's job is to build and preserve this environment, but also to insure that each child engages in a meaningful activity. Here the infant perceives nature, recognizes his or her perceptions and knows the truth of existence. The topic and its behavior is slowly developed into the imagined universe by turning reality, building a universe of its own with the own rules and chosen playmates. Free games can be created independently or in communities, facilitated by a child or children's community. The truth is, several children can enter if it appears important.

In respect to the academic setting unique to Montessori academic, it is important for the preschooler to have all the information he wants in order to be easily included in all sorts of activities undertaken by children.

Analyzing the meanings given and the basic facets of the play in the developmental alternatives mentioned, we notice that most relate to the implications it provides for the child's growth, the growth phases, parental interaction levels and the resources used. To explore this topic in a detailed manner, we consider: the socio-cultural context of the infant, the disparities between the sexes, the affinities of various peers and, overall, the adult's dependence / independence in the generated setting. We should clarify the criteria by introducing the underlying ideas relating to them momentarily. Therefore, pre-school children or pupils decide the preference of the form, habits of the family and cultural objects and specifically define how they function. There are variations in children's free play in urban and rural regions, but also due to the social standing of the communities in whom they derive. While every child's family member's everyday actions can trigger his immature games. However, small behavioral improvements may arise due to imitations of other people's actions, thereby promoting social dynamics. In rural areas, for example, children's playgrounds grow outdoors in a large play area near the house with toys created by them. Free play is, however, influenced by different job tasks that these children have to perform (feeding the livestock, supporting parents to tidy up their houses, etc.). Within metropolitan settings, play indoors mostly takes place today as play fields within blocks of fiats are not secure (in the eyes of parents) so children can either run out in the woods, or other play areas.

Sex gaps also render a major impact to children's sports. The psychologist researched the way pre-school children in an urban kindergarten describe themselves as boys and girls. We also found that there are various guidelines for what and one will do, due to gender, and thus set up separate games for boys and girls. The preferences are attributed in particular to family traditions, but also to instinctive patterns. Rare are cases in which a child plays girls or vice versa. In general, kids favor constructing plays, role-plays, every day works, while girls prefer role-playing, drawing or painting games, etc, but never design plays (except girls' unique legoes). As a result, we argue that there are multiple valences of free play due to the aspects the instructor pursues. We will therefore present them through his theoretical and realistic research, but also articulate our point of view. With respect to the research parameters chosen, we agree that the improvement areas relevant to pre-school education have been applied to, with an expansion to primary school pupils as the targets are focused on various competencies. From a **socio-emotional point of view**, fair play;

- Reduces anxiety
- Creates positive mood
- To moral determinations, to exhaustion
- This promotes calmness, flexibility and capacity for coping
- To foster teamwork and co-operation with unforeseen incidents, and to facilitate persevering and concentration
- To nurture self-discipline

- To allow children to make errors; Learning from errors
- To play through does not feel the burden of failure

From a **cognitive point of view** we describe the benefits of this kind of play on mental growth as: it is focused on:

• Creative thinking; encourages diverging thoughts;

• fosters thinking through testing carried out by children during

•free play; strengthens brain neuronal connections;

•develops the self-realization of thought;

•defines test- and error-related learning; Children 'imagine, perceive and foresee, communicate their ideas through means of words and pictures and maybe also through acts that go beyond playing. Creativity thus developed strengthens their capacity to understand, perceive, and interact with others more complexly. 'Develops the intrinsic desire (the child plays in his/her needs for self-satisfaction and therefore the child is in a different place, requiring complete devotion to the game; cultivates the will because of the absence of The bulk of kids speak to someone during free play, without restrictions or the fear that everyone is watched and corrected. Kids often discuss what they openly did in kindergarten or school with friends.

From **functional point of view**, free play has the following attributes:

- Positive feelings during play decide the state of the immune system, the endocrine and the cardio-vascular system, the weakness and tension,
- Improving stamina, flexibility and exhaustion;
- In order to minimize their detrimental effects, the time allocated by the parent must be measured judiciously and the value of play in the spare time underlined.

Ways to arrange and improve free play

In both pre-school and primary school, open play can be found. If the time allotted to this play is greater at pre-school level, elementary school students can play freely in school breaks, in the classroom or at the yard. The games they create are not focused on a rich subject, but they promote team sports, teamwork, socialization and role-playing in particular. How students play free games may provide personality details. To this point, primary or school teachers may aim to track certain events in a given preparatory class pace as a possible aid in the completion at the end of the preparatory class of the student's appraisal study. The instructor will spend some spare time in the regular schedule, since the teaching-learning-evaluation exercises occupy 30-35 minutes, the remainder of the day for pre-chosen recreational activities. Class II, III and IV occupy 45 minutes of teaching-learning-evaluation tasks, while the rest is generous for these things. Throughout this case, the instructor will allow students to make better use of the material in the classroom. At an early school age, the attention of children is based on cultural, literature, reading, or writing, performing roles, or debating other topics.

The daily conference will be another perfect opportunity to incorporate open play. Therefore, children thrive and produce greater outcomes in school. In this aspect, I began a final trial within the class I guidance (in the instructional alternative Step by Step): I spent 15 minutes free play during the week during the morning meeting, after which I spent the students learning in open centers. For 85 percent, students concentrated more on their work activities than on the same period during which free play was not enforced. The students affirm these optimistic results, who said they liked working in centers because they had worked and had fun before. It has to be said that, as an instructor, I did not intervene explicitly in the activity, unless requested to do so, according to their own preferences or conditions, the activities preferred by the boy. The students could use all the resources in the classroom instead, so that they were willing to put them in place after the game had ended and to "trade" them with others. We have told children to use voice indoors throughout the session. As a consequence of the above, it is evident that young school children's free play is one of the most popular types of play. With respect to children's daily schedules, free play can be seen both in the first part of the day and after their rest. In the first example, we are concerned about how long the child lasts from his entrance to the nursery to the meal, during which he decides what and how he wants to play. This form of play is used before leaving home during the afternoon activities. However, despite the many facets it has, the free time allotted to the kindergarten curriculum is inadequate.

While children love free play, organized programs (based on learning experiences) involving infants, concern over children's school performance, rigid structuring of pre-school / school curriculum, etc. have limited it. A simple examination of the everyday practices of children allows one to conclude that they are often organized through "professional coaches." There are unusual circumstances in the community where children play ("hinter the block") and parents arrange their regular schedule in conjunction with themselves. Overworked adolescents, with planned, in-house or outsourced tasks and insufficient free time, have long-term consequences, including lack of sleep, treatment, irritability, unexpected mood changes, etc. While the value of play for the growth of adolescents and particularly free play is encouraged by experts in early education.

As I have previously claimed, the instructor will not need any special initiative to plan free play at all pre-school and primary stages. The instructor intervenes to a very limited degree, being chosen and appointed by kids according to their own desires, conditions, and inclinations. To ensure its efficacy, though, pre-school children need to be well-arranged with resources for various uses and the classroom area. The Playful ecosystem as an ensemble of individual, content, ergonomic and temporal capital dictates the efficacy of free play organization and creation. In the community space, the works, toys and artifacts and the different centers of focus may be useful instruments for doing so (cubes, mugs, plastic cups, assorted containers, tubes, building parts, etc.). The usage of toys may be the traditional but also a modern, creative one that demonstrates the imagination of the boy. For e.g., the child will get a musical instrument to use in his free play from a box and a few grains from the role play centre.

This condition was stated during a doctoral internship held in Hungary, where I found in the kindergarten the utility of using free play, but also a range of issues concerning its growth. Therefore, the length of the practice was of the children's discretion, in certain instances the trainer indicated the end of the free play time from his actions. The instructor did not participate in the play of the girls, except where asked or when a specific circumstance occurred. The educational room was also designed to suggest a miniature house with specific furnishings and amenities. For this cause, children skillfully used toys that were household objects (dishes, sweatshirts, vacuum cleaners, laundry shelves, etc.), which naturally lead to the growth of realistic household skill. The whole team was distinguished by an aura of well-being, such that smiles and good-mood occupied the community room. Open play was compulsory in the regular curriculum, irrespective of atmospheric circumstances, in the kindergarten too, and the instructor maintained the children's physical dignity. In each community space there was a gateway to the outside courtyard where a "play field" was created which children valued in order to escape hazards. Creating a playful environment defines the pleasure of the practice, engaging children in this activity based on this dimension.

Chapter 3: Montessori and Positive discipline

Any person who cares for children is responsible for leading, addressing and socializing children into healthy behaviors. Such acts of adults are also called infant supervision and training. Positive reinforcement and supervision are important as they foster self-control for children, reinforce accountability for children and help children make wise decisions. The most successful adult parents are at promoting positive infant activity, the fewer energy and attention adults expend on addressing misbehavior at infants.

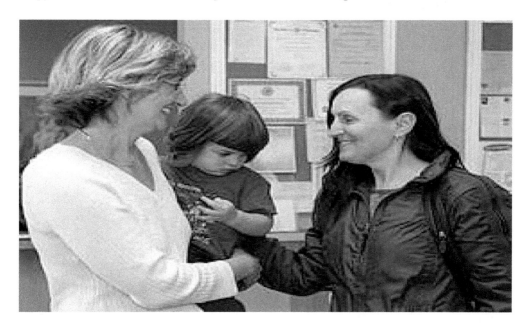

3.1 What is positive discipline?

Good Training is a curriculum intended to educate teenagers to grow to be conscientious, polite, and resourceful community citizens. focus on fastest-selling books on Strong Discipline by Cheryl Erwin ,Dr. Jane Nelsen, Mary Hughes, Mike Brock, Kate Ortolano , Lynn Lott , Lisa Larson and others, it incorporates critical emotional and life lessons in a way that is profoundly compassionate and empowering for both adults and children (including instructors, parents , community workers ,child care professionals, and others worker). New work shows us that kids are "genetically programmed" to interact with others from conception, and that child who experience an intellect of attachment to their culture, families, and kindergarten is less probable to be misunderstood. Children need to develop the requisite life skill and community to be effective, to become members to their society. Good training resides in the belief that training needs to be learned and that it improves training.

Family specialists always accept that there is no perfect solution which addresses all disciplinary questions. Children are special and so are the households they are raised in. A technique of punishment which may work with one child may not work with another.

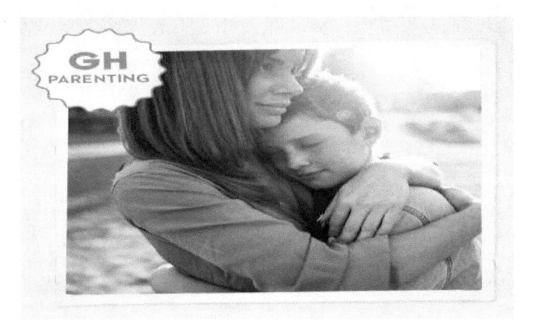

The child's growth is focused on positive instruction and training. They protect the self-esteem and integrity of the child too. Acts that offend or disrespect are likely to lead children to look poorly at their parents and other relatives, which may hinder learning and may encourage the child to be unkind to others. Nevertheless, acts which consider the accomplishments and success of the infant, no matter how slow or weak, are likely to foster healthy growth.

It is a challenging job to teach children self control. It needs caution, careful consideration, cooperation and the child's clear comprehension. It also needs understanding of one's own abilities and addressing behavioral issues. Unfortunately for certain parents the only practice is their own parental knowledge. These childhood encounters can not necessarily help to develop the children of today.

How to Start With Positive discipline

•**Certified Constructive Attitude Teachers are available**, and they offer courses and seminars around the world.

•**Take note on how the family treats stimuli**. "I suggest that you listen more than you talk," says Zeichner. "If a kid feels a sense of identity and purpose, he or she is far less likely to misbehave and far more inclined to listen and participate. It's also good to realize that our children learn how to control and regulate their feelings through controlling and regulating ours, and it's necessary to model the same actions we want to see." Good Reinforcement is also seen as a means of handling teacher actions in the classroom. "This occurs when teachers are moist and strong, setting students reasonable ideas about what needs to be achieved, having consistent instructions about what actions are inappropriate, engaging with students to fix their issues, and encouraging good actions or punishing bad habits in a very straightforward and transparent way," says Dr. Rodman. If teachers can do it with thousands of kids in a school, so you should definitely do it at home.

•**Choose a family target**, and formulate a roadmap to accomplish it. Recall giving you plenty of options!

Five conditions for successful discipline

1) Helping children to feel linked. (Significance and Belonging)

2) Being polite and helpful of one another. (Classical and strong simultaneously).

3) is successful in the long run. (Think what things the child assumes, learns and prefers for itself and its world – and how to foresee in the coming years to survive or thrive.).

4) Teaches essential cognitive and life skills; (Respect, empathy for others, teamwork and problem solving, and an opportunity to belong to the home, school or larger society).

5) Invite children to learn if they are capable. (Encourages the positive usage of personal resources and self-reliance)

The styles of Constructive Reinforcement Classroom Management and Parenting seek to build partnerships that are equally reciprocal. Strong Training encourages adults to equally practice compassion which firmness, and is nor coercive neither permissive.

Positive Disciplinary methods and principles include:

1. Mutual love and support. Young's shape determination by honoring oneself and the social needs, empathy by considering the child's needs.

2. Identify the conviction following the activities. Good punishment understands the motives why children and whatever they want and tries to alter certain values, rather than simply attempting to modify their actions.

3. Efficient listening capabilities and crisis solving.

4. Discipline instruction (and not permissive, not punitive).

5. Focusing on options, rather than retribution.

6. Encouragement (and not praise). Encouragement recognizes commitment and change, not just performance, and creates self-respect and confidence over the long term.

The Positive Discipline Model's special characteristics often include:

1. Teaching by experiential experiences to adults and pupils. Develop different techniques and have entertaining learn by playing.

2. Classroom training initiatives and clear teacher awareness systems. Childcare, teachers and parents provider can work collectively to provide children with a safe, reliable atmosphere.

3. Inexpensive preparation and continuing help so that group leaders can show positive lessons of discipline to each other.

4. Countrywide accredited teachers that can collaborate with neighborhoods and schools and.

Precautionary steps

Part in utilizing constructive reinforcement is to avoid circumstances where harmful habits will evolve. There are various strategies that instructors may use to discourage inappropriate behavior: pupils who "misbehave" display "mistaken" behavior. There are several explanations why a student may demonstrate wrongdoing, i.e. lack of awareness of appropriate behavior or feel unwelcome or unaccepted. The instructor should prescribe correct behavior for students who actually do not realize what acceptable actions they will be displaying. For e.g., a child who struggles drastically with a product will be confronted by a instructor who will seek to establish a rational compromise by promoting feedback from the child and thinking about their issues in order to prevent another dispute. For students who feel rejected or unaccepted, a healthy interaction between the instructor and the student needs to establish before any sort of discipline works.

If the students had a good bond with the person in charge and understood that the instructor valued them, punishments would be less required. Teachers must be willing to develop such relationships. For some of them, just asking them to display appreciation and interaction with students is not enough, since they might still lack information of how to do so.

Teachers must treat each pupil as an account; they must deposit good interactions in the student before allowing a withdrawal from the pupil at the moment of discipline. Teachers will make deposits on the back through recognition, special events, enjoyable classroom work, smiles and appropriate pats. Any kids never received good exposure. Children are hungry for recognition; when they gain constructive feedback, they will display actions that would draw adverse interest.

Teachers should recognize classes of students that aren't functioning well together (because they're buddies or don't get along well) and isolate them at the outset to avoid circumstances that contribute to unpleasant behavior. Many teachers use the "boy-girl-boy-girl" technique of lining or circling up (which, depends on your viewpoint, could be patriarchal or effective) to hold groups of friends apart and enable the students to make new friends. The classroom's physical structure will influence classroom behavior and instructional effectiveness.

Another strategy will be to be straightforward about the laws from the start, and the repercussions for violating certain guidelines. If students have a good understanding of the rules, they will be more obedient as their actions ultimately have repercussions. Sometimes a set of 3 alerts are used before a tougher result (detention, time-out, etc.) is used, especially for smaller annoyances (for example, a student may obtain warnings for calling out, rather than having an immediate detention, as an alert is generally fairly effective). Any alerts for more extreme actions (hitting another pupil, swearing, intentionally disobeying an alert, etc.) severe penalties will arrive. Teachers should feel justified in not "pulling a fast one" on the students.

Students would be most inclined to obey the guidelines and standards as explicitly defined and early defined. Most students ought to learn and grasp what the problematic habits are before unintentionally showing up with it.

Involving the students in creating the guidelines and preparations for punishment will help discourage other students from behaving. It promotes accountability to the students and provides knowledge about what positive habits are vs. negative ones. It often helps the student feel honored and encouraged to obey the rules as they were interested throughout the process of their formation.

3.2 Positive discipline historical introduction

The Positive Parental Behavior and Classroom Leadership Model were focused on the research of Rudolf Dreikurs and Alfred Adler. In the 1920s, To U.S. viewers Dr. Adler first brought the concept of parental instruction. He promoted fair care of infants, but still claimed that pampering and spoiling infants did not promote them and contributed to behavioral and social issues. Throughout the late 1930s, Dr Dreikurs took the teaching methods, which were first developed early 1920s throughout Vienna in to the United States. Adler and Dreikurs refer to the compassionate and strict method to parenting and teaching as 'self-governing.', Jane Nelsen and Lynn Lott in the 1980s attended a workshop led by Taylor John. Lynn began educating interns to instruct experientially and published the first Teaching Parenting Manual (with the aid of her intern). The founder of Project accept was Jane (Techniques Adlerian Counseling to Encourage Teachers and Parents), a federal supported initiative that had achieved iconic recognition through its growth process. Jane in 1981 wrote and released him Good Discipline. It was first released in 1987 by Ballantine. Lynn and Jane in 1988 agreed to work on the book of teenagers now titled, Teenager Positive Discipline s, and started experientially teaching leadership and communication strategies in the classroom. Jane and Lynn both published in Classroom Positive Discipline and created a textbook for students and their teachers packed with experiential experiences. Good Training series has evolved since year to take account of title covering various age ranges, social dynamics and unique circumstances. Good discipline is administered through professional Accredited Successful Behavior Associates to the students, adults, and teacher educators. Group leaders, teachers, and caregivers are empowered to become qualified launch pad and to communicate in their own classes the principles of constructive discipline.

Parent education positive Discipline courses are conducted around the world, and in public elementary schools, social and ethnic. Positive Discipline is widely utilized as the standard for classroom management. A curriculum for the demonstration school is currently under growth.

3.3 Evidence of positive discipline

Comparing Successful Punishment Programs of programs with certain training schemes, systematic assessment is only starting. However, Positive Discipline methods application trials have demonstrated that Positive Discipline strategies can yield meaningful outcomes. A review of the district-wide introduction of classroom meetings in a lower-income high school in Sacramento over a four-year cycle found that suspensions declined (from 64 annually to 4 annually), violence declined (from 24 incidents to 2) and teachers recorded change in the environment, behavior, behaviors and academic success in college. An analysis of parent and teacher intervention interventions engaging parents and student teachers with "maladaptive" actions incorporating Constructive Disciplinary strategies found a statistically substantial increase of student conduct of system schools relative to control schools. (Nelsen, 1979) Smaller experiments investigating the impact of different methods in Positive Discipline have demonstrated encouraging outcomes. Studies have shown consistently that the sense of a pupil being part of the school group (being "related" to school) reduces the occurrence of socially unsafe activities (such as mental anxiety and suicidal thoughts / attempts, usage of tobacco, alcohol and marijuana; aggressive behavior) and improves academic success.

There is also strong proof that teaching social skills to younger students has a beneficial impact that endures into puberty. Children who have been learned social strategies are more likely to excel in school and less inclined to participate in activities causing difficulties. While detailed tests of the parenting system Positive Discipline are in the early stages, initiatives related to Positive Discipline have been tested and have been found to be successful in improving parent behavior. Researcher observed in a sample of Adlerian adult education programs for adolescent parents that parents performed more problem-solving for their teenagers and became less autocratic in decision taking. Positive training gives caregivers both compassion and firmness at the same moment. Numerous research suggest that teenagers who view their parents as both good (responsive) and strict (demanding) are at lower risk of smoking, drug usage, alcohol consumption, or violence, and subsequently having sexual intercourse. Many findings associated the teen's understanding of parental style (kind and strict or autocratic or permissive) with better success in academics.

3.4 Positive discipline in Toddlers (18 months to 3 year)

Children aren't raised with social skills — to continue with a survival-of-the-fittest mindset is human nature to them. That's why you ought to show your kid how to behave responsibly and properly — while you're home and you're not. In a nutshell, the task is to install in her brain a "normal person" memory chip (Freud named this the superego) which will inform her how she will act. It's sort of like killing a wild animal, but if you do it right, you won't kill your child's spirit.

Why do you not listen and misbehave your Child Conduct Tantrums?

Disciplining a kid is difficult, since you have to consider his brain growth period to do so successfully. The 1 to 3-year-old kid has not yet received an adult person's critical thought. He can't grasp nor recall laws quickly yet. He also dislikes the idea of empathizing with others, being sweet, and even keeping himself free. His interpretation of reasoning, and the consequence of his acts, is still simplistic.

A kid also starts building his sense of self and continues to want to do something for himself. Sometimes he tries to do something he's not even ready to achieve and it makes him feel anxious. And while he often lacks the coping ability, he expresses his emotions by tannery and unruly behavior.

A kid can not necessarily intend misbehaving, either. It is just his reaction to his condition; the only way he knows how to grow underdeveloped. That's why you ought to be empathetic or compassionate when finding the most acceptable approach to your child's abuse. You ought to be conscious of what your child is going through in its developmental growth to help you adapt correctly and control it.

You ought to consider some of the main triggers of the misbehavior of your toddler:

1. **Severe exhaustion, appetite, physical pain, nausea** – this may contribute to temperature tantrums for your kid. They're a call for support, and at times his only way to tell "Enough!". In the only way he understands how, he communicates his emotions – of cries, contortions, sitting on the floor of flailing arms and moaning.

2. **Frustration**-Despite his shortcomings, the kid always feels helpless. These are also activities he needs to do physically but he's too frail or too uncoordinated to do, such as correctly holding a doll. Sometimes a major source of anger is not being able to communicate what he needs orally. He then channels this into outbursts of rage, hostility and antisocial behavior. He is always at a point where he has trouble managing his anger.

3. **Not receiving everything he needs** – Toddlers are having a tough time managing their urges and emotions, so they want to get what they want. When parents reply "no," it is tough for children to handle the frustration and do not grasp why they are refused it. Even today elders have no idea of "delayed gratification" yet.

4. **Curiosity** -The kid actively tries to learn about the world, and sometimes it leads him to cross the line with inacceptable behavior. To see how it responds, he can pull the cat's tail, or pound a spoon on things to hear the different sounds it creates.

5. **Checking-** The toddler is more and more conscious of his own strength. He is seeing what cap he will get away with.

6. **Need for love**-A kid has a deep desire for treatment. He would rather be faced with the implications of his misdeed than dismissed.

7. **Changes** – Changes in major life, such as getting a different sitter, or small adjustments, such as quitting the park, cause your kid feel mentally confused or frustrated.

Why is it necessary to teach your kid in a positive way?

While you may recognize why a kid misbehaves, this doesn't imply he can disregard his misbehavior. Toddlers will be regulated, ensuring that, from an early age, he becomes conscious that something like right and wrong happens. It should be an ongoing effort to punish your baby, not just something you do when your kid is misbehaving.

These are some of the items you can do by disciplining your child positively:

- Teach him right from wrong, and appropriate moral expectations.
- Correct inappropriate behavior, promote good behavior.
- Impress upon him the boundaries of what he should do.
- Let him conscious of the rules that make possible and not challenging his existence.
- Hold him in risk.
- Let him know how to control himself growing up.

Age-appropriate Child positive discipline

Here are few generic strategies to positive disciplining your infant, depending on his age:

Age 1

Your one-year-old to 18-month-old baby has no influence of his internal reaction because of his already undeveloped frontal brain lobes. Among other roles the frontal lobe of the brain is responsible for many facets of the feelings of the infant. Your toddler should feel intense emotions at this point. When he's stressed, exhausted, afraid, needing something, sick, or even need a change of diaper, he can whine and act out

The important thing to note is to remain careful when responding to the child. When he appears to like something, you ought to find out what that is as soon as possible. Sometimes, diversion is the only way to deal with whether your kid is behaving or "misbehaves"

Age 2

The 2-year-old baby is also unable to think objectively and his reasoning is not too intelligent to anticipate the implications of his actions. He also continues to grasp and use the words. He may obey basic commands, but often he forgets what he wants to do at halfway. He has a small anger tolerance, and can be short-tempered, show hostility, and have no control of impulses. He may choose not to do such actions because it is related to adverse consequences, such as a reprimand or penalty. He also continues to claim his power over other facets of his life, and starts to give commands.

Since your kid really does not grasp the reasoning and justification very much at this point, it is still easier to deflect focus or use comedy anytime your kid tries to do something that you don't want him to do. Disable things you might not like to contact him. When he wants to do stuff you don't want him to do, politely advise him "no." Create quick, aggressive reactions even for conduct that has significant repercussions including burning the stove or unexpectedly rushing into the driveway. Echo the laws time and time again. Ignore unwelcome actions like crying and tantrums because there is something serious to it.

Age 3

The child is more able to express its desires and expectations at year 3. While his language skills are more advanced, he is still not improving his critical thought. He can recall basic laws, but his urges are still provided in. It is the era he learns by repetition, that's why he likes regular patterns, and constantly hears the same songs and tales.

Say laws over and over again in order to punish your 3 year old, and make him say them to you. It's a vital period to remain calm. Should not be inclined to alter your reaction to his moaning or throwing a tantrum, if you say no. Rather of scolding him, start avoiding harmful items and other temptations. If he has done something negative or violent, pull him out of the environment for a few minutes. Keeping him without communicating or having eye contact because he doesn't remain there by himself. If the attempt to punish him is frustrated with him, do not give consolation until he calms down.

Right way to handle the toddlers positively

Here we discuss the following ways to handle the toddlers positively:

1. Know what you want from a kid you have to familiarize yourself with and empathize with the stage of your child's mental growth. Your one-year-old, for example, could not stay still for fifteen minutes, or your 2-year-old did not often tidy up after herself. If you want your toddler to hit the stage of advanced development, you'll probably be disappointed. Yet heighten your hopes as your child develops. Learn your kid too, and see what is best for disciplining her. Toddlers do not react to the training in the same way. Many kids react best to happy or friendly rebukes and some reply best to harsh reprimands.

2. To be successful, send your kid a gentle yet clear order to stop the behavior, remind him its wrong (why it's wrong if he's old enough to understand), what the result is if he continues doing it, and what he can do then. For e.g., for a child who takes a friend's toy, you might tell, "Roland, avoid catching Kathryn's toy. Grabbing is not pleasant. When you carry on doing so, you will no doubt be playing with her. Wait till she's done, so you can have your change. "Get along, tell his name, talk to him at his eye level, contact him, and get him to look at you. You should wink at him, after the reprimand. When he keeps on misbehaving, then carry up on the outcome you warned him about.

3. Consider arguing with older children, who are more vocal. These that help your kid begin to appreciate the thoughts and desires of others, as well as the impact of his actions on the big picture. For instance, instead of telling a plain "no" and "because I'm telling so," inform your older kid that she can only drink her juice on the table, because if she takes it to the living room, the juice might spill and create a mess on the floor. Any meaning, constant reprimand renders the child reluctant to do something different or angry peers.

4. Using non-verbal punishment when appropriate for small misdeeds. A facial gesture that expresses anger, raising your head or some other language of the body will be as powerful as physical reprimand for slight misdeeds if your child listens to it.

5. Whenever you may, keep your child from misbehaving. When an event or circumstance is likely a cause of misbehavior, when necessary avoid the catalyst in advance. For starters, providing her a daily routine of eating and sleeping will avoid hunger- and fatigue-triggered meltdowns. Sometimes, as your child has a poor memory, inform her of the laws anytime she might be misbehaving. Of example, you might say "Please drink your juice at the table" when you offer your child milk, or "Don't spill water on the tile" while you bathe.

6. Distract the child from difficult circumstances. The kid has a really limited period of time and then you can quickly switch his focus away from something that could trigger problems. There is less tension for both ends, this way. The more the diversion is tempting, the stronger, like an attractive gift, or a change of scenery. It's a smart idea to have a relief stock when you carry your kid to the public.

7. Any abuse is largely dismissed. General moaning, signs of poor mood and irritability, and other non-big deal actions should be overlooked as long as no one gets injured. You should use the technique with tantrums. Miss the kid before your tantrum runs out. Save the resources for harmful activities and those that may create unsafe precedents such as kicking,

scratching, manipulating hazardous materials and being physically dangerous. Give the most focus to your child while she is a cooperative. Offer the smallest focus when she is busy.

8. Place guidelines and restrictions, and then remain strict on them. Your child can continually challenge you to see how far he can expand the limits of what you'll let him do. He wants to find out what's good and what isn't. Let him realize about inacceptable conduct. Indeed, your child requires and desires well specified boundaries to keep him comfortable on how the universe works. If you've defined your boundaries, remain firm and don't compromise unreasonable conduct. Inconsistencies would only confuse him, and prevent him from knowing.

9. Do not lose your composure in remaining strong. Don't lose control there. Your kid can understand the message of punishment faster if you convey it respectfully and rationally. If you get incredibly angry and start screaming, then you can actually allow your child to react in the same way. If you're really upset with your kids, count to ten before you question them. Note your rage is not the same as restraint and venting.

10. Using simple instructions, and be short. The baby reacts best to the message and orders quick, simple and to the point. Using the fewest and shortest practicable terms to inform her, for example, what you want her to do, "Go inside now!"Or" Never fly! "It's 11. Render meaningful paths. Consider asking your kid what to do, rather than just advising him what not to do. Word the orders respectfully, for example "Roll gradually" or "Eat on the bed." Using "Yes" or "Off" less often, and reserve them to severe cases. (You should even make "no" emphatic by using a clap to gain your child's focus and stress on her the severity of the situation.)

12. Build a bond of love with your kids. Sit down and speak to your boy, and console him. Teach him to stop, and reflect about his actions. It's not an opportunity to punish the baby, but opportunity-out isn't the right approach to control a small kid at an early age. First attempt the friendly

corrective approaches such as compassionate demands, respectful appeals or even a kiss.

13. Don't give way to moaning. Whining is a transitional phase in the middle of moaning and being able to talk. Toddlers are banking on creating this sound to convey their anger and to show their wishes. Parents feel obligated to respond to moaning, so the irritating sound is prevented. This impresses the toddler, though, that moaning exists, and can become a routine if left unchecked – and the behavior may also continue to adulthood.

14. Be a strong example for your son. Be a role model for your kids. If you tell your kid not to strike you don't hurt your child. To your child your behavior talks clearer than your voice.

16. Look for ways to praise the kid for positive behavior – and not simply to punish or condemn him for poor behavior. Discipline isn't all about discipline; it may be a great lesson to improve positive conduct. Your kid enjoys your show of affection, and whether he is greeted with an embrace, a smile, an approval or a compliment, he will be well behaved. Try to applaud the actual action because, for example, it's acceptable to suggest "It's good to pick up your toys."

3.5 Positive discipline technique

Here I discuss the constructive strategies of discipline that I am familiar with these are following;

1. Give Options

You are less likely to wind up in the traditional power struggle scenario when you offer your children options instead of orders that they will use a 'no' response. This tend to evade both know for a reply and complete defiance. Children are empowered by choice.

And you're comfortable with all options, of course. Don't give your children a decision that you can't stick to, as that will only render you weak in their minds. The decisions don't should be so complex-it can be very helpful to only ask them if they want to do it. Instead of commanding "Move it, we get late" a gentle "Would you like to wear your shoes first, or the jacket first? "It's going to make them move with much less fuss.

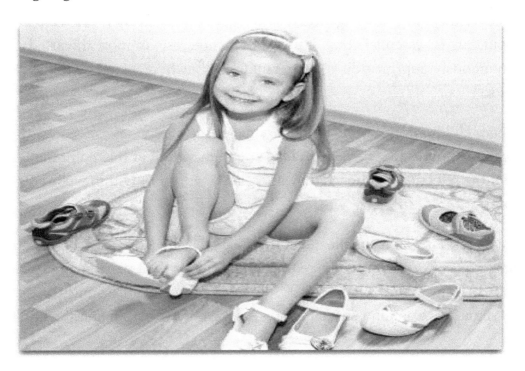

I will never forget my background as a very successful pre-school teacher employed in classroom. During the moment of circle one boy declined to comply. He followed the instructions of the instructor, punished himself and did his own little thing. One day, a couple of weeks into the year, the instructor wanted to test out a "newfangled" option theory. She called the little Mr. Independent in and offered him seats to sit at circle time. He happily took up his spot, and perfectly cooperated for the remainder of the year. The Teachers face expression of surprise was priceless. "I hope there's something different that everybody should know," she whispered.

The good thing about this much-recommended constructive method of training is that you encourage freedom, but also keep the reins. Kids enjoy flexibility and you're going to appreciate it working — win-win.

2. Build an atmosphere for YES

Children are born with a healthy curiosity, so they need the opportunity to discover their surroundings freely and figure out what their universe is all about. It is essential that this normal interest is not thwarted by continuously reprimanding your child for touching objects around the house.

When children grow older their innate inclination is showing their creativity and testing their boundaries. It is important at this point that you offer them the independence they are searching for but within well-defined limits.

Child proofing for smaller children e.g. placing out of control any dangerous or breakable items reducing tension for both parents and babies. Your kid isn't going to have to say "no" all the time because you're going to get some peace of mind ensuring he doesn't get into anything he shouldn't.

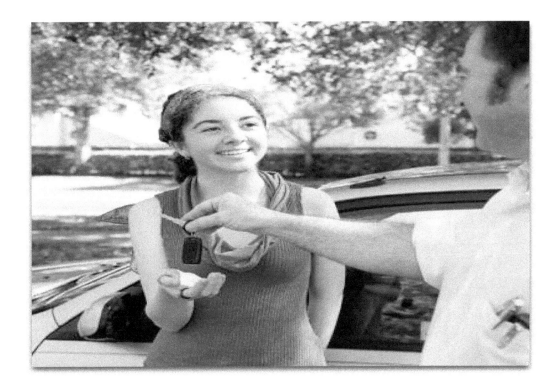

Positive Teaching Techniques: Creating a Yes Atmosphere for older children, clarifying what is and is not appropriate is important. For examples-" Yeah, you can start driving. However, we would then have to settle to a driving policy that any time you break that, you forfeit the driving right for a complete month" is far more likely to encourage the teen to drive responsibly than threatening to prevent him from driving (in which case they might be tempted to "borrow" their mates' vehicle to drive that without insurance!) or persistent lecture/haranguing.

When you sparingly use the term "no," as you do it, the kids will be more apt to pay attention. So make a concerted attempt to use constructive words wherever possible to avoid questioning behavior.

3. Teach emotions

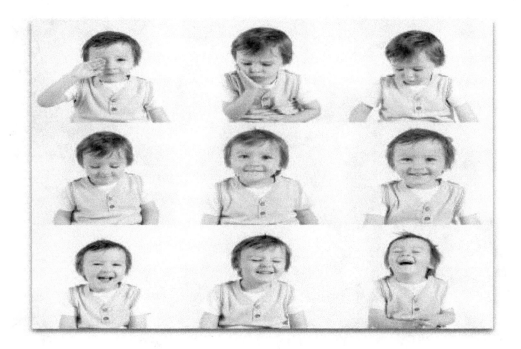

A clear map of the emotions may be perfect for younger people. You may also build your own by picturing the emotional expressions of your kids.

Teach them terms from this meaning language chart to expand their repertoire of feelings for older ages, so that they can convey themselves properly.

Rachel Wagner Sperry said in the book Flip It, "Feelings are the origin of all behavior," and then, "We will be conscious of what they feel, until we expect them to regulate it."

4. Ignore abuse

You have to choose sides and select fights. Most of the time, as a high school teacher dealing with teens, mother says she often pretends not to hear or see certain behaviors. Although this isn't one of the optimistic methods in training to employ very much, it fits extremely well with small issues.

Here's the thing we're not a cop, so we're behaving like one would drain. So, let's take a break for ourselves and our babies. Children are going to be children and frankly, don't we deserve any rest room as well? We can create and enjoy a more relaxed atmosphere in our homes, as long as we use this judiciously.

Children often get derogatory publicity. They strip away the pleasure of it by avoiding the negative conduct and the desire to indulge in those actions in the future.

5. Using Third Party Fictitious Mediators

For little ones, using a doll to model constructive behavior, or mediate battles. A third party will help make things calm down and disperse the stress. Choose a peaceful time to model good actions for a short puppet display. It doesn't have to be a sophisticated puppet but fits perfectly with plain handmade spoon puppets, Popsicle puppets, or paper plate puppets.

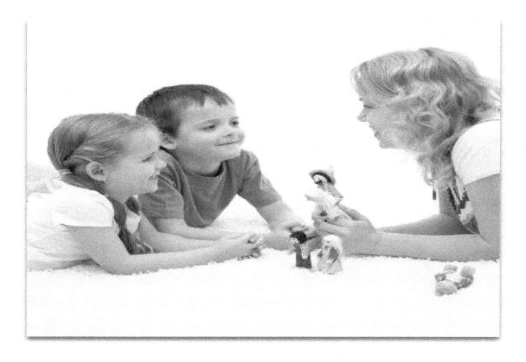

My buddy uses supper time with a doll to create healthy eating patterns. The kids enjoy the imaginative performances and they act during the series and supper as a treat!

Using the news reports or social affairs as mediators to encourage tough discussions for older children. Speak to your teenagers regarding the Ferguson, Missouri protests for starters. It's a smart place to bring up sexism, ethnicity, rioting and other troubling issues. Address things by exploring a range of views – from the point of view of the families and the ideals that you hold dear, from a wider viewpoint on what that entails within a society, the balancing between authority and duty etc. No one wants to be lectured all the time. A third party will bring a message out a lot more easily and with far less opposition, particularly a fictitious character or someone in the internet.

6. Detective Play

Why does the kid act out? Are there hours of the day or particular events more likely to cause stressful behavior? Might it be a warning for other children or adults nearby? Are there any environmental factors which may be a factor? (Example: too dry, cold, noisy, much noise unpredictable and the weather). Or will all of these conditions be a factor: sickness, allergies, food shift, drug shift, obesity, parties or crowds, caregiver transition, exhaustion, routine improvement?

See if the root of the tantrum can be identified before you leap to conclusions. Circumstances can affect behavior, and you should prevent potential outbursts by dealing at exterior problems.

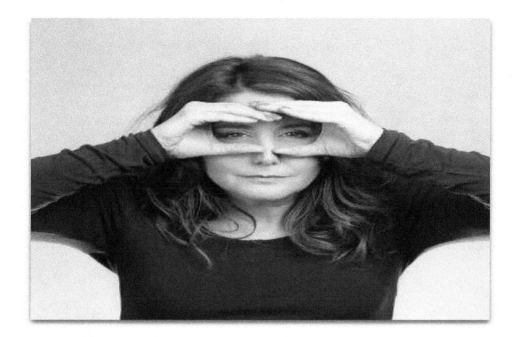

Another smart approach might be to document what time of the day the activity takes place. You may use the log ABC (precedent, action, consequence) to see whether a trend is developing.

You should have them for older children in the process of finding out what's troubling them.

7. Be compliant with this

Make sure you hold your training clear. Your child wants to learn what is appropriate, and what is not. And they judge, yesterday and the day before, on what was and was not all correct.

When they don't get a clear answer, so they actually not know how to act. This will make your child feel scared and insecure.

Seek daily to stick to the same timetable. That means having regular nap times, meals and bedtime, as well as free time for your child to have fun.

It helps warn your child in advance when you need to make a change. It will brace her for a completely changed schedule, and potentially discourage a scene from forming.

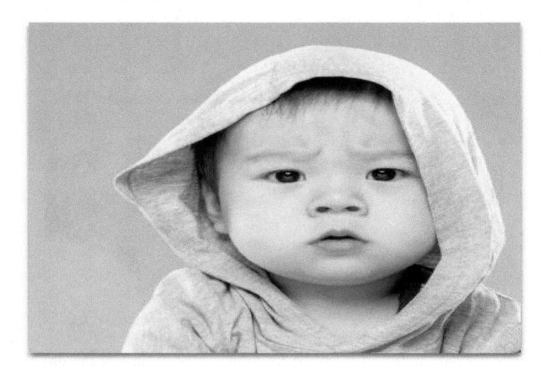

A quick handwritten book that the kid will re-read can be incredibly beneficial with a big transition, such as a relocation, new sibling or death. Place a photo of the old home, community, and current building, if you are moving. Write down what happens. This will give the child an understanding of what is going on, and will prevent myriad discipline problems.

8. Switch and Steer

Diversion is a perfect resource for juveniles to utilize. Little ones have a limited range of time so that should be exploited to your benefit. You might divert them from everything they worry over. Find something fun to do or speak about that could be of interest to your boy, rather than giving in.

3.6 Example of positive discipline

If you've never been good with conventional punishments for your kids, maybe the sort of discipline that you want to pursue could be constructive discipline. Positive parenting seeks to incorporate methods such as avoidance, diversion, and substitution to discourage the kid from doing something that you don't want him to do.

Good discipline proponents say this approach will help strengthen the relationship and improve trust between parents and kids. This also reduces the battle between you two and shows your child that it is important to react to tough moments without intimidation, bribery, yelling or physical discipline.

You should integrate four positive discipline examples into the parenting techniques such as;

1. Redirection

Little ones have a small period of concentration and when they act up, it's not too hard to divert them to another task. If your kid is playing with a harmful tool, add another item that will grab his eye. Bring him to another place or head outside to distract his mind if that doesn't work. Ask an older kid what they should achieve, and not something they can't. And instead of asking him that he should no longer watch TV, remind him that he should go outside and play or that he should focus on a puzzle. Focusing on the optimistic will every certain complaints and stubborn behavior.

2. Strong Reinforce

Praise positive behavior for your kids. When your child and a friend or sibling share a gift, remind her how sweet she is. When your kid expresses compassion to another, find out what a wonderful job she has accomplished.

It brings her more focus to everything she's done well; instead of highlighting the stuff she's achieved that go against the law. Explain how she will make a different decision in the future when the kid does violate the law.

3. Using time-in rather than time-out

Time-out may be an important tool, but sometimes it is overused. When a kid is put in frequent timeouts, he will shoot back to have him behave ever harder and attempt and gain your love and affection.

When the child is misbehaving, settles down and read a book instead of sending it alone before the child has cooled down and is willing to apologize for his actions.

4. Using Single-Word Files

Instead of telling your child (stop playing Take off your hat! Fire the toy!) Say a word in a relaxed tone: stroll. Dress. Dress. Swap. Swap. She'll not be angry about this subtle note, but realize what the correct action is. And occasionally you have to pick your fights. This may be seen as a failure of discipline, rather than a discipline process, and you ought to rely upon it wisely.

Chapter 4: Positive and Gentle Parenting

Parenting approaches are frequently discussed, as they may vary from tiger parents' strict techniques, to a gentle strategy, for example, for permissive parents and supportive parents. Here we discuss the facets of gentle parenting and the effect it has on both adults and babies.

Gentle parenting is a respectful and constructive attitude towards parenting, separate from the conventional strict parenting model of 'old school.'

It is a kindergarten characterized by empathy, respect, understanding and limits.

"Gentle parenting" is also used interchangeably with the concept of "relation parenting," although the two parents are somewhat distinct, both should be seen side by side.

Parenthood is a form of parenthood that encourages a connection with your children focused on desire and desires, rather than parental expectations and laws.

It teaches children what is healthy, rather than intimidation or anger, utilizing positivity and courage.

Sarah Ockwell-Smith is a parental expert who is a supporter of gentle parenthood and the author of The Gentle Parenting Book.

Sarah says: 'Gentle discipline just doesn't have to use these approaches. It's an ethos and it changes the way you think. It's more a way to be than a way to do. Approach all parenting circumstances with concern for the child and seek to understand the causes behind its behavior, work together to improve it positively and to acknowledge that which cannot be improved.'

Why can I find soft childhood?

Parents will strive to adopt the four core concepts of gentle parenting:

Kindness and compassionate parenting

Parenting when you are still conscious of the thoughts and needs of your kids. Usually, complicated behavioral circumstances arise where an infant is confused. Instead of denouncing a child as "manipulative" or "naughty" a parent will seek to consider the source of the child's abuse. A parent may prevent this in the future by discussing the underlying cause of the negative behavior.

Respect

Another main aspect of gentle parenting is consideration for your child as an adult. Parents also feel the urge to set out laws and expectations – to tell a kid what to do and what not to do. However, gentle parenting means respect for the feelings and personalities of the parent and the child learn to respect its parent over time.

Comprehension

The gentle technique of parenting understands that children have not fully developed and thus have no identical control over their conduct. With this in mind, parents will change their 'natural' or misbehavior standards. This is critical when a child has a sob or sleeping problem.

This interpretation must always be recognized by an adult. For example, when they feel the need to shout or lift their voice aggressively towards their child. Modifying our own actions is important to children's role models.

Limits

There is a myth that gentle parenthood is identical to a parenthood that allows children to get away with anything. Boundaries, though, play a critical function. The limits are not long sets of laws or legislation instead; the limits are about showing children a safe way to do stuff.

4.1 Golden rule of parenting

The Golden Rule is usually stated as, "Do to others as you would to you." It is present in every major religion and, also, in most modern life ideologies. The fundamental ideas behind this well-known rule are humility and reciprocity, recognizing that people will feel for you conscientiously and expect the same care for themselves.

Many parents teach the Golden Rule to their babies. Yet the basic spiritual message of the Golden Rule, where parents are adamant about improving their babies, is still a guidance that can be taken to mind by parents and potential parents. Children, wit: Respect your own mother, like your children should regard you later in life. This variant of the Golden Rule may be named the Intergenerational Golden Rule.

When talking regarding parenthood, parents prefer to understand how they educate their children rather than how they handle their own parents; however the latter is heavily affected by the former. Kids are committed listeners and brilliant impersonators, and the lessons they adopt are transformed into unconscious patterns as they mature. So far so comparisons are concerned, the experience of the own parents' kid would have a significant impact on how your children view you.

Everyone is flawless, and no one was the ideal father. It is quite enticing for parents to attach themselves to the chain of responsibility without knowing that they are prepared to continue their children in this practice. If you talk about your father, and your children are listening to your grievances, your children are likely to talk about you. Our culture is full of stories of people separated from their parents over alleged child injustices.

Below are a few items for parents needing specific guidance.

Walk the walk first and foremost. It must be nothing than a mere pretext: if you wish your children to show the same conduct, you truly must honor and support your parents. This may be challenging, particularly if your parents mistreat you, but someone has to break the chain of negativity. If nothing else, sever the destructive chain for the sake of your babies. Keep in contact with your parents and have your children speak to their grandparents. If it is important to repair fences, fix certain fences. Unconditional redemption in all but the most profoundly unfortunate situations can contribute to unconditional devotion.

Have social outings for your friends. Arrange your travels or invite your parents to come. Naturally, holidays provide wonderful incentives for intergenerational interaction.

Love your kids. Work about your friends. Do not only plan for or compensate for your parents' aged treatment, but share in the caring cycle. "Senior care problems such as depression and illness create significant challenges for elderly persons," says Justin L. Scott, Bratton Scott Estate and Elder Care Procurators counsel. "Strong encouragement from caring family members is a vital factor in reducing these difficulties."

Live close your house, or sometimes in the same home as your mother, if possible. This alternative is less common in our modern American society, but perhaps the most powerful way to reinforce the links between your families.

Stop quarrels with your parents or at least spare your kids the sight of these quarrels. Nothing refers to disagreements or conflicts – just hold the kids out. Seek the counsel of your parents and seek their guidance. It's part of the process to love your ancestors.

Explain to your children how, given their faults, you love and support your mother. You don't have to make lies, but you should be forgiving and imaginative.

When your parents died or no longer stay for whatever cause, seek to include your presence in your family's everyday existence. And if your schooling is less than good, teach your children happy things and respect their knowledge of your mother.

4.2 Positive discipline and parent child relationship

For all aspects of child growth, supportive parent-child relationships are significant. You will improve your bond with your child by investing quality time and displaying love, consideration and appreciation.

Positive parent child relationship

Positive partnerships between parent and infant establish the basis for the development of children. With responsive, attentive and consistent caring for parents, young children improve their life skills. Early parent-child interactions have major impacts on the social well-being and children's intrinsic ability to manage and fix challenges and their potential ability for relationships. During these experiences, children learn to collaborate alongside others and experience achievement in different settings. We know how to control feelings and conduct and develop stable interactions with adults and peers. They also learn how to adjust to different circumstances and settle conflicts. Parents are more likely to maintain healthy interactions with their children whether their peers, peers, community leaders and service providers maintain dry, comfortable and stable interactions.

• To offer relational and practical assistance to parents;

• To insure that parents accept diverse types of parenthood;

• To appreciate cultural variations and languages in the home;

 • To affirm the role in fathers and other partners;

• To help parents communicate with other parents and community leaders and services, and

• To strive for a successful parent-child connection result;

Positive parent-child ties improve infant growth and training for schools

The regular experiences between infants and young children and their parents lead to their social, physical and intellectual growth.

Parents that are receptive and attentive to children's signs lead to structured contact between parent and infant.

Such experiences allow children to establish a sense of self and model various emotional gestures and cognitive management skills (self-reassuring, self-control). Families, including very small children, should participate in everyday learning experiences to help them cultivate lasting inspiration, resilience and the joy of learning. For starters, parents should engage in early literacy activities with their children, including pointing and naming things, sharing stories, and reading. Early Head Start services projected fifth-grade mathematics and reading skills for the child to encourage connections among mothers or fathers and their babies. When school continues, parents may encourage positive changes and resilience through the involvement of children in shared literacy activities, such as reading and having enjoyable discussions on educational matters.

Creating healthy connections between parents and children from the outset

The move to parenthood may be a period of anticipation, tension and confusion for many parents and co parents.

Before the infant is raised, often parents plan for treatment by pouring a lot of time into worrying about the kid they intend. Expectant parents tend to become parents as they see their unborn baby growing and evolving.

People who tend to see themselves as parents and improve relationships through breastfeeding, have greater empathy for their babies, become more active in day-to-day caring and experience greater relationship satisfaction. Single parents and orphans, adoptive parents and other parents who don't have a parental or paternity connection with their children may of course often establish healthy partnerships and good relationships with their babies. Building a stable and balanced maternal atmosphere is another early phase in cultivating a good partnership between parents and babies.

Work on the consumption to prenatal compounds is nuanced. The consequences of cigarettes, drugs and alcohol are hard to understand from the effects of poverty, abuse, neglect and inadequate access to health care, sometimes compounded by the use of medications while pregnant. The required programs and legislation will tackle these problems. Shortly after conception, parent-child safety services may reduce the consequences of these exposures. Breastfeeding, for example, is a supportive influence in stronger ties between parents and children during childhood. Active and receptive feeding – through breast or bottle – leads to the shared connections between parent and child and encourages the development of healthy attachments. Attachment is the mechanism by which cares and babies communicate sensitively with each other from conception. They use visual appearance, facial gestures, body movements and vocalizations to build clear and enduring relations.

When a sleepy infant cries, a parent responds softly and lullaby, for instance, the infant confirms the parent's responses by calming and resting. Via the attachment cycle, parents are relaxed and committed to the well-being of their babies. Babies understand that their environment is a secure and trustworthy place to communicate desires and anticipate consistent replies.

Attachment and engagement studies contributed to a broad variety of expertise and a new area of science, infant behavioral wellbeing. The research of Mary Ainsworth and her colleagues has shown how attentive parenting improves children's mental wellbeing and protection. It also demonstrated how various types of discipline lead to all kinds of relationships.

Parents must not be completely attuned to their children at all times nor must they react perfectly to every of the children's questions. Daily, responsive responses are necessary wherever possible. When parents and children misinterpret the signs of each other, as they do from time to time, their relationship may be momentarily interrupted. This offers them both an ability to practice how to cope with quick stressful periods and reach out to bond again.

But if misunderstandings are the rule and the infant cannot depend on the attention of a parent, the child's growth may be halted.

Parent-child relationships are often influenced by the unique traits of growing infant and the match of the personality of the child to the adult. For starters, a very quiet child may be challenging to comprehend even an extroverted adult. Every parent, particularly one who is already overwhelmed, may be exhausting for a very active boy. These facets of childhood personality and other genetic characteristics, along with the unusual reactions of the infant to different childhood habits and styles, often influence the connection between parent and child.

Different cultures, various kinds of successful ties between parents and child.

In separate cultures, successful parent-child relationships can look very distinct. A broad variety of caring types, positive experiences and emotional reactions promote the balanced growth of infants. This can rely on your own personality, your personal experience, your existing living circumstances and your cultural goals and beliefs. Your answers will also differ with your gender. Moms and dads have considerable impact on the social and emotional growth of their children and potential academic achievement. Families of all sorts will raise successful babies. That involves households of two adults, single parents and families with many family members participating in care. It also requires people who are sole cares of the same and separate sex, siblings or grandparents. It is the essence and consistency of the relationships that is most important for the safe growth of children in any family.

Obstacles

Poverty actively and implicitly influences the growth of infants, the relationship between parents and children and the dynamics of communities. Poverty households are more likely to have low schooling and become homeless, rely on public services, and raise their children as single parents.

If households become lonely, lack money, and cope with increased tension and uncertainty, the likelihood of detrimental infant safety and behavior is higher. Child growth will be thrown off the track if parents feel anxious or need social care, or if they perceive the personality of their child as challenging.

Any such danger will present a challenge. When the threats are mixed, there is a danger to family treatment. This accumulation of risk factors will adversely affect the relationship between parent and infant. It may also adversely influence the vocabulary, cognitive and social emotional growth of infants. If preventive factors occur, they may also serve to offset the dangers – such as tangible assistance, social networks, improved leadership abilities and services such as Head Start and Early Head Start.

Promoting good ties between parents and children from the outset

Head Start and Early Head Start services offer practical resources and foster healthy child experiences while addressing the expectations of children. For starters, services encourage parents to find employment and safe homes, apply with school opportunities and link to neighborhood groups that assist them more. This form of support will improve the interaction of parents with their children by rising tension.

Head Start and Early Head Start services often offer psychological resources to caregivers and provide a significant impact on the interaction between caregivers and the mental and emotional effects between children. Parents involve their children more regularly and become more receptive with improved social interaction and less tension. Head Start and Early Head Start Home visits will provide social support whilst encouraging faith and successful growth results among children and parents.

Social help is one of the most significant safety factors against parental tension, distress and inefficiency (competency sense) Social reinforcement and the general sense of mental wellbeing also predict beneficial consequences for caregivers, such as:

• feeling confident as a parent (parental auto effectiveness),

• Constructive approaches to interpret the child's anger and growth and

• Overall parental satisfaction

Efficient parenting may also make parents feel less anxious, happier and less isolated. The feeling of confidence of parents will be enhanced by calling on the parents to:

• express their awareness about their children and friends,

• invest time interacting and studying with their children in the school,

• interact with their children about their houses,

• exchange home experiences.

Workers may also hear from communities regarding the societal principles and expectations that form their children's goals at different ages. Such priorities can influence how parents are receptive and react to their babies, children and elderly children.

In all these cases, Head Start and Early Head Start workers reinforce the connections of parents with their babies. It increases the effectiveness of the system, family involvement and learning outcomes for infants.

Important approaches to strengthen and maintain healthy connections with parents and children include:

• note and encourage the multiple ways parents help school preparation and

• alleviate parental tension by pleasant interactions with friends, encouragement from peers and individuals, as well as assistance to satisfy specific material needs.

Another approach to foster healthy parent-child interactions and to support households whether their children display problems or are identified with developmental disabilities. Late Start and Early Head Start schemes. Head Start and Early Start workers are also the first ones to speak to households regarding such growth issues. Their function is vital, skills and social assistance are given and children are linked with early intervention programs.

Head Start and Early Head Start staff will not be qualified or skilled to offer such services for children with serious difficulty or slow growth. However, they will serve as mentors, help children build their own leadership skills and collaborate with parents together. Staff will also help parents navigate regional services that promote the safety and wellbeing of their children.

Parent child relationship

Adolescence is a period where adolescents mature on many levels, eventually affecting parental relationships.

In puberty, children will respond to these improvements as they develop physiologically, and gain new cognitive and social skills. Social and cognitive developments can arise from alterations in social interaction habits and quality of near relationships. Impact is not unidirectional. Some work indicates that connections with parents tend to be valuable social and emotional tools well after childhood years, given altered habits of contact. However, this assumption must be reconciled with the common understanding of a decrease in consistency and power in parent-child ties during adolescence.

Theoretical accounts of the effect on parent-child relationships of teenage growth

Conceptual paradigm of relationships between parents and teenagers differ in the degree to which they stress transition or consistency. The prevailing view suggests that the physical, emotional, and social maturation of teenagers threatens the norms of children's contact. The results of adult transitions vary from one scientific viewpoint to the next, but they have a similar emphasis on teenage volatility and uncertainty compared to adolescents. However, recent trends illustrate characteristics of parent-child relationships that are persistent in the face of teenage development. The lasting relations between parents and children have been created.

The basis for consistency in the functional properties is expected to be the partnership which transcends age-related changes in participants' characteristics and changes in their content and mode of interaction.

Relationship shift in youth development answer

While there is no consensus on the consequences of such disturbances, most human growth models expect instability and uncertainty in ties during the younger years. Freud's psychoanalytic ideas suggested that hormonal shifts in adolescence offer rise to unhelpful sexual desires, promoting impulsive behavior and fear, which in effect hasten rebelliousness and alienation from parents. Later updates to the principle illustrate problems resulting from the promotion of individuality and the creation of ego identification. Parent-adolescent relationships are projected to deteriorate when increased tensions and declined proximity accompany pubertal maturation; disputes will reduce in late adolescence and attempts to regain proximity can be made. The cycle of separation and reconnection is intended to fundamentally alter the ties between parents and teenagers, such that children engage in relationships with parents as adults.

Evolutionary theories of teenage growth often begin with pubertal maturation, but here the focus is on competition from beyond the family to choose a sexual spouse.

Proximal structures are expected to help the ambition and individualization of youth, which raise tension with and decrease closeness to parents. More flexibility and independence from parents decreases the gap between the young person and the parent in order to improve the probability of the youth marrying with the unknown. While evolutionary views do not provide for the eventual restoration of parent-child closeness, as a previous record of responsive parenting suggests, parental engagement in the child may provide a foundation for warmth and affection to promote reconciliation in particular where parents give resources which help to improve the reproductive success of the child.

Many maturation models relate parent-adolescent interactions to neural mechanisms that mediate behavioral behavior. Wide development in the critical understanding of young people encourages an awareness of the individual gaps and a more balanced perception of parent-adolescent interactions. Conflict occurs and closeness declines when parents refuse to embrace young people's desires for a horizontal reversal in their vertical affiliations. Parents and teenagers must renegotiate partnership positions and obligations in order to maintain peace. When partnerships are effectively reconnected, tensions will subside and parents and adolescents may maintain closeness inside a can autonomy system. Children with such traits or actions generate different reactions from parents in child-driven models. Individual variations in teenage traits decide evolving relationships between parents and adolescents. One indication is the creation of delinquent or temperamental babies. Parents appear to react by removing intimacy and decreasing control to noisy, violent and undesirable babies. Child-driven approaches for adolescents usually concentrate on the effects of temperament and emotional control, although recent theories suggest that maternal behavior varies as well as adolescent issues linked to negative affective behaviors and internalization. In summary, models focused on child growth reflect systemic transition in young people and the consequent impact of this shift on ties with parents. These models demonstrate that improvements in family relationships rely primarily on the maturation of the teenager. This refers to a shift in the parent-child relationships of adult adolescents.

Link Consistency in Teenage Development Reaction

Models that stress family partnerships rely on stabilizing factors. The leading explanation, the principle of connection, illustrates the close interpersonal bonds between parents and infants. Parents and children function together in a jointly controlled mechanism to sustain the bond, in a manner compatible with cognitive experiences generated from their experience of contact. Adolescent attachment is different from earlier age attachment, but roles are identical. Protection offers young people a sense of faith when discovering worlds outside of the home, particularly new partnerships. These positive traits will be preserved in puberty by children and parents with a background of receptive, attentive relationships and deep emotional linkages. Children and parents with a background of unpleasant experiences will still perceive consistency, albeit in satisfactory, in the standard of their experiences.

Models of interdependence often demonstrate lifelong bonds between parents and adolescents. Throughout an interdependent partnership, spouse's trade affects each other and holds the belief that their bonds are mutual and permanent. Interconnections are internalized by participants and incorporated into conceptual structures that decide possible communication preferences. In puberty, greater control enables young people to affect parent-to-parent relationships. The way ties with parents shift depends on the degree to which participants see their interactions as mutually beneficial and which are directly related to expectations of connection efficiency. There could be growing tensions in low performing partnerships and a decrease in closeness as adolescents show growing frustration with care that is considered to be unfavorable. High quality partnerships can alter little or strengthen as partners draw on mutually beneficial communication trends. In brief, theories based on partnerships indicate that parent – adolescent bonds are immune to transition as they maintain a system of interdependence and lasting cognitive structures.

When teens are attempting to evaluate relationships with parents, transition takes place gradually and in ways that usually prolong the partnership consistency trajectories from earlier times.

Theoretical account of the effect on youth growth of parent-child ties

In this portion, we outline philosophical models that discuss the supposed effect of parent-to-child ties on the creation of young people. Most models believe, in the child growth processes, that parents (and relationships with parents) form youth development through intervening and overlapping interactions with Adults. We will continue with a summary of the various modes of influence and an outline of the proposed mechanisms of influence.

Predictors, Mediators and Editors in Parent – Child Partnerships

The primary paradigm for research into parent-young relationships is still models which expect participant-led results, usually from parent to offspring. However, relationship-driven frameworks are not uncommon and work designs represent this viewpoint increasingly.

Early perceptions of family control were primarily based on parenthood. This insight is more currency than analytical model as a study model. Most experiments also require simple estimation of teenage activity outcomes. Parental research, parental behaviors and parent psychological influence are significant in this regard.

Parenting approaches describe partnerships between parent and child dyad. Authoritative parenting relates to a mixture of acts that emphasize the interests and abilities of the infant while preserving the sophistication of age requirements. Authoritarian behavior is marked by utter carelessness in favor of the child's parental goal, strict expectations for enforcement, and rigid control strategies. Permissive parenting ensures low parental demand and child-centered indulgence.

Uninvolved parenting relates to infant carelessness and negligence. Findings show that strict parenting decreases in early adult years, lenient parenting rises and hierarchical parenting is persistent during adolescent years.

Parent style must be separated from parent practice. The parenting styles are global behaviors and relational roles, while parenting methods are particular techniques for children to obey, monitor and enforce standards. Parenting styles and activities are not an indication of the quality of connection, but rather are representative of the parent's perception of his position. Parenting types and behaviors draw on the traits of parents, but they are not characteristics. Parents adopt different types and activities for multiple babies. Parenting shifts as adults change their attitudes about parenting. Parenting preferences shift through familiarity of individual activities within different interpersonal relationships.

Parents are posited as causal factors in parent-driven models. Changes in the actions of adolescents are believed to be liable for parent or father-child ties.

Paths of power can be direct or indirect. Clear mechanisms suggest improvements in parent / teenage attitudes or interactions as a consequence of shifts in teenage results, such as improved adult supervision quickly rise in children's lies. Indirect pathways indicate parent variables influence proximal variables which in effect have effects on youth development, as could be the case when parent warmth facilitates an environment of moral optimism that allows family members to express feelings. Mediated models were often suggested in which parent variables function as mediators, normally between circumstances (e.g. community distress) and youth outcomes. The severity of the association between community anxiety and negative transition outcomes may, for example, be greatly decreased by a supportive parent-child interaction.

Parent variables are used as moderators in another layout. Usually such models begin with the assumption that qualitative disparities occur between classes. As a consequence, correlations between the indicator variables and the outcome variables vary among those observing various forms of relationships with parents and babies. Parenting approaches function as an indicator. Authoritative parents vary in a set of characteristics, which help to create specific childcare settings, from oppressive parents. Common parent activities will elicit specific outcomes. For e.g. adolescents with dominant parents are less likely to lie with oppressive parents than teens. Parent moderators will increase the danger for some young people and increase the chance of hardship for others. Some claim that oppressive parents can protect against negative peer effects for young people residing in disadvantaged areas, but the same parents can alienate the young people in stable situations.

These models evoke parent-child interactions at any stage in a causal chain as a significant impact. Models with direct effects suggest that parents contribute to teenage outcomes. Mediated model results indicate that parents alter an intermediate entity, which in turn contributes to improvements in teenage outcomes. Moderated models interpret the parent-child partnership as a source of adolescent control, impacting ties between environmental demands and youth transition.

Parent-child partnerships and peer interactions have a quantitative impact

A prevalent myth that is not firmly founded in literature is opposing parent and peer pressures. Because parent-child relationships are setting the way for the choosing and control of all partners, parent-child relationships are more of a norm than an exception. Relations have been recorded between characteristics of family connections, friendships and romantic relationships. Relationships with kin, acquaintances and intimate partners often have roles that overlap. Of starters, in maturity, but even with peers and intimate relationships, these roles are increasingly more common than the responsibilities of parents, but not removed.

For other households, parents approve of the preference of peers and intimate interests for their offspring, which ensures that there is nothing in the way of big cross-pressures. The growth from primary relationships to expanded social networks with friends to involvement in intimate partnerships shows how parents and peers appear to act as cooperative factors rather than as opposing powers. Parents have a stable framework for the first journeys of the infant into the peer social environment from which friends arise. Parents and acquaintances are inevitably the foundation for establishing interaction with future sexual partners.

Recent research toward parents showed that the latter was increasingly affected at the detriment of the former. The subsequent research illustrated the drawbacks of this paradigm and demonstrated that the relative effect varied through domains. For potential problems (e.g. education and career), the impact of parents remains stronger than that of peers during puberty, but, in contemporary lifestyle concerns (e.g. clothing and leisure activities), the effect of peers during adolescences decreases and eventually outweighs that of parents. In this way, there is potentially significant cultural variation. Compared to some in conventional cultures contemporary west culture will have an outsized control on leisure time. Aside from cultural differences, ties with parents remain the most dominant of all adolescent connections and form much of essential decisions facing teens, even as the relative control of parents over the situational specifics of adolescents' lives wanes.

Continuity and transition in relationship between parents and teenagers

Closeness implies love, unity, friendship and trust. Given altered patterns of contact, there is significant consistency between beneficial facets of interactions during adolescence and earlier ones. Surveys consistently indicate that interactions with each other are viewed by most parents and young people as cozy and friendly. Closeness terms differ between parents and between stages of puberty.

Developmental differences in relation between parents and teenagers

Confirming the concepts of commitment and interdependence hypotheses, social love throughout the first decade of life is the strongest indicator. Most families focus on enhanced teenage maturity by the development of experiences that promote interpersonal closeness, which is no longer related to interaction frequency. Families with a background of relationship difficulties, though, can be unable to respond during a period of relative isolation to different ways of closeness. Young people who record high parental warmth at the outset of their puberty undergo little to no decrease in perceived support over puberty, whereas those who indicate weak initial warmth rates show significant decreases in perceived support subsequently. In all but a few exceptional situations, however, perceptions about teenagers who are not communicative are alienated or disassociated from communities exaggerate the situation.

Of example, there is a major difference in proximity of parent-child relationships during adolescence. The time spent together by parents and young people falls in a longitudinal manner from pre-adolescence to late adolescence. Accordingly, in contrast with preadolescents, teenagers encounter fewer parental affection and familiarity and show declines in parents' approval and maternal fulfillment. Both young people and adults show fewer regular signs of optimistic feelings than elders and pre-teens. Daughters 'temperature reduces faster than sons' energy, partially because the former begins at a point greater than that of the latter.

Such patterns tend to be moderated by the birth order. First-born children show warmest interactions with mothers and fathers in puberty, but first-born children register the steepest temperature decreases from early to mid-teens. Not all patterns are negative: even in the middle and late teens, friendliness and beneficial impact between parents and young people continue to grow to pre-adolescent rates.

Individual variations in proximity between parents and teenagers

There is general understanding that family friends have specific backgrounds. How does that mean? What does that mean? For example, it implies that moms, husbands, and teens have various perceptions of their ties. Fathers consider the family to be a respite from work; mothers anticipate family responsibilities to be a significant source of tension and enjoyment. Differences between views of connection exist when experiences in form and substance are different between members of the family: Mother's interactions with children are more routine than fathers and much higher in this group are mother-to-child interactions than father-to-child interactions. In comparison, fathers commit more energy to social sports for young men. Participants view these experiences in their relationship schemes; fathers, trying to relax, try to minimize difficulty with their offspring, while mothers, who often experience negative emotional disturbances from work, can spend significant emotion in otherwise worldly behavior.

Parents and teenagers are especially characterized by their separation in early adolescence. Kids usually see the family very differently than their peers. Mothers and mothers agree more with each other than one adult does. Where mothers and fathers see special partnerships, young people see monolithic relationships. Parents, especially mothers, seem to respect the family more favorably than young people. Mothers show more love and appreciation within their families regularly than teenagers. It is important to note that at the onset of puberty, contrasting expectations of unity, expressiveness and encouragement are higher; parental and child opinions slowly evolve over time.

Young people have more time with their moms and are more inclined to express their thoughts. In comparison, teenagers typically see fathers as comparatively distant individuals who are mainly approached for knowledge and material help.

Sons and girls have equally warm interactions with moms, but sons are typically closest than females to husbands. Such patterns are growing with age. Pubertal maturation was correlated with declining closeness, particularly for fathers and daughters, and also a decrease in sons' time spent with mothers and fathers. However, some of these gender disparities might be embedded in past phases of the partnership. A longitudinal research has found that childhood parental engagement projected teenage closeness with greater relations for girls than for women.

Marital strife and divorce have a significant effect on the closeness between parents and babies. Divorced mothers continue to demonstrate less love about their children and start handling their children worse by increasing the usage of intimidating orders.

Divorced fathers appear to be indulgent and permissive. For split one-parent families, affection and familiarity are somewhat stronger than single, two-part households, but this closeness, when the parent remarries, often precipitously decreases. About 2/3 of children with divorce parents will undergo remarriage from their parents and almost 2/3 of such remarriage incidents would also contribute to divorce. Mothers and mothers, particularly in the first year, are usually less successful parents directly after the divorce. But finally there is a strong trend of strengthening interactions between parents and babies. Latest researches demonstrate the role of cultural diversity in the aims, principles and expectations of socialization. Research has shown that there are significant and persistent cross-cultural differences across class, family structure and socioeconomic backgrounds. For e.g., weak parental control means parental warmth for Korean teens whereas loose parental control means repression for North American middle-class teens. Furthermore, disparities in the focus on family obligation tend to be associated with discrepancies in positive results, but there is no indication that these ethnic distinctions produce significant group differences in the course of teenage growth. Even in cultures that promote teenage individuality and sovereignty, often children hold a large proportion of the beliefs of their parents surrounding family duties. Moreover, it does not seem that upholding such ideals has a detrimental effect on teenage growth. Any differences can be due to the condition of immigration. There may be a significant number of families in some ethnic groups where parents and children do not have the same cultural experience. As a consequence, refugee children are frequently socialized at home in one community and outside the household in another. This division of generational status contributes to sociocultural shifts in the family that have important consequences for the environment of the household as well as the developmental results of the infant. Recent research has shown that such various socialization platforms do not have harmful effects on the development of children and may have particular adaptation characteristics. However, they are also a cause of major conflict in immigrant families between children and parents. A particular difficulty for immigrant families occurs as parents require information about the new community from their babies. Children are cultural negotiators and alter conventional intergenerational ties as the infant becomes gradually interested in the family's problems and concerns.

Continuity and improvement in the tension between parents and teenagers

Disagreements in family partnerships are omnipresent at all levels. However, in teenage years, there is a peculiar obsession with confrontation as common beliefs find it especially uncomfortable. Surveys of young adults clearly showed that differences are more prevalent with families, followed by parents, peers and intimate relationships, followed by sons. Disagreements between parents and teenagers usually involve trivial things, commonly alluded to as 'garbage and galoshes' by John Hill. In contrast to polite disputes, disputes with the parents frequently include a mixture of common concepts and manipulative methods including strong negotiations, furious and hostile consequences and lack of performance. Much parental conflict is settled by compliance (on the part of the teenager) or disengagement. This should be remembered that disputes between parents and young people rarely have a detrimental effect on their partnership.

Development patterns in tension between parents and teenagers.

It has long been believed that tension between parents and teenagers requires an inverted-U pattern with tension levels increasing in the early teen years, peaking at the middle of adolescence and then declining in late teenage years. Nevertheless, a meta-analysis showed that this surprising pattern is an artifact of the absence of a differentiation between the level of confrontation and its affective tenor. The number of disputes between parents and children actually decreases from early to mid-adolescent and again between mid-adolescence and late adolescence, whereas in such conflicts the frustration rises from early youth to mid-adolescence and then varies little. Disputes are therefore less common yet more severe. Some indicated that late childhood and early adolescence could be the most contentious time for parent-child interactions, second only to younger years, but that no scientific evidence has been given.

None of the problems that precipitate tension between parents and children nor the outcome of the confrontation differ consistently with the young person's generation. There is however some evidence that settlement will shift over the years, as submission rates decline and disengagement rates increase. In late puberty, the usage of mediation to settle conflicts can often be significantly enhanced. In gestures of indignation, there is significant consistency. Negative effects create resentment, which results in interchanges between families engaged in oppressive disputes that deteriorate gradually. Changes in views regarding the validity of parent authority and decision-making are perhaps more significant. Parents and children need to renegotiate realms of authority over the years, but particularly during early teens. Teenagers see a growing number of personal problems beyond parenting, while adults tend to see the same subjects as concerns within their own authority. According to a maturational model theory, tension continues before positions are reconsidered. Adults see puberty as especially divisive because young people can seem too willing to deny the ways of their parents in the course of gaining control over previously controlled territories.

Parents and teens experience a distinctly specific interpersonal tension. Compared with the experiences of non-family members, findings from professional sources frequently suit young people, but not adults. While the fathers are stereotyped as the member of the family who is least aware of interpersonal complexities, the analysis of data suggests that mothers more frequently overlook and overestimate the frequency of parent / adolescent conflict. Moms almost unsurprisingly show the most detrimental consequences of disputes with underage children. Mothers may respond to a perceived power loss in the family. Youthful position renegotiation ultimately decreases maternal (but not inherently paternal) power. Parent and child dispute records intersect at long last in late adolescence, leading to the claim that differences play a significant role in aligning priorities and promoting contact. The level of confrontation in mother-child relations declines rather than in father-child relations. Conflict is recurrent and negative effect rates are higher in relationships between the mother and the daughter than in other interactions between the parent and the infant. Compromise is more popular with mothers than husbands, and retirement is more characteristic of sons' conflict than of daughter conflict.

Specific Parent-Adolescent Dispute Gaps

Connections between the tension between parents and teenagers and adolescence are greater than that of confrontation and adolescence.

Pubertal progression relates to the maturity stage of the infant relative to its peers. Pubertal status relates to the total maturity stage of the fetus. Pubertal status has little relation to conflict duration, but higher adolescence is related to moderate rises in negative effect during war.

Pubertal growth was proposed to promote the renegotiation of ties between parents and adolescents. Observational evidence suggests that fathers disrupted children through disputes at the height of adolescence and effectively retained their influential position in parent-adolescent decision-making.

Unlike the moderate results for adolescence, broad and comprehensive studies merge parent-adolescent disagreements with pubertal timing. Early-grow sons and daughters encounter more severe and serious disputes between parents and children than teenagers that grow in time. Such results have been discussed many times, several of which relate enhanced disagreements to parents' failure to acknowledge the opinions of adolescents that physical growth is a necessary foundation for autonomy.

4.3 Physical discipline and technique

Specifically, physical discipline includes employing brute pressure, such as beating a child with a stick, to force a child to feel some form of pain or distress in order to change the behavior. Typically, corrective punishment involves beating an infant with open hands on the buttocks or limbs to alter his or her actions without risking actual harm.

Training of an infant at any age is a challenge for caregivers. Most parents aspire to raise responsible, healthy and respectful children. There are many programs for children to be educated. Both will use training by instruction and the other will punish a child forcibly to fix unacceptable behavior. "To advise anyone to follow laws or to act in an organized or regulated fashion," is the Encarta Concise English dictionary. Physical punishment is focused around the utilization of intimidation as a motivation to alter the actions of an infant. 'Components without serious physical damage (i.e. spank, slap) are called corporal punishments, whereas conduct which includes potential injury (i.e. kicking, punches, burning) is called physical violence.' Parents who use such physical discipline of children ought to recognize the negative effects of their actions on the mental, spiritual, and social growth of a child.

Mental growth

The self-esteem of a child is built by caregivers who support, understand and cultivate their emotions. "Emotional awareness is especially significant because it reflects the early usage of psychological data from which children's future impressions and behavioral reactions rely." The idea that psychologists utilize physical punishment as a motivation to change a child's actions impacts their emotional resilience. The usage of disciplinary action is in clear contrast to what is used for punishment and may impact the growth of an infant. "To hit or strike is a terrifying and intimidating experience, which creates intense negative feelings such as embarrassment, depression and rage." "Children can be sluggish in meeting social and physical growth goals." Physical punishment impacts the emotions of approval of the infant and is more likely than to be optimistic to react with aggressive urges. "Children and adults affected by violence have been taught to use their senses to interpret or communicate constructive signals through their contact processes." Parents and cares ought to support children build competence, competence and control. Children who understand their own usefulness by providing easy options continue to gain moral understanding.

Moral development

Discipline, whether constructive or harmful, creates a child's self-perception and determines the spiritual awareness of how it will behave. An infant who knows how to strike can be puzzled, because hitting is inacceptable in many other areas of his life; schools, daycare and leisure activities. It undermines what they know in their families, which in effect is an advantage. Furthermore, adolescents who are subject to excessive punishment are on prone to become offenders. Parents who are not armed with correct discipline devices become irritated and furious at regulating the actions of their children. Researchers claim that spanking has its origins in two societal misconceptions, one is Fine if it is performed by a caring adult, and two is ineffective because all such punishment approaches collapse. Parents who recognize the tendency of their children to internalize all corrective action are often mindful that they are establishing the beliefs of their children. "The internalization of the confidence of children is expected to be improved by policy of parental control, limited parental influence, preference and flexibility and a justification for acceptable behavior." The short-term effects of physical punishment hinder the creation of a spiritual awareness of the infant and further disrupt its social growth.

Social development

The concept of violence of an excessively controlled infant becomes evident when its contact with other children shows itself. A kid with excessive punishment becomes traumatized at school. Studies say that adolescents become more socially aware and vigilant regarding nearby dangers. The resultant hostility is then mistakenly applied to everyone with whom the child comes in touch outside of the room, which is typically college, for example. Across a recent review by scientists focusing on pre-school students, students who are aggressively punished become more violent than children who have not been harmed and are more likely to be controlled by teachers. Kids who cannot deal with their pent-up anger respond in the school atmosphere in a destructive way. "The absence of social sensitivity is even increasingly apparent for the neglected infant." The emotionally controlled kid who matures and heads through high school for many behaviors, shows much psychological and cognitive impairment. "Insecure maternal relationships, lower intelligence, language deficiency, poorer emotional competence and motivation for intervention, more negative effects and less positive effects, less pro-social behavior and violent and inconsistent behavior." The initial relationship between child and parent is therefore essential to the child's development. "A good child-to-parent partnership is necessary as children are more likely to embrace parental constraints and to obey parenting expectations when there is a connection with the parent." Bonding and relationships are tensioned when the confidence is reduced to a primary source, namely contact between parent and infant. There is a great deal of concern regarding a child's relationship with other girls, parents, and even family members.

Children's effect with physical discipline can be negative in the long term, APA Resolution says

Resolution endorsed by the American Psychological Association suggests physical punishment to children by parents and other cares may impair children's emotional wellbeing and likely improve their potential for violent behavior. Alternatively, alternate types of punishment are advocated, which are correlated with more beneficial children's performance – such as organized parenting, consistent conduct, positive engagement and constructive dispute resolution.

"Evidence indicates that physical punishment is not successful in the long-term goals of parents to eliminate violent and disruptive activities in children or to encourage disciplined and socially responsible attitudes in children." "Research on adverse disciplinary effects reveals that any potential short-term advantage of physical punishment does not dominate over the downside of this type of punishment."

The resolution states that children learn about their parents' actions and, according to experts, "physical punishment will impart inappropriate dispute management behaviors." There is also evidence that physical punishment will lead to physical violence by caregivers.

The proposal was adopted at its meeting of Feb. 15 by the Governing Council of the APA. APA's Committee on Infants, Youth and Families adopted the bill, the representatives of which focused on a thorough analysis of scientific literature. They were checked by the APA boards and committees until a vote was held on the council.

The agreement encourages APA to increase general consciousness and teach about the effect on children of physical punishment and the value of alternative approaches. This calls for APA to promote culturally sensitive awareness and instruction for alternate curriculum approaches and their efficacy. This also encourages APA to promote study programs in the US and other countries on the reasons behind why parents embrace and depend on physical education.

"For the last 50 years, the usage of physical discipline for children has declined in the US," said APA President Rosie Phillips Davis, PhD. "We expect that this resolution will warn more parents and cares that alternative interventions are successful and much more likely to contribute to their children's behaves." A supporting argument referencing comprehensive studies into the usage and effects of physical punishment for children was included in the resolution.

"While physical punishment provides an efficient way to eradicate inappropriate child behavior, or to encourage children to cooperate with demands of parents, there are no clear empirical findings that physical training allows children more or less likely to stop undesirable behavior, or to indulge in acceptable activity in a short time," the supporting statement says. "Research also shows that physical punishment is not different than other forms of training and will not improve the beneficial effect of parenting, such as the growth of awareness or good behaviour. It predicts that even when regulating cultural, gender and socio-economic class, the usage of physical discipline may contribute to increased difficulties with conduct in children." Although cultural and religious variations in attitudes to and beliefs about physical punishment that lead to its usage, evidence indicates that the negative effects are the same.

According to the declaration of help, effective leadership strategies-such as structured modeling, consistent conduct, constructive engagement, and mutual mediation-" are more likely to create beneficial outcomes and promote a more productive and welcoming family atmosphere.

The statement accepted the restrictions on physical discipline study, stating that it is immoral "to allocate children arbitrarily to a situation under which they undergo physical punishment from the moment they are raised." Recent work has utilized rigorous experiments using many approaches and analyzed different samples. "For this reason, results from these methodologically validated experiments suggest that the usage of parental physical punishment may be negative and that certain interventions lead towards better child behavior over time," he says.

The proposal is being adopted by the APA, which comprises the American Academy of Infant and Adolescent Medicine, the American Academy of Pediatrics, the American College of Emergency Physics, the American Medical Association, and the US Centers for Disease Prevention. The proposal calls for the APA to discourage the usage of physical punishment. In fact, the universal convention on the inefficiency of physical training has contributed to the abolition of the activity in several nations.

Both children are incorrect. No children are false. Growing parent is faced with the task of disciplining its infant. It can be stressful anytime a kid has issues with behaviour.

Children require guidelines and laws. There are several approaches to control and improve children's behaviour. Examples cover constructive reinforcement, pause, loss of rights and physical discipline. Physical punishment, also defined as a body discipline, is performed in reaction to the actions of the infant to inflict harm or distress.

Examples of physical discipline involve cutting, dragging or pushing with an item such as a rope, belt, hairbrush, chain, or stick. Having others consume soap, hot sauce, hot pepper or other irritating material Parents who are violently disciplined as adolescents are more inclined to violently punish their offspring.

Physical punishment may impact short-term actions. Physical punishment strategies may, however, contribute to the following effects for the child:

- Bullying other children
- Violent behaviour issues
- Fear of their parents' weak self-esteem
- Hitting is all right

Physical punishment can contribute to more serious and abusive actions towards children in extreme circumstances. Abuse will trigger harm, lack of control, incarceration, arrest and even a child's death.

Many Behavior Modification Methods

There are several ways to foster positive behavior for your kids. A stable, pleasant and positive partnership with your child is the most important place to begin. The easiest way to handle your child's actions is to let your kid realize upfront what you want of him or her. Clear limitations include a sense of control, continuity, predictability and protection for children. Make sure that you always appreciate the positive behaviour of your kids. Healthy behavior is considered moral reinforcement which contributes to more of it.

As a teacher, a successful form of punishment may be daunting. Try utilizing alternative strategies for fostering positive behavior in your kid if you utilize physical discipline. When you have issues with other methods, address the child's developmental concerns, a child's and teen therapist, or another trained mental health specialist.

4.4 Strength and personnel growth

Self-esteem is the central conviction of an individual about himself or herself. The self-esteem of an individual is expressed in their behavior and in what they do and in what they say. While self esteem differs from time to time, it typically depends on a positive or negative self-vision. An individual is more likely to thrive in life with positive self-esteem.

While building self-esteem is a lifelong cycle, childhood is the base of self-esteem. The structure will do a lot to support a kid cope with tough life issues.

Adults have the greatest effect over a child's confidence in itself. When you let your kid feel that it counts, it goes well and allows him or her to build positive self-esteem.

Have these issues in mind as your child is born.

- Kids know like they are aware of their parents' way of communicating and behaving about them. Show your kid that you value him or her, and that you feel about him or her.

- Children know how well they respond to their actions from their parents. Praise children for their good actions and warn them when errors are made.
- Children know how to communicate with people when living as a team. Offer your child those duties for age-appropriate household.

How do you encourage your child to build positive self-esteem?

Developing a sense of identity, caring and supporting your child will help you establish positive self-esteem. The following are ways you will relate to your child's success.

Identity

By messaging us, we realize we are cherished, valued and belong to each other. Use the following suggestions to help your child know that he or she is part of your family.

1. **Display your devotion**. Demonstrate your affection. Let your kid realize that you value him or her because of who he or she is, not because of what he or she is doing. Making it a routine of expressing your child's affection in at least two respects every day.
2. **Let your child know it's unique**. List at least three of the positive attributes of your child and put them on your fridge. Attach such values sometimes. Celebrate the positive attributes of your child always.
3. **Praise your husband**. Your kids. Give encouraging remarks regarding the actions of your kids. Note the qualities of your infant, even when he or she is misbehaving. When you focus on what you want, the behavior of your child will improve.
4. **Listen to your dad**. Listen to your kids. Offer him or her undivided attention and listen closely as your kid discusses something with you. Don't offer advice unless you are told or believe like the health of your child is concerned. Don't insult your kid or taunt him.
5. **Have personal days**. Social hours. Provide daily activities for friends, including playing boards or table games to have fun together. Seek to

get as many family dinners as possible together. Do not speak at these occasions about issues or worries with your child unless it is absolutely necessary.

6. **Fosters constructive peer interactions**. Search for events of adults where your child can feel achievement and recognition, such as taking part in an activity or entering a club.

Caring

While learning takes place all the time, focus on providing your child with a learning opportunity at least once a week.

1. **Choose an aspect in studying**. Choose an experience that is beneficial that draws on your child's strengths. If the task can be risky or challenging, please let your child know without overdoing it. Enable him or her to learn of how such challenges should be dealt with. You can ask your child to help one of your tasks or hobbies. If so, make sure you don't feel hurried during the process. Let's have a nice time.

2. **Let your child seek**. Make your child seek. Even if your child has difficulty with a new task or talent, do not step control immediately and teach them how to do it. Let your child seek, be careful.

3. **Break up a tough mission**. Simple measures enable a child develop nuanced skills and make improvement. Don't shame the kid if he or she tells other people to perform tough activities.

4. **Lovely accomplishments**. If the job done does not reach the expectation, at least one aspect you may claim is optimistic.

5. **Foster work**. Do not demand success for the first time that your child discovers a new talent, such as riding a bike. Support your child not give up the first attempt. Encourage the child to exercise and speak during through exercise about his or her development.

Supporting

It strengthens our sense of identity and offers the foundation for continued learning and self-esteem. Using the following tips every day to make your child know like he or she contributes.

1. Family traditions allow children to recognize that the family aims for everything and allows them access to structure and tradition. Get as few social laws as practicable and regularly follow them.
2. Welcome collaboration. Daily family gatherings are a means for children to learn and work together. Family gatherings are a location where family leaders speak about problems and complaints.
3. Expect obligations. Through giving him or her household jobs, you will encourage your child to learn to be responsible. Make sure the activities are appropriate for your child's generation. As your child grows up your child must be accountable for his or her decisions and actions that will have inevitable or rational implications for your family.
4. Express thanks. Let your child realize that you value his or her assistance with jobs, like household labor.

Chapter 5: The Impact of Strong Parenting Discipline on Montessori Toddler

Parenting styles influence adolescents in the fields of behavior, risk-taking, emotional wellbeing and academic success Researcher identified three parental types as parental role patterns: strict, passive and permissive parenting. Such types of parenting are distinguished from each other based on their level of demandingness and sensitivity towards children. The degree, to which parents exert authority, influence, and oversight on their children, and place boundaries on their children, is overwhelming. Responsiveness is to the degree parents display affective warmth and approval to their babies, offer encouragement and justification with them.

Developmental psychologists have long been involved in the way parents influence the development of infants. Nevertheless, it is very challenging to identify clear effect-and-cause connections regarding parents' individual acts and children's subsequent behaviours. Several children born in radically different environments can grow up later to have strikingly close personalities. On the other hand, kids who share a household and are grown up in the same community will develop up to quite different personalities. Despite of these difficulties, there are connections between parenting styles and the impact these styles have on adolescents, studies have proposed. Some say that these consequences spill over into adult behaviour.

5.1 What work reveals about forms of parenting

Psychologist Diana Baumrind performed a report on over 100 preschool-age children during the early 1960s. She established several essential aspects of parenting utilizing naturalistic assessment, parent interviews and other methods of study.

Such measurements include corrective techniques, compassion and caring, contact modes, competence and management standards.

Based on those measurements, Baumrind indicated that most parents exhibit one of three distinct types of parenting. Further work by Maccoby and Martin has proposed introducing a fourth type of parenting to the three originals.

5.2 Parenting Forms

Let's have a deeper look at each of these four parenting types, and their effect on the actions of an infant.

1. Authoritarian parenting

The hierarchical model was one of three main types described by Baumrind. Children are required to obey the stringent guidelines set down by the parents in this parenting method. Failure to obey these laws usually contributes to discipline. The logic behind such laws is not clarified by oppressive parents. If asked to clarify, the parent the clearly respond, "Because I said so." Whereas these parents have strong expectations, they are not particularly receptive to their children. They want their kids to act beautifully and not make mistakes, but they have very little guidance about what their kids can or should prevent in the future. Errors are disciplined, sometimes very severely, and they often leave their children asking just what they did mistake.

Such parents "are conformity- and status-oriented, and require their commands to be followed without justification," according to Baumrind. Parents that display this style are also characterized as authoritarian and dictatorial. Their method to parenting is one of "spare the rope, spoil the child." They are doing nothing to explain the logic behind their petitions, despite having such stringent rules and high expectations, so they simply expect kids to comply without doubt.

2. Authoritative Parenting

The authoritative style was one second main style defined by Baumrind. Like oppressive parents, those with a strict parental style put down laws and instructions to be followed by their children. The parenting method, though, is much more egalitarian.

Authoritative parents are able to respond to concerns and attentive to their babies. These parents are demanding a lot of their kids, but they also have love, encouragement, and proper care.

Those parents become more caring and compassionate rather than harsh when children refuse to fulfill the standards.

Baumrind indicated that these parents "track and impose consistent standards for their children's behaviour; they are assertive, but not restrictive and invasive; their parenting approaches are constructive instead of punitive; they need their kids to be confident, socially responsible, cooperative and self-regulated"

3. Permissive Parenting

Now, the final form that Baumrind described became what's regarded as the permissive parenting model. Often mentioned as indulgent parents, permissive parents have little demands to make of their babies. Such parents never regulate their kids because they have comparatively low standards of competence and self-discipline. According to Baumrind, these parents "are much more sensitive than they demand; they are non-traditional and lenient, they do not need adult behavior, they provide for significant self-regulation and they prevent conflict."

4. Uninvolved parenting

Now in comparison to Baumrind's three main types, educator John Martin and Eleanor Maccoby suggested a fourth type, known as neglectful parenting or uninvolved. A parental style that is not active is distinguished by little requests, poor sensitivity and very slight contact.

While these parents meet the essential needs of the infant, they are usually disconnected from the life of their infant. They can make sure their children are fed and protected, but give little or little in the way of instruction, structure, laws, or even assistance. In serious situations, some parents can also ignore or overlook their children's needs.

5.3 The Effect of parenting discipline

What impact will these types of parenting have on results of child development? In addition to Baumrind's original analysis of 100 preschool students, several experiments have been undertaken by scholars that have contributed to a range of findings regarding the effect of parenting styles on infants.

The conclusions of these studies:

- Authoritarian styles of parenting usually lead to kids who are skilled and obedient, but rank junior in, social skills, confidence and happiness.
- Authoritative parenting styles appear to produce healthy, competent, and productive babies.
- Permitted parenting also contributes to children ranking poor in self-regulation and satisfaction. These kids are more prone to have leadership problems and continue to do badly in school.
- Uninvolved types of parenting list lowest in all spheres of life. Such kids appear to lose self-control, poor self-esteem and less ability than their peers.

Why does authoritarian parenting give certain benefits over certain styles?

Since authoritarian parents are more likely to be perceived as rational, decent, and just and their kids are more willing to cooperate with the demands made by those parents. Kids are often much more prone to internalize these teachings as certain parents have guidelines as well as reasons for these laws.

Instead of merely enforcing the rules as they avoid retribution (as they would do for oppressive parents), the kids of dominant parents are willing to consider that the rules apply, recognize that they are reasonable and appropriate, and aspire to obey certain rules in order to fulfill their own understanding of what is wrong and right. Of note, different parenting approaches often converge to form a special mix within each unit. The mother, for example, may exhibit an authoritative way whereas the father likes to favor a permissive approach.

This may also contribute to conflicting messages or even circumstances when the permissive parent wants permission from a child to have what they want. Families must strive to collaborate in order to establish a consistent method to parenting, as they incorporate different aspects of their individual parenting styles.

Parenting Work Shortcomings and Critiques

However, there are several significant shortcomings that should be acknowledged in the parenting style study. Ties among parenting styles and actions are focused on association analysis which is useful in discovery of relationships among variables but can't create conclusive relationships between effect and cause. Although there is proof that a specific type of parenting is correlated with a certain form of behavior, certain significant factors such as the personality of a child may also play a vital role.

There's also some evidence which behavior of a child can impact styles of parenting. One research released in 2006 showed that child's parents who had problematic actions have begun to show reduced parental influence over time. These outcomes suggest that children may not disobey as their parents are so much permissive but these parents with troublesome or violent children may only give up trying to take control over their children, at least in some cases.

Also, the researchers also indicated that associations between parenting types and attitudes are at best often low. The predicted child results don't materialize in certain cases; parents with dominant styles may have children that are rebellious or engaging in disruptive behavior, whereas parents with permissive styles would have children that are academically productive and self-confident.

All four parental types may not automatically be common, however. Also cultural factors play an important part in outcomes for children and parenting styles.

Conclusion

Montessori Child & Toddler programs delivers a curriculum that derives from growing child's unique talents and desires. The teachers develop new resources and exercises focused on everyday experiences that promote thinking and pique interest. At this age, your child's learning priorities include improving language skills, communication skills, problem solving, facial sensitivity and physical coordination.

The Montessori Methodology promotes systemic, self-motivated success for children and teenagers in all facets of their emotional, behavioral, social and physical growth

In this book we conclude that specific type of parenting, their way of talking, and their positive relationship, is connected with a certain form of behavior, certain important factors such as the personality of a child may also play a major role.

References

1. What is pedagogy?. Retrieved from
   https://www.tes.com/news/what-is-pedagogy-definition

2. Six Strategies for 21st Century Early Childhood Teachers. Retrieved
   from https://www.earlychildhoodteacher.org/blog/six-strategies-
   for-21st-century-early-childhood-teachers/

3. Book Review- Chapter 2- Tools for Engaging Cooperation. Retrieved
   from https://www.thisindulgentlife.com/chapter-2-tools-for-
   engaging-cooperation/

4. 8 Discipline Strategies That Are More Effective Than Spanking.
   Retrieved from https://www.verywellfamily.com/alternatives-to-
   spanking-1094834

5. Old, H., Toddler, T., Delay, I., & Toddler, H. How to Discipline Your
   Toddler: Age-Appropriate Tips for your 1 - 3 Year Old - Raise Smart
   Kid. Retrieved from https://www.raisesmartkid.com/1-to-3-years-
   old/3-articles/discipline-toddler-teaching-good-behavior-1-3-year-
   old-child

6. The little toddler that could: autonomy in toddlerhood. Retrieved
   from
   https://www.canr.msu.edu/news/the_little_toddler_that_could_au
   tonomy_in_toddlerhood

7. 4 Positive Discipline Strategies to Change Your Child's Behavior.
   Retrieved from https://www.verywellfamily.com/examples-of-
   positive-discipline-1095049

Potty Training in A Weekend

The Step-By-Step Guide to Potty Train Your Little Toddler in Less Than 3 Days. Perfect for Little Boys and Girls. Bonus Chapter with Tips for Careless Dads Included

CALEMA DUMONT

Table of Contents

Introduction

Congratulations on purchasing <u>Potty Training in A Weekend</u>: The Step-By-Step Guide to Potty Train Your Little Toddler in Less Than 3 Days. Perfect for Little Boys and Girls. Bonus Chapter with Tips for Careless Dads Included and thank you for doing so.

The following chapters will discuss the step-by-step instructions to potty train your child in just three days. Going beyond the bare minimum, this book covers not only just the physical steps that will need to be taken but also the mental preparation that will ensure that both you and your child are set up for success! This book will dispel the myths and misconceptions surrounding the potty training process and will outline how parents and caregivers can use psychology to make the potty training process more teamwork and less brute force. By following the system outlined here, potty training will be a shared goal that both parents and/or caregivers and their children will want to achieve together!

Not only will parents and caregivers benefit from learning how to create a spirit of teamwork during the process, but parents and caregivers will also learn how

to handle the potty training outliers when potty training is not going as it should. Learning how to best support children in a variety of scenarios is an important part of potty training successfully and in a healthy manner.

To set the reader of this book up for success, it is important to begin with a strong knowledge base of the physiological and psychological processes behind potty training, or potty learning from the child's perspective. In other words, parents and caregivers need to know the physical and emotional processes at work during this period of time in order to best support their children through it. A brief note to the reader: Be prepared to hear some "potty talk" in this book! It is both necessary and healthy to be able to use accurate bathroom-related terminology during this process. Ultimately you will choose what terminology you use with your child, but for the purposes of this book it will be important to use bathroom-related language, so be prepared.

In addition to the real-life advice found throughout this book, there is also a bonus chapter that includes potty training tips and tricks from real-life dads fordads still in the trenches! All too often, books aimed at parents and caregivers forget that fathers are an Important

part of this team, and the unique relationship they have with their children can be utilized in specific endeavors like this for ultimate success for everyone.

There are plenty of books on this subject on the market, thanks again for choosing this one! Every effort was made to ensure it is full of as much useful information as possible, please enjoy it!

Chapter 1: In the Beginning

As you prepare yourself to begin the process of potty training with your child, there are techniques that you can use to prepare both yourself and your child to set yourselves up for ultimate success during this process! A significant part of this preparation will be the mental preparation because the mindset that both you and your child enter into this endeavor with will largely determine how quickly you are successful. The process of preparing yourself and your child mentally for the new journey you are undertaking is called priming, and it is going to play a huge part in helping your potty training process run smoothly.

To begin, you must prime yourself to approach potty training in a healthy and practical manner. Sadly, according to the American Academy of Pediatrics, the premier children's health governing body in the United States of America, the developmental experience that has the most potential for abuse of children is potty training and it is easy to imagine why. Frustrations are understandable during potty training as pressure is high for everyone: parents, caregivers, and trainees! It will be important that parents and caregivers

understand how to best manage their expectations and any frustrations that may come up during the process.

Parents and caregivers are understandably anxious during the potty training process as there is truly only so much that a parent or caregiver can do. It is always ultimately up to the child if they are ready to ditch their diapers or not, and this is not likely an intentional choice on the part of the child as much as it is just the result of their developmental reality at that moment.

In addition to this, parents and caregivers are also under the additional burden of the actual work involved in potty training. While most parents and caregivers are more than ready to shuck the diapers to the curb for the additional ease and freedom of having a toilet-trained child, the reality is that there will be much more work coming down the pike before the child is fully potty trained. Before the child is fully potty trained, there will be plenty of accidents and additional laundry, as well as the extra mental and physical work of setting timers and organizing and developing a game plan that involves potty schedules and schematics for rewards and reinforcement!

Children feed off of this anxiety and pressure as they

often recognize the importance of this monumental task being placed in front of them. This has the potential to create power struggles around toilet use, and nobody wants that! It is understandable that children will act out and push back against this pressure and anxiety, and this is what can lead to unacceptable and even dangerous uses of force from parents and caregivers as unnecessary and unproductive punishments intended to manipulate their children's behavior.

Careful examination of the expectations that parents and caregivers hold over their children's capabilities as well as a solid game plan to complete the potty training process will help to set the parent and/or caregiver up for success with their children.

Some of the expectations that parents and caregivers hold around the potty training process are a result of myths and misconceptions around the practice that have been around for many, many years that we will cover now.

Myth #1

There is a magic potty training age that if a parent and/or caregiver begins, the child will be more successful in the potty training process.

Fact

Every child develops according to their own schedule! Potty training is not an exact science because every child will have their own distinctly unique timetable as to when their mind and body is ready will be ready to begin the process. There is no need to put extra pressure on the process by ignoring the signs and signals your child is showing you as to whether or not they are ready to begin potty training just because the calendar says so!

Most children potty train sometime between the ages of two and four, with outliers that begin younger than two and those that are still training beyond the age of four.

Myth #2

Potty training is something parents do to and for their children, not with their children.

Fact

This is as wrong as wrong can be! Potty training is not something that a parent and/or caregiver can do for their child, it is an interactive process that requires cooperation and teamwork from both parent and/or caregiver and child. You want your child to be your

partner in this venture!

Myth #3

Your child is being willfully disobedient if they won't potty train according to your schedule and expectations.

Fact

While it could be true that your child is willfully pushing potty training away, this does not necessarily mean that your child is being disobedient. As was discussed in the introduction, there are many reasons why you cannot force a child to potty train before they are ready. There are physical and mental processes that must be developed before a child can fully learn the skill of proper toilet use.

Myth #4

If you've already potty trained an older sibling using a specific method, then the younger siblings should also be able to train using that method.

Fact

Each child is their own unique and individualistic person with their own personal needs and capabilities. Each child develops in their own time and what may have worked for their older sibling (or their cousin, or neighbor, or playmate) may not necessarily work for them.

Myth #5

Once my child potty trains, there is no looking back!

Fact

This is a very common myth. It is not accurate, however. Most children do go on to have accidents for some time after potty training. The window for becoming a potty pro is quite wide for small children, with some children having accidents up to a few years after they officially "potty train" and ditch their diapers. This is very normal. There is much to distract small children and it can be very easy to forget all about their bodily functions when they are learning so much every day about this dazzling new world all around them!

Myth #6

If we potty train our child to use the toilet during the day, we should potty train our child to stay dry throughout the night, too.

Fact

There are schools of thought regarding potty training that believe that potty training should be an "all or nothing" sort of experience, and this includes getting rid of any sort of diaper or pull-up type of training pants at nighttime. However, potty training at night is actually a completely different process than the process for potty training during the day because a child's ability to stay dry throughout the night has less to do with learning proper toileting habits and bodily signals and more to do with night time hormones related to urine production and the degree to how heavily your child sleeps. Most doctors and urologists agree that nighttime bladder control is not an issue until the child is around seven years old.

As you can see, there are many myths and misconceptions surrounding the potty training experience that can set a parent and/or caregiver up for expectations that can't be met. Sometimes this is a result of failing to recognize what potty learning truly is for the child.

For a child that has been diapered since birth, learning how to ditch their diapers requires a whole world of

complexity that parents and caregivers often do not take the time to consider. For their tiny little bodies and minds, they have never had to pay much attention to their elimination habits. They've always just had their waste products exit their bodies when it needed to, without any real consideration or effort on their parts. To begin the potty training process, parents and caregivers must realize that they are essentially starting from scratch!

The child must first learn to be aware of her body and its functions. This requires an awareness that what is consumed will need to then exit the body as a waste product eventually. For some children, this is a surprise! Taking the time to help teach them this connection is an important building block in the potty training process. They need to understand that the juice box they just drank will be ready to come out within the next hour or so, and this will be an important part of the methodology in Chapter 2 when you are introduced to the steps of the three-day potty training method.

In addition to being aware that what comes in must go out, children must then learn to be aware of what it

feels like *before* they need the toilet. Again, they have never needed to be aware of the sensation of a full bladder in need of emptying in their life, their bodies have just released whenever they needed to without any help or awareness on the part of the child. This process of paying attention to the body and learning to associate the sensations of their body with the need to sit on the potty chair is often one of the most aggravating aspects of potty training for both the child and their parents and/or caregivers.

One way to facilitate your child's learning about their bodily functions and the awareness of when they need to visit the restroom is to model this for them with your actions. This would include announcing to your child when you need to use the restroom and using descriptive language that they will understand. You will know your child best, but this could sound something like, "Oh, I think that glass of water I just drank is ready to come out! My bladder feels full, I need to pee/urinate/whatever terminology you choose," and you would say this while perhaps poking one finger into your lower abdomen over your bladder. Or perhaps you might say, "Oh, my stomach hurts a little bit down here,

I need to poop/defecate/whatever terminology you choose," and you would also say this while motioning to your lower abdomen. The point here is to help your child learn where these parts of their body are so they can begin to associate these areas with making a trip to the potty. You are also teaching them the language they will need during their potty training experience.

The other crucial element here is in modeling the actual process for our children. Children are visual creatures, and they love to do what they see others doing! For most children, their primary caregivers and/or parents are their primary models of behavior and being allowed to see a parent and/or caregiver sit on the toilet and go through the process themselves can give them a clear example of how they're supposed to do it. It is also important here to narrate the process for your little one, like this: "Okay, I have to pee now so I'm going to the potty. I'm going to pull my shorts down and sit here on the potty. Okay.... Now I just need to let my pee out! There it is, can you hear it? That's my pee going into the toilet! Alright, now I can grab a little bit of toilet paper, just like this, and wipe myself clean. Now I just need to toss it in the potty, pull my shorts back up, and

flush! Ready to hear the toilet flush? Here it goes and WOO! Alright, now I get to wash my hands! I like this soap, it's blue. Pretty cool, right?"

Notice in the narrative above that the parent and/or caregiver is not only narrating each part of the experience, but they are also making the entire experience sound like fun! Children will want to also be able to mimic this experience, especially aspects like flushing the toilet. The entire experience needs to be described like it is something that is a great part of growing up. This is a part of priming the experience for your child. If the experience is primed as something fun and attractive, your child will join you in this quest rather than resist you.

In addition to this physical learning about the parts of your child's body and their awareness of them and what they do, there is a cognitive aspect that is required in potty training. Children must be able to not only feel the sensation of a full bladder or a bowel movement, but they must also be able to reason and rationalize with themselves to a certain extent. Young children often struggle with this part of the potty training process because it can be difficult for them to

understand and engage in delayed gratification or time awareness. If a child is playing with their favorite toy in the living room, it won't matter too much if they feel the pressure of a full bladder and understand what that means if they don't have the cognitive skills yet to understand that they can set the toy down to go to the restroom and then come back for the toy again. For young children, they live in the moment, every moment. This cognitive awareness is one of the most crucial aspects of potty training and one of the reasons why so many of the "potty training tips and tricks" geared towards young toddlers do not work. A very young toddler simply will not have this cognitive awareness down enough to be able to make this choice, and this can lead to serious bladder and bodily issues when they are trained to hold their waste anyway.

This is why pediatrician and urologist groups caution against enforcing any potty training protocol before a child is displaying at least the following signs of readiness: able to communicate their need to use the toilet either verbally or nonverbally, can physically get themselves to the restroom safely and efficiently by either walking or crawling, can dress and undress themselves to use the toilet, and can sit safely on a

toilet seat unassisted. Enforcing a potty training program before a child is ready can result in urinary tract infections, kidney damage, constipation, and a lifetime of poor toileting habits.

Parents and caregivers can assess if their child is cognitively prepared to begin the potty training process by gauging how much interest and self-awareness the child has around all things potty related. Ask yourself the following questions to see if your little one is cognitively prepared for potty training!

- Does your child express interest in the toilet by following family members into the restroom or commenting on "going potty" when it is mentioned?

- Does your child express interest in "being a big kid" and want to do what older siblings and older children do?

- Does your child express when their diaper is soiled by pulling on the wet/dirty diaper, trying to remove it or even removing it themselves, and/or announcing that they need a diaper change?

If you answered yes to all three of these questions, then

it is very likely that your child is cognitively prepared to begin the potty training process! Ask yourself the following questions to see if your little one is physically prepared for potty training!

- Is your child able to verbally and nonverbally express their physical needs, such as by asking for something to drink when thirsty or by stating they are cold and need a sweater?

- Is your child able to physically get themselves, without assistance, to the toilet and back by crawling or walking?

- Is your child able to dress and undress themselves efficiently enough to do so in the restroom largely unassisted?

- Is your child able to safely sit unassisted on a toilet or potty chair?

If you answered yes to all of these questions, then it is very likely that your child is physically prepared to begin the potty training process!

Once your child is demonstrating the cognitive and physical signs of readiness for potty training, then you can safely move on to the three-day potty training

system! But first, a few words on the mental preparation moving forward.

You and your child will need to be a team in this endeavor. Not only is this necessary because one person cannot force another person to use a toilet (not safely and respectfully, anyway!) but it is also a matter of simple psychology.

Toddlers want to please their parents and caregivers- although it may not always seem like it! This perception happens because, for so much of those early childhood years, children have little to no bodily autonomy or control over where they go or what they do. This leaves them very few opportunities to assert their independence and capabilities in a healthy and constructive manner. This often translates then to what adults often view as being "petty" demands and tantrums, such as may occur over what color cup the child wants to drink out of or whether the child wants to put on their shoes or not.

Step back a moment and try to look at it from this tiny person's perspective for a moment: If you had no control over what time you woke up in the morning, what you had available to eat, no capabilities to perform

the majority of the tasks being performed around you (cooking, driving, talking on the phone, etc) and little to no choice over how you spend your days, wouldn't you also on occasion feel the need to make a choice of your own, on your own terms, no matter how trivial it may seem to others? This is the perspective of the small child, and the more that parents and caregivers can explore and understand this, the better they will be able to work with their child's psychology so that everyone can experience a win.

This is where the psychology behind team building comes in. Parents and caregivers don't need the potty training process to be any more difficult than what it already will be and should take all the help they can get! This includes the help of their small child, and it begins with how the child is approached with the process of potty training.

The child should never be made to feel as if potty training is an event that is coming up that they will be forced to be a part of, but rather should feel as if they are making the decision to begin potty training. This is easy enough to do for most children between the ages of two and four because this age range is typically in

the "I want to do it all by myself" mentality as they are looking to develop more of the autonomy and independence, they see being exercised by older people around them.

A note to parents and caregivers on how they speak to one another about the potty training process: Watch how you are wording your conversations within earshot of your small child. Keep in mind that children are almost always listening, even when they appear busy at play.

Comments that may not seem like much of a big deal can play into negative perspectives about the potty training process when heard by young ears that don't entirely understand what it all means. An example of this might sound something like, "We plan on <voice dropping conspiratorially> *potty training* this weekend," or "I just hope it's nothing like <insert name of child's playmate here> because their mom told me it was absolutely miserable! They spent months fighting it." This is even more of an issue for those comments that are made between parents and caregivers where there is visible negative body language such as head shaking, eye-rolling, or whispering behind hands.

Children are more aware of these social cues than parents and caregivers often assume, and this is not a good way to prime the potty training experience for your child!

In the interest of setting up the experience of potty training as a shared goal and shared effort, look around for examples of meaningful models that your child may use for potty training. Is there an older sibling that they look up to? Is there maybe an older neighbor that is close to the family? Or perhaps a favorite cartoon character?

Remember, you want your child to *want* to potty train, otherwise, it will be you trying to *force* your child to complete this developmental process, and this rarely works. Think about other developmental leaps that children take such as crawling, walking, and even talking. Has any parent and/or caregiver ever succeeded in forcing a baby to crawl? Is there any physical way to force a baby to walk when they simply don't have the leg and core strength and coordination between their body parts? How about forcing a baby to walk that simply doesn't have any interest in it yet because they still prefer to crawl? No, of course not.

Just as we encourage our children to learn to talk by modeling it for them and engaging with them verbally in a fun way, we can do the same with the developmental process of potty training.

Keeping this in mind, enlist the help of the meaningful models that you know your child will look up to and want to emulate. If it is an older sibling, ask the older sibling to join in on the modeling of bathroom behavior by both physically modeling the process and narrating in a fun and upbeat way. The older sibling can even say things like, "someday you will be able to do the potty just like me! Isn't that cool?"

If your child's meaningful model is a neighbor, you can ask the neighbor to announce before they have to run to the restroom, saying in an excited voice, "I have to go to the potty now, I'll be right back to keep playing with you in just a moment!" This would model both the process of making the decision to go to the toilet and also the idea that you can take a quick break from playing to go to the restroom and come right back to it.

If your child's meaningful model is a beloved cartoon character, then use that! There are a variety of ways that you can make this happen. There are many cartoon

character toys that demonstrate the potty process and even sing cute little songs about going to the restroom, and they are available from major retailers; a quick google search will reveal what is available in that department.

There are also several cartoon episodes dedicated to teaching children how to go to the potty, and these are available in many different streaming services such as Netflix, Hulu, Amazon Prime, and PBS Kids, to name a few. They are also largely available via a quick google search, so do take advantage of that!

One children's show that is renowned for its successful induction of children into the potty training experience is PBS Kids' Daniel Tiger's Neighborhood and their episode, "Daniel Goes to the Potty." This episode features the beloved main character, Daniel Tiger, learning to go sit on the potty. The song that Daniel sings every time he feels the urge to go to the potty is incredibly catchy and memorable and has been used successfully by many a parent and caregiver to remind a child that they need to go sit on the potty!

If you are a screen-free family and have no interest in using media to help during the potty training process,

then feel free to be creative and make up your own potty training song for your little one to sing! The catchier, the better. Make it something fun and upbeat that your child and you enjoy singing every time they need to go sit on the potty. This is a part of keeping the experience fun and upbeat. It's amazing what our children will do in pursuit of light-hearted fun with their parents and caregivers!

To further prime the potty training experience for your child, you can determine how to best set up your restroom for your child. Many parents and caregivers choose to use an independent potty chair, which is the small, child-size potty that can be purchased at any major retailer/big box store or online. An advantage of this is the safety feature of it being their perfect size and situated firmly on the ground. There is also a feeling of pride in ownership that many children feel when they have their very own little potty, just for them to use. Some parents even take their children with them to the store to pick out their very own potty chair or give them stickers to decorate the potty chair and make it their own.

Another option is to purchase one of the seat modifiers

that are also available through any major retailer and big box store or online that either attaches to the regular toilet seat or can be easily placed on top that makes the toilet seat a more child-friendly size. There are a few advantages to this, such as if bathroom space is limited and there is simply no room for another potty chair in the same room. Some children even prefer this option over the standalone child-size potty chair because they feel like more of a "big kid" with this option, and this seems to be the case more often when there is an older sibling as the child's meaningful model.

Another option that is similar to the seat modifier is to simply add a safety stool for the child so they can more easily get up on the regular toilet themselves. Often times this option can even be found with a hand-rail so they have something to keep their balance while climbing on and off. An advantage of this particular option is that it fulfills the same desire of the child to feel like a "big kid" in using the regular potty, and it also teaches them the necessary skills to navigate the regular-sized toilets they will find outside of the home. This can be very helpful for some children that may be uneasy about moving from the child-size options at

home to the regular size toilets that they will find while using the restroom outside of the home.

Whatever potty option you choose, be sure to tailor it to your child and their needs. If you know that doing it "just like the big kids do" is going to be a big motivator, then perhaps it might be best to go with the options that modify the standard size toilet. If you know that your child doesn't like sitting on full-size chairs as well as smaller child-size chairs, then perhaps the child-size potty chair is best. If you know your child is always excited to sit in regular-sized chairs to be "like a big kid" then using the regular toilet with a safety addition might be the right incentive for them.

Your shopping trip also needs to include some favorite beverage options for your child. This is important because you will need to have your child drinking plenty of fluids during the three-day potty training weekend. This is to ensure that your child is experiencing a full bladder and the sensations that come along with it as you teach your child to associate that sensation with the need to go sit on the toilet. Parents often opt for both regular favorites and "special" beverages that the child rarely gets so there will be no question as to if the child will be interested in drinking them. You know your child best, but fruit juices, lemonades, or any sort of sweet beverage is usually always a hit with any small child!

The next thing to gather in preparation for your three-day potty training process is the underwear that your child will be replacing their diapers with! Many children really get a kick out of picking out their "big kid" underwear, so take them shopping with you. This also plays into the pride of ownership psychology, in which you want your child to feel like they have some control here, too. Really have fun with this, talk it up at the store and make it exciting and fun to get to pick out underwear with their favorite characters, colors, and patterns on them. Remember, this is all a part of priming the experience for your child!

Pro tip from a parent that has been there, done that: However, many pairs you think you need to start off with, double it. At the very least, double it! It is very likely that you will need them- and then some- during your potty training weekend extravaganza, so prep yourself well here!

Another important shopping trip that must take place

before the three-day potty training process is the trip in which you procure the treats and rewards that you will use to keep your child associating potty use with celebration and reward. Parents and caregivers will know their children best, but whatever you do, diversify your treat and reward supplies!

Some common ideas for treats and rewards that are often used during the potty training process are small candies such as skittles, smarties, or M&Ms that allow for sweet, exciting treats to be doled out just a couple at a time. Stickers with favorite cartoon and storybook characters on them and little puzzle and workbook-style books that your child can interact with are always a big hit! Some parents and caregivers like to create a treasure box of sorts for the potty training experience that the child gets to pick out after they've had a successful trip to the potty, and this is often filled with a variety of sweet treats and small prize style toys. Dollar stores often provide a great value for this avenue, as you can buy many little exciting "treasures" for the child that won't break the bank! Anything that is new and different is typically enough to incentivize a child to want to participate in the potty training process so they can earn their rewards!

Some parents and caregivers choose to share the treasure box with the child the day before the potty training process kicks off by letting the child take a peek and know that tomorrow, they will get a chance to check it out and pick items out for themselves when they use the big-kid potty. This gives them an element of excitement to associate with the big day!

Before the child heads off to bed the night before the potty training weekend, you can let them know that tomorrow you will be throwing away the diaper they are wearing and they will get to wear their big kid underwear and try the big kid potty! Let them know they will get to pick prizes out of the treasure box every time they pee or poop on their potty and that you will be right there with them to celebrate with them. Make sure they hear that you are excited for the next day and you are confident that you guys will have a great day. Let your child drift off to sleep imagining the exciting things awaiting them the next day!

In order to successfully utilize the Potty Training in A Weekend methodology, it is important to have a three-day long weekend devoted exclusively to the potty training process. This means that there need to be

three days dedicated to the potty training process. No trips to the park, no running to the grocery store, no guests in the house to distract the parent and/or caregiver, and if you can swing it, siblings either 100% on board with helping be a part of this process or spending the long weekend out at a friend's house. The only thing you and your child should be doing over the course of this three-day weekend will be sharing this potty training experience!

Parents and caregivers that have been there and done that during this process recommend ensuring that you have the laundry and other household chores caught up, including meal planning and prepping so that your mind can remain exclusively focused on the task at hand. There will be accidents- make sure you're not the cause of them because you were distracted taking care of some household chore!

The Potty Training in A Weekend method has gained steadily in popularity over the course of the last decade, particularly in Western countries, with varying degrees of difference in each guide. The guide provided in this book is set up in such a way that you can learn about the many variances to this methodology and choose to

adopt what you believe will work best for you and your little one. Just as every child is uniquely individual, so too is the home setup and the pattern of each individual household. View the guide here as a buffet of sorts: choose what you like and leave the rest.

Your results will vary because every child is an individual, but Potty Training in A Weekend method, when approached in a focused and mindful manner on the part of the parent and/or caregiver, is guaranteed to provide a bedrock foundation for your child's potty training prowess. Your goal should not be a 100% accident-free, potty using a child at the end of this weekend, but rather a child who is well on their way to becoming one.

Now that you have done the setup work to prime both yourself and your child to have the best mindset going into this process, you are ready to begin to delve into the step by step guide of potty training in a weekend.

Chapter 2: Potty Training in A Weekend

Day 1: Welcome to the Big Day!

Wake up and get yourself set up immediately with timer reminders before you even wake your child up for the day. Most people choose to use their smartphone for this, but if you do not have a smartphone, then any clock, watch or another electronic device that has a timer and alarm capability will do! It is best if it is a timer that is portable and you can move around with you as you move around your home, but if you are using a stationary alarm such as a microwave or stovetop, then just be aware of keeping the volume down on other electronics and outside noise throughout the day so you can hear the alarm.

The alarm will cue you to each and every time that you will need to take your child to sit on the potty. This should be approached as an exciting, fun thing for the first day. Every time the alarm sounds, react as if you are thrilled to be hearing it. Your child will catch on to this and be happy to hear it, too.

Your first alarm needs to be set for exactly 15 minutes after your child gets set up for the day, so set that up

as you go in to get your child out of bed. Building on what you began the day before, get your child out of bed in a fun and playful manner, reminding them of the exciting day you two have planned!

Keep your language here simple and direct so as not to confuse your child too much on what the day will contain. A sample script might sound something like this: "Today you get to start using the big kid potty just like <insert meaningful model here>! You get to wear big kid underwear and when you go big kid potty today, you'll get to pick a prize out of the treasure box! Let's take off this soggy diaper and pick out some big kid underwear!"

A lot of parents make a big production out of tossing this "last wet diaper" into the trash with their child and some even have the child toss it out and say something along the lines of "bye-bye diapers! I'm a big kid now!"

Let your child pick out their own underwear to wear and be sure that you comment on how fun it is to have underwear with their favorite character, pattern, or print on it. You can comment on the softness of the

material or the colors found on it. At some point during putting the underwear on, remind your child that underwear is not a diaper and that it is not meant to be peed or pooped in. Be sure to include something along the lines of, "do you feel like such a big kid with your big kid underwear on?"

Regarding the type of clothing your child should wear during this intensive potty training weekend, the only real requirement is that it needs to be something that your child can easily remove to sit on the potty. Many parents choose to just use an underwear and t-shirt combo, but anything that slides down and then back up easily will work. You don't want anything complicated that requires buttoning, zipping, or even Velcro because you don't want there to be any additional steps that your child will need to take to sit on the potty. You want to encourage as much independent movement as you can for your child around the potty. You want to help foster any associations between feeling capable and in control and use of the potty that you can.

Once you have gotten your child into their big kid underwear, it is time to begin the potty training process in earnest! Going into breakfast mode, allow your child to help you pick out what they would like for breakfast

and announce to them they get to have a special drink since it is the morning, they begin their potty training process. Give them one of their favorite beverages that you have picked out from the store and encourage them to drink up. Let them know that they are going to fill their belly up with their special drink and then be able to go sit on the big-kid potty. Once your child begins to drink, set the alarm for 15 minutes. This will be the first time you put your child on the potty, and hopefully, the sugary drink will have done the trick. Let your child know that when the alarm goes off, they will be able to go in and sit on the big kid potty!

Once the first fifteen-minute alarm sounds, this will be your time to really play up the event. React to the alarm as if it is the most exciting thing you have ever heard. Lead your child into the restroom (or depending on their excitement level, they can lead you!) and narrate the process as you go. "Alright! Here we go, off to your big kid potty. I'm so excited for you! This is great. Here we are, to the bathroom. Okay, can you pull your big kid underwear down, *all by yourself*? Awesome! Okay, now you can climb up to sit on your potty. Okay! Now let's check-in, see if there's any pee-pee in there that you

can put in the potty! <Show your child how to gently poke and put pressure on their lower abdomen, above their bladder> Do you feel some pee-pee in there? Let's see if you can put it in the potty!!!"

The cycle of drinking a beverage and then heading to the restroom will be repeated throughout this first day, but one of the most important aspects of this ritual will be in the narrative that you provide during this process. You want to continue to provide the child with the physical cues of where they will be feeling the pressure of their bladder, so they will make the association between the sensations of a full bladder and going to sit on the toilet.

For this first day, you will react with a celebration during every single visit to the potty. You want your child to experience a positive reinforcement of the association that going to the potty equals fun and happiness. It is not necessary that your child actually uses the potty chair, today you are celebrating just making the trip! You will celebrate each and every time they sit.

Allow your child two to three minutes to sit each time. During this time, stay with them. You can read a book about using the potty, listen to or sing a song about

using the potty, or watch one of the episodes about potty training available on various forms of media. Again, you are working to train your child to associate the sensations of a full bladder and pressure in their abdomen with the experience of sitting on the potty. Remember that you are building these connections from the ground up because they have never had to build them before! They have to move from mindless and passive elimination to conscious and mindful recognition and decision-making.

Again, this first day your child will get to pick a new treat from the treasure box each and every time they sit on the potty, regardless of if they go to the bathroom in the toilet or not. This first day is only for creating positive associations and teaching both toileting habits and how to be aware of their bodily sensations.

An Important Note About Accidents

Accidents will happen over the course of this weekend, especially on the first day. Do not be discouraged! Treat each accident as a neutral incident and keep your emotions level. Do not react as if it is a disappointment or a failure of any kind. A sample script for this scenario might be, "Ooops, it looks like you didn't make it to the

big kid potty. Let's go take this wet/dirty underwear over here and get all cleaned up. Next time, we will try to make it to the potty in time!"

Keep your narrative around potty accidents neutral and matter of fact. This is going to be a normal and natural part of the process and your child will be learning that when they go to the bathroom in their big kid underwear, it is a different sensation than when they went to the bathroom in their absorbent diaper.

Your child is making lots of new connections this weekend, one connection that they do NOT need to make is one of shame, disappointment, and disgust surrounding the toilet learning process. Keep your reactions neutral and matter of fact and they will adopt that same reaction.

In order to minimize your own stress and anxiety over accidents and the potential mess that can be made on furniture, some parents choose to either keep all activities for the day on the floor with a towel beneath the play space. Some parents even invest in some of the puppy pads that are available for dogs during crate training! These can even be put on furniture with regular bath towels over the top of them for both the

added protection of your furniture against accidents and also for the extra comfort for your child! Be sure to do the same for the child's spot at the dining room table, as well. Mealtimes can sometimes be an extra tricky time for new potty learners to navigate paying attention to their bodily sensations and signals while enjoying their meals!

Day one will proceed with the fifteen-minute intervals to sit on the toilet, keeping it an experience that the child wants to have with reading, singing, or media watching every time they sit on the toilet. Many catchy little jingles have been created surrounding potty use and they are helpful because children love catchy, rhyming, sing-songs phrases to begin with, and delivering helpful potty information is a way of reinforcing the potty experience for them. If you don't want to use one that has already been made, make up one for your family that you know your child will enjoy!

During the course of this first day, any time your child does actually pee or poop in the toilet, be sure to make a giant fuss over this! You want your child to feel proud and accomplished and to always reinforce that experience of elimination on the toilet with celebration and acknowledgment.

Going to bed that evening, be sure to tell your little one how very proud of them that you are, even if they didn't pee or poop in the potty a single time. Explain to them that because they will be asleep and unable to tell when they need to go potty, you will be putting special training pants on them (NOT their regular diapers, but something absorbent like a pull up) but will begin their awesome work on the potty again in the morning. This training takes a lot out of children, so be prepared for your kid to sleep like a log!

A Quick Note About Nighttime Potty Training

After a long day of visiting the restroom every fifteen minutes, you and your child will be exhausted! It can be tempting to introduce nighttime training at the same time but do be aware that this is not really something that can be trained but rather just something that a child outgrows and develops into. If your child often wakes up from their naps and their nightly sleep stretches dry, then nighttime training and trials with underwear have a great shot at success! However, it is very rare for a child to be dry during naps and nighttime sleep stretches but unable to control their bladder during the day. Typically, bladder awareness and potty training come before nighttime dryness.

By the age of six, approximately 85% of children will be able to stay dry, but children can continue to have nighttime accidents on occasion up until the age of 12 without it being considered an area of concern. Parents and caregivers know their children best and will be able to determine if nighttime toilet training should begin at the same time.

If you do choose to go this route, you will essentially continue the interval training as you do during the day, only with longer lengths in between. Instead of every fifteen minutes, you will set your alarm for every three hours and will pick up your child (because they will be half-asleep!) and carry them in to sit on the toilet. Some parents use audio cues to help their children use the restroom in the middle of the night by turning on a nearby faucet. Once the child has gone to the potty, return them to their bed.

In order to decrease some of the time spent dealing with nighttime accidents, it will be important to use a waterproof mattress protector underneath the regular sheets. Some parents even choose to do additional layers of waterproof mattress protectors and sheets so that way when an accident occurs, the wet layers of sheets can be easily stripped away and there will be a

dry layer already on the bed below. This can decrease nighttime sleep disruptions during the training process but do be aware that most nighttime potty training will be full of accidents if the child is not already mostly dry throughout the night. Again, this isn't really a training opportunity because nighttime bladder control has more to do with hormone production levels and those are produced on different timetables and have nothing to do with training.

Onward to Day Two!

Day two is much like day one, with one important difference. You will explain to your child that today, they will only be able to pick a treat out of the treasure box if they actually pee or poop in the potty. Do NOT mention accidents and be very careful about how you frame this information. You don't want your child to feel like they are being punished for having accidents, you want the emphasis to be on the reward for making it to the toilet!

Keep your spirits up and don't let up! This three-day potty training process is a *process*, not an event!

Day Three, Finally!

Day three is the day where big changes can often be seen. Explain to your child that today, you will be focusing on paying attention to your body and checking in. You will adjust your timer to half-hour increments, and rather than immediately traveling to the toilet to sit, you will instead encourage the "check-in."

"Let's stop and see if we need to go potty! <cue the gentle poking of the lower abdomen> Is there pee or poop in there that needs to come out? Should we go to try?" If it has been over an hour and your child still says they do not need the toilet and they have remained dry, encourage more drinking of fluids. Today is the day to really let your child figure out what these bodily sensations mean!

Chances are, your child is beginning to really connect the dots between what the feelings in their body mean and what they need to do about it. Day three is the day for them to really practice taking charge of this. You will still be checking in every half hour- and encouraging fluids- but you need to let them work out some of the cause and effect here, too.

Even if your child makes it to the toilet 100% on day 3, this does not mean that there will not be accidents moving forward! Small children are easily distracted and will still require some cueing and reminding the adults in their life. This is normal!

Read on for the next chapter if you find you have a Potty Training Outlier!

Chapter 3: Potty Training Outliers

Some children will potty train earlier than their peers and some will potty train later. This is just a normal part of this developmental process! If you have a child that has potty trained earlier than two, then you still may have some potty work coming in the future.

Potty training regression is when a child who was fully potty trained for a significant period of time begins having accidents consistently. If this is the case, you need to look at potential reasons why such as if there is an emotional or traumatic event occurring that needs addressed (toilet accidents are often present during times of abuse) or if extra support is needed day to day. Consult with your medical professional to rule out medical reasons such as a urinary tract infection or constipation.

For children who are beyond the age of four and still not interested in the potty or successful after an extended period of consistent potty training efforts, then this is also a scenario in which you might want to check in with a medical professional to see if there are any health issues at play that are causing the delay.

There are children who will potty train early and those that will potty train much later, but outliers exist on both ends and are typically not a cause for concern. Children who are not successful with potty training programs between the ages of two and four can spontaneously train themselves seemingly overnight when they decide that they are ready. Again, there is very little that children are able to have complete control over in their lives and the toileting process can be one of those things that children for reasons that adults may not understand. This does not mean your child is being manipulative or trying to be difficult; it means that they are trying to meet their own needs in the best way they know-how and support during this time means more emotional support than physical force.

Again, always speak to your child's doctor if you have any questions at all about health or well-being.

Bonus Chapter: Tips for Dads, From Dads

The relationship that a child has with their father is very unique and these are some tips and tricks that dads have shared with us:

"My little guy loves to do target practice in the toilet. I set him up with a few cheerios in the toilet and tell him to hit them as many times as he can and he is getting very good aim now!"

"My daughter loves to "show me how" so I like to pretend that I forgot how she uses the potty and she will walk me back to "show me how" and even sportscast the entire process!"

"I was worried about potty training and being away from home, but it's worked out really well so far. My son is really interested in all public restrooms, so anytime we end up at a store or restaurant, he immediately "has to go potty" which just means he wants to go see their restroom. It's working out though, not a single accident outside of the house!"

"Don't tell mom, but I still use Skittles. For pee on the potty, she gets two and for poop, she gets three. She never has an accident when I'm around."

"I let my daughter pick out a special foaming soap that she only gets to use after she's used the potty. It's sparkly blue and purple foam, so she makes sure that she makes it to the toilet so she can use some of her fancy "unicorn" soap!"

"I let my son pee in our backyard by our maple tree. We have a privacy fence so no one can see anything, and he LOVES it. I'm not sure what we will do in the winter, though..."

A lot of these dads have created playful ways to make the potty experience fun! Use your imagination to think of ways to do the same with your little one. Find ways to make this process tailored to you and your child and the this you like best.

Conclusion

Thank you for making it through to the end of **Potty Training in A Weekend:** *The Step-By-Step Guide to Potty Train Your Little Toddler in Less Than 3 Days. Perfect for Little Boys and Girls. Bonus Chapter with Tip for Careless Dads Included,* let's hope it was informative and able to provide you with all of the tools you need to achieve your goals in potty training your child.

Remember, potty training is a process and not an event. The three-day potty training method is intended to give your child a strong baseline knowledge of how to pay attention to and interpret the signals of their body and use the toilet properly. This doesn't mean that children will not have accidents as they go about their days, because children are easily distractible and after the fun of the three-day potty training method, going to sit on the potty won't seem quite as exciting as it did when they had a cheerleader on standby!

Continue to provide support for your child on their potty training journey and repeat the process as many times as you feel you need to. Remember that the potty training process requires a lot of your child: it is as

much a cognitive process as it is a physical one. Be sure to tell your child each and every night that they are doing a great job in learning how to use the big kid potty and that you are proud of all their hard work. Children that feel supported for their efforts, even when their efforts don't yield perfect results, will be far more likely to persist with determination than a child that is given the signals that because they did not do something perfectly that they have failed.

If you have been consistently potty training for an extended period of time with no results, consult with your child's doctor to rule out any possible medical issues. If none are present, then consider pausing the potty training process and revisiting it later. Keep your child in the loop of what is happening with as neutral language as you can. A sample script might sound like, "It seems like maybe you aren't quite ready to begin the big kid potty yet. We will try again in one month, okay?" It isn't a failure, just a standard part of the process involved in this major developmental leap! Kids that seem resistant at first may just need a little while longer to fully understand and grow comfortable with the process.

Besides, you can always be rest assured that everyone learns how to use the potty eventually. You will not be sending your child off to college in diapers, guaranteed! Just as some kids walk later than others, some will potty train later, too. The day will come, believe it or not, you might even miss the days when your little one was in diapers.

Finally, if you found this book useful in any way, a review on Amazon is always appreciated!

Potty Training for Newborn Superheroes

Say "Bye Bye" to Diapers in 72 Hours. The Perfect Guide for Busy Parents That Love Their Baby Genius.

By

CALEMA DUMONT

If you love listening to audio books on-the-go, I have great news for you. You can download the audio book version of this book for FREE just by signing up for a FREE 30-day audible trial! See below for more details!

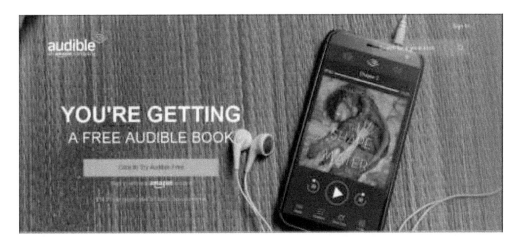

Audible Trial Benefits

As an audible customer, you will receive the below benefits with your 30-day free trial:

- FREE audible book copy of this book
- After the trial, you will get 1 credit each month to use on any audiobook
- Your credits automatically roll over to the next month if you don't use them
- Choose from Audible's 200,000 + titles
- Listen anywhere with the Audible app across multiple devices
- Make easy, no-hassle exchanges of any audiobook you don't love
- Keep your audiobooks forever, even if you cancel your membership
- And much more

Click the links below to get started!

For Audible US

For Audible UK

For Audible FR

For Audible DE

Table of Contents

Introduction

Parents play a key role in toilet training. Parents need to provide their child with direction, motivation, and reinforcement. They need to set aside time for and have patience with the toilet training process. Parents can encourage their child to be independent and allow their child to master each step at his or her own pace. WHEN TO BEGIN TOILET TRAINING YOUR CHILD There is no right age to toilet train a child the approximate time is between 15 months to 30 months.

Readiness to begin toilet training depends on the individual child. In general, starting before age 2 (24months) is not recommended. The readiness skills and physical development your child needs occur between age 18 months and 2.5 years.

Potty training might seem like a daunting task, but if your child is truly ready, there's not much to worry about. "Life goes on and one day your child will just do it," says Lisa Asta, M.D., a clinical professor of pediatrics at University of California, San Francisco, and spokesperson for the American Academy of Pediatrics. "When kids want to go on the potty, they will go on the

potty. Sometimes that happens at 18 months, sometimes it doesn't happen until close to age 4, but no healthy child will go into kindergarten in diapers." So don't stress — your child will ultimately get on the potty and do his thing, but you can help guide the process along. If you're ready to make diapers a thing of the past in your house, experts recommend following these seven easy steps.

Your child will show cues that he or she is developmentally ready. Signs of readiness include the fol-lowing:

• Your child can imitate your behavior.

• Your child begins to put things where they belong.

• Your child can demonstrate independence by saying "no."

• Your child can express interest in toilet training (e g, following you to the bathroom).

• Your child can walk and is ready to sit down.

• Your child can indicate first when he is "going"(urinating or defecating) and then when he needs to "go."

• Your child is able to pull clothes up and down (on and off).

Each child has his or her own style of behavior, which is called temperament. In planning your approach to toilet training, it is important to consider your child's temperament.

• Consider your child's moods and the time of day your child is most approachable.

Plan your approach based on when your child is most cooperative.

• If your child is generally shy and withdrawn, he or she may need additional support and encouragement.

• Work with your child's attention span.

Plan for distractions that will keep him or her comfortable on the potty chair. All this and many more on how to get your kid on potty will be explain in this ebook.

Chapter 1 What is potty training?

Potty training is teaching your child to recognize their body signals for urinating and having a bowel movement. It also means teaching your child to use a potty chair or toilet correctly and at the appropriate times.

1.1 When should toilet training start?

Potty training should start when your child shows signs that he or she is ready. There is no right age to begin. If you try to toilet train before your child is ready, it can be a battle for both you and your child. The ability to control bowel and bladder muscles comes with proper growth and development.

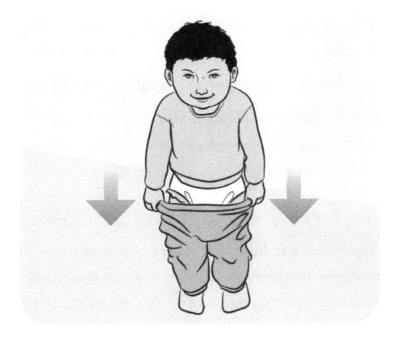

Children develop at different rates. A child younger than 12 months has no control over bladder or bowel movements. There is very little control between 12 to 18 months. Most children don't have bowel and bladder control until 24 to 30 months. The average age of toilet training is 27 months.

If you think your child is showing signs of being ready for toilet training, the first step is to decide whether you want to train using a potty or the toilet.

There are some advantages to using a potty – it's mobile and it's familiar, and some children find it less scary than a toilet. Try to find out your child's preference and go with that. Some parents encourage their child to use both the toilet and potty.

Second, make sure you have all the right equipment. For example, if your child is using the toilet you'll need a step for your child to stand on. You'll also need a smaller seat that fits securely inside the existing toilet seat, because some children get uneasy about falling in.

Third, it's best to plan toilet training for a time when you don't have any big changes coming up in your family life. Changes might include going on holiday, starting day care, having a new baby or moving house. It can be

a good idea to plan toilet training for well before or after these changes.

Also, toilet training might go better if you and your child have a regular daily routine. This way, the new activity of using the toilet or potty can be slotted into your normal routine

1.2 General Knowledge of potty for children

You may (happily) have noticed that you're changing fewer diapers lately and your little one is usually staying dry during nap time. These, along with other signs, indicate that it's time to dive into the world of potty training. The key to potty training success is patience and an awareness that all tots reach this ever important milestone at their own pace. Different strategies work with different children, but these tips generally get the job done.

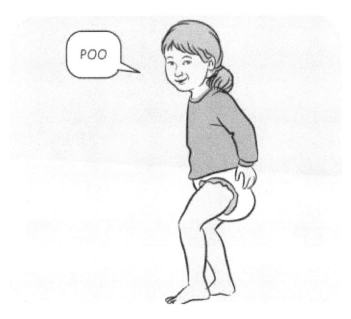

Since kids typically start potty training between 18 and 30 months, start talking about potty training occasionally around your child's first birthday to pique interest. Keep a few children's books about potty training lying around your house to read along with your child. And bring up the subject of the potty in conversation; saying things like, "I wonder if Elmo [or your child's favorite stuffed animal] needs to go potty" or "I have to go pee-pee. I'm headed to the potty." The idea is to raise awareness about going potty and make your child comfortable with the overall concept before he's ready to potty train.

If your child is staying dry for at least two hours during the day and is dry after naps, this could mean she's

ready to give the potty a shot. Before you head to the bathroom, know that she can follow simple instructions, like a request to walk to the bathroom, sit down, and remove her clothes. Also make sure she's interested in wearing big girl underwear. Then consider if she's aware when she's wet: If she cries, fusses, or shows other signs of obvious discomfort when her diaper is soiled and indicates through facial expression, posture, or language that it's time to use the toilet, then she's ready to start the process.

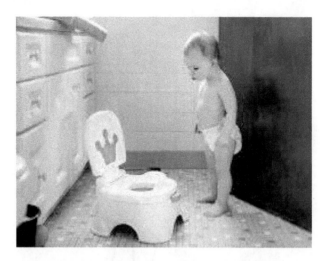

Some children are afraid of falling in the toilet or just hearing it flush, If your child is comfortable in the bathroom, try a potty seat that goes on top of your toilet to reduce the size of the bowl's opening. If not, you can buy a stand-alone potty chair and put it in the playroom or child's bedroom, where he'll become comfortable with

its presence over time. When he's ready to give it a try,

experts suggest you move it into the bathroom for repeated use, so you don't have to retrain your child down the road to transition from going potty in other rooms. Also get a stepstool — if he's using a potty seat, he'll need it to reach the toilet and also to give his feet support while he's pooping. "People can't empty their bowels and bladders completely unless their feet are pressing down on the floor.

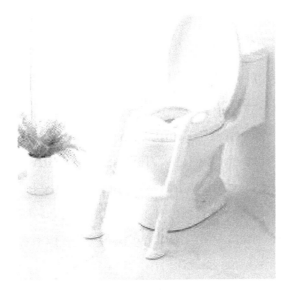

Even if your child seems ready, experts say to avoid potty training during transitional or stressful times. If you're moving, taking a vacation, adding a new baby to the family, or going through a divorce, postpone the potty training until about a month after the transitional time. Children trying to learn this new skill will do best if

they're relaxed and on a regular routine. You might prefer to get potty training over with as soon as

possible—maybe you're curious about the 3-day potty training trend. That's fine but do not always believe it, experts because you might find it frustrating not. "I often see parents who boast that they trained their 2-year-old in a weekend, and then say that the child has accidents four times a day, This is not the same as being potty trained. When kids are truly ready, they often will just start going on the potty on their own."

When you do decide it's time to start potty training, you'll want your child to go to the bathroom independently, day or night, so make sure she has transitioned out of

the crib and into a big-kid bed. "Kids need access to a potty 24/7 if they're potty training so they can reach it on their own when they need it. Keep a well-lit path to the bathroom so your child feels safe and comfortable walking there during the night. Of course, if you think you're child isn't ready for a big-kid bed (or, let's face it, if you're not ready), there's no harm in keeping her in diapers at night for a while longer. Talk to your child's doctor about the best time to potty train your child; the

answer will range greatly by child, though most kids should be out of diapers during the day by age 3. When you're ready to start training, let your child sit on the potty fully clothed when you are in the bathroom to get a feel for the seat. Then create a schedule: "The key is having times throughout the day where you ritualize using the potty so it becomes more of a habit," Dr. Swanson says. You might want to have him sit on the potty every two hours, whether he has to go or not, including first thing in the morning, before you leave the house, and before naps and bedtime. Tell him to remove his shorts or pants first, his underwear (or, if you're using them, training pants) next, and to sit on the toilet for a few minutes (allot more time, if you think he has to poop). Read him a book or play a game, like 20 Questions, to make the time pass in a fun way. Then, whether or not he actually goes potty, instruct him to flush and wash his hands. Of course, always praise him for trying.

It's not uncommon for a child who has been successfully using the potty for a few days to say he wants to go back to diapers. To avoid a power struggle or a situation where your child actually starts a pattern of withholding

bowel movements, which can lead to constipation, you might agree to a brief break. But try to build in a plan to resume by asking your child, "Would you like to wear underwear right when you get up or wait until after lunch?"

When you're potty training, accidents are part of the process; some kids still have accidents through age 5 or 6, and many don't stay dry at night until that age (or even later). Never punish your child for wetting or soiling his pants; he's just learning and can't help it. In fact, doing so might only make your little one scared of using the potty, and that, in turn, will delay the whole process even further. Instead, when your child uses the potty successfully, offer gentle praise and a small reward. You might want to use a sticker chart—your child receives a sticker every time he goes potty; after he's earned, say, three stickers, he gets a small prize. "However, don't go nuts!" Dr. Goldstein says. "A lot of toddlers will react to excessive praise as they react to punishment—by getting scared and avoiding doing the thing that they were excessively praised or punished for." In other words, stick with stickers, a trip to the local park, or even a surprise cup of hot cocoa— no need

to go on a shopping spree to Toys 'R' Us. Less tangible rewards, like finally living up to the promise of "being a

big kid" are enough for some kids. Remind your child about the benefits of "being a big kid," like if he wore underwear, he would never have to stop playing in order to get his diaper changed.So this should result to setting children up with good hygiene habits that will last a lifetime, washing hands should be a routine from Day 1, along with flushing and wiping, regardless of whether your child actually went in the potty. The Centers for Disease Control and Prevention recommends wetting hands with cool or warm running water, lathering up with soap, and scrubbing for at least 20 seconds. Make hand washing fun by buying colorful kid-friendly soaps, and make it last long enough by singing a favorite song, like "Happy Birthday to You" or the "ABC Song," so the bubbles work their germ-fighting magic. Yes, toilet training can be stressful—for the parents, that is! But if you follow your child's lead, it won't be stressful for him.

1.3 Dealing with the emotions

In this step-by-step guide, we are going to take you through some really in-depth training and information that my I have put together over the years on potty training. Additionally, When it comes to potty training, most parents and most people think it begins with the child. The reality is that potty training is begins with you, the parent or the grandparent, the relative or the daycare worker.

When we get testimonials from our clients and they say, "Thank you, thank you, thank you," I always like to say, "No, thank you. You are the one that did the hard work, so you are the one that deserves the congratulations." With that being said, we are going to start with you, the parent, or you, the person who is going to be doing the training.

You must be prepared and know that this is going to be a trying time, for some parents more than others. This can be a very stressful time because it tends to be a very stressful situation. What I want to make sure you understand is that nothing that is going on with your child with respect to potty training is your fault.

You have not done anything wrong. It may be as simple as the information you have received (or lack thereof). As an adult, what you know is that kids are not born knowing what to do and we are not born knowing how to be parents. Potty training, like many other lessons is something that is learned and you've taken the right steps in trying to acquire that information. So, the first step is to prepare yourself mentally for this project. Remember that your child has spent two or three years going to the bathroom in his or her diaper.

Now, you are going to ask them to do something that is completely out of the norm and, essentially erasing two or three years of habit. Saying that this is going to be a challenge may be an understatement as some children may battle and butt heads with you.

But being mentally prepared will help you in coping with the challenge itself. How do you get prepared? First, take your time, and get relaxed. Do whatever it takes to help you get into a relaxed state of mind. Its better if you can start the potty training process when have had a good amount of sleep. Being tired and trying to potty train makes it just that much more difficult.

You will also want to make sure your child is rested as

well. This is just as stressful for them and being cranky while learning a new technique is not a good combination. Also, practice counting to 10 and then counting backwards from 10. This is a practice that you will find calms you down during periods of frustration in the process. In addition to being relaxed, you will need

to ensure that you have a good support system. Talk with your husband or your wife or friends, and make sure that everyone is on board with what you are going to do so you are all heading in the same direction and can be a sounding board for each other.

This is critical because if there isn't a support system, the person doing the potty training will have a more difficult time and experience feelings of their own relating to the responsibility, frustration, and in some cases, failure (at least in the short run). If you are able to start this process on a weekend, it is highly suggested because you won't have the stress of work and you can have the dedicated focus needed to get this done right the first time. This can be applied to any period of time when you can get yourself a good three days to focus and concentrate.

1.4 Using motivation for the training

A lot of products out there will tell you that to motivate your child, you need to go to the store and pick up a toy or something like that. And while that's good, I want to give you something even better when it comes to motivation. Here's the problem with giving them toys or

saying, "I'm taking your toys away," and actually taking the toy away and hiding it so that they don't see it. When children are between the ages of 2 and 5, out of sight, out of mind, the average attention span at that age is about 7 minutes. So, if you take the toy away it only takes 7 minutes before they never even realized they had a toy in the first place. So, that motivation does not go very far. What I like to do is instead is use fear of loss versus fear of gain. Now, let me explain the difference to you between fear of loss and fear of gain. Most people even as adults think about it today. We work harder to prevent ourselves from losing things than we do to gain things. Fear of loss is a bigger motivator than fear of gain. So if you are saying, "If you behave, you will get..." or, "If you use the potty, you will get..." Although it can be a good thing for motivation, I think you can get a better response by saying, "If you don't

use the potty, you will lose this." In other words, if they don't use the potty, they're going to lose something.

Let me give you an example of one of the motivations we used to use with my youngest son. We had to "outsmart the fox" as I call it. I used to have to say something like, "Lorenzo, do you want to go to

McDonald's?" And he'd say, "Yes, let's go toMcDonald's." So, then I would say, "Okay, great. Go get your coat. Go get your shoes. Let's go to McDonalds." He'd go get his stuff and we'd open the front door and get ready to walk out. And then I would say, "Oh, you know what Lorenzo, let's use the bathroom before we go because you don't want to have an accident at Ronald McDonald's house." So, what did I do it at that point? Using a fear of loss, I defuse the potty. At that point, losing McDonalds was way more important to him than the toilet. So, he went without any issues at all. Now, granted, going to McDonald's means you have to spend money, but there are other ways that you can use the same methodology inside the house. For example, you can use their favorite cookie or their favorite snack.

Let's say they like pudding. You might say, "Hey Lorenzo, do you want some pudding?" And the answer of

course is going to be, "Yes." You then take the pudding, you put it on the table, you put the spoon in the bowl, you actually let them grab the spoon, get ready to take a bite and you say, "Wait a second, wait a second. Before you take that bite, let's go use the potty." At this point, the pudding and the reward are so real to the child that the potty is nothing. They'll use the potty just so they can come back and get that reward. You can do this with the toys as well.You can also do it with television. If it is a television program that they really like, then I would wait until the show is getting ready to start and I'd say, "Hey, let's go use the bathroom before we have an accident watching the show." If they said, "Oh the show is starting. I don't want to use the bathroom." Then, your answer is, "Well, we better go quickly if you want to see that show. Until we use the bathroom the show is not going to be on." Then, you can literally turn the television off. So, that is the way to motivate getting to the results. You don't want to use the same old, "I'm taking the toys away." You hide the toys and they don't see the toys for months, and to them, they never existed in the first place.

1.5 How will I know my toddler is ready to be potty trained?

If your little one isn't developmentally ready for potty training, even the best toilet tactics will fall short. Wait for these surefire signs that your tot is set to get started: You're changing fewer diapers. Until they're around 20 months old, toddlers still pee frequently, but once they can stay dry for an hour or two, it's a sign that they're developing bladder control and are becoming physically ready for potty training.

Bowel movements become more regular. This makes it easier to pull out the potty in a pinch when it's time. Your little one is more vocal about going to the bathroom. When your child starts to broadcast peeing and pooping by verbalizing or showing you through his facial expressions, potty training is on the horizon.

Your child notices (and doesn't like) dirty diapers. Your little one may suddenly decide she doesn't want to hang out in her dirty diapers because they're gross. Yay! Your child is turning her nose up at stinky diapers just like you do and is ready to use the potty instead. Kids are generally not ready to potty train before the age of 2, and some children may wait until 3 1/2. It's important to remember not to push your child before he's ready and to be patient. And remember that all kids are different. Your child is not developmentally lagging if he's far into his 3s before he gets the hang of potty training. Potty training success hinges on physical, developmental and behavioral milestones, not age. Many children show

signs of being ready for potty training between ages 18 and 24 months. However, others might not be ready until they're 3 years old. There's no rush. If you start too early, it might take longer to train your child.

1.6 Is your child ready? Ask yourself:

λ Can your child walk to and sit on a toilet?

λ Can your child pull down his or her pants and pull them up again?

λ Can your child stay dry for up to two hours?

λ Can your child understand and follow basic directions?

λ Can your child communicate when he or she needs to go?

λ Does your child seem interested in using the toilet or wearing "big-kid" underwear?

If you answered mostly yes, your child might be ready. If you answered mostly no, you might want to wait especially if your child is about to face a major change, such as a move or the arrival of a new sibling.

Your readiness is important, too. Let your child's motivation, instead of your eagerness, lead the process. Try not to equate potty training success or difficulty with your child's intelligence or stubbornness. Also, keep in

mind that accidents are inevitable and punishment has no role in the process. Plan toilet training for when you or a caregiver can devote the time and energy to be consistent on a daily basis for a few months.

1.7 How to know when its time for a child with special need

While parents often complain of difficulty potty training their children, for most families, potty training is a fairly easy experience. Even when there are problems or children show signs of potty training resistance, usually, they will eventually become potty trained.

1.8 Signs of Potty Training Readiness in Children With Special Needs

However, this is not always the case for children with developmental delays or disabilities, such as autism, Down syndrome, mental retardation, cerebral palsy, etc. Children with special needs can be more difficult to potty train. Most children show signs of physical readiness to begin using the toilet as toddlers, usually between 18 months and 3 years of age 1, but not all children have the intellectual and/or psychological readiness to be

potty trained at this age. It is more important to keep your child's developmental level, and not his chronological age in mind when you are considering starting potty training.

Signs of intellectual and psychological readiness includes being able to follow simple instructions and being cooperative, being uncomfortable with dirty diapers and wanting them to be changed, recognizing when he has a full bladder or needs to have a bowel movement, being able to tell you when he needs to urinate or have a bowel movement, asking to use the potty chair or asking to wear regular underwear.

Signs of physical readiness can include your being able to tell when your child is about to urinate or have a bowel movement by his facial expressions, posture or by what he says, staying dry for at least 2 hours at a time, and having regular bowel movements. It is also helpful if he can at least partially dress and undress himself.

1.9 Potty Training Challenges

Children with physical disabilities may also have problems with potty training that involves learning to get on the potty and getting undressed. A special potty chair and other adaptations may need to be made for these children.

Things to avoid when toilet training your child, and help prevent resistance, are beginning during a stressful time or period of change in the family (moving, new baby, etc.), pushing your child too fast, and punishing mistakes. Instead, you should treat accidents and mistakes lightly. Be sure to go at your child's pace and show strong encouragement and praise when he is successful.

Since an important sign of readiness and a motivator to begin potty training involves being uncomfortable in a

dirty diaper, if your child isn't bothered by a soiled or wet diaper, then you may need to change him into regular underwear or training pants during daytime training. Other children can continue to wear a diaper or pull-ups if they are bothered, and you know when they are dirty. Once you are ready to begin training, you can choose a potty chair. You can have your child decorate it with stickers and sit on it with his clothes on to watch TV, etc. to help him get used to it. Whenever your child shows signs of needing to urinate or have a bowel movement, you should take him to the potty chair and explain to him what you want him to do. Make a consistent routine of having him go to the potty, pull down his clothes, sit on the potty, and after he is finished, pulling up his clothes and washing his hands. At first, you should only keep him seated for a few minutes at a time, don't insist and be prepared to delay training if he shows resistance. Until he is going in the potty, you can try to empty his dirty diapers into his potty chair to help demonstrate what you want him to do.

1.10 Tips for Potty Training Children With Developmental Delays

An important part of potty training children with special needs is using the potty frequently. This usually includes scheduled toileting as outlined in the book Toilet Training Without Tears by Dr. Charles E. Schaefer. This "assures that your child has frequent opportunities to use the toilet." Sitting on the potty should occur "at least once or twice every hour" and after you first ask, "Do you have to go potty?" Even if he says no, unless he is totally resistant, it is a good idea to take him to the potty anyway. If this routine is too demanding on your child, then you can take him to the potty less frequently. It

can help to keep a chart or diary of when he regularly wets or soils himself so that you will know the best times to have him sit on the potty and maximize your chances that he has to go. He is also most likely to go after meals and snacks and that is a good time to take him to the potty. Frequent visits during the times that he is likely to use the potty and fewer visits to the potty at other times of the day is another good alternative. Other good techniques include modeling, where you allow your child to see family members or other children using the

toilet, and using observational remarks. 4 This involves narrating what is happening and asking questions while potty training, such as "Did you just sit on the potty?" or "Did you just poop in the potty?" Even after he begins to use the potty, it is normal to have accidents and for him to regress or relapse at times and refuse to use the potty. Being fully potty trained, with your child recognizing when he has to go to the potty, physically goes to the bathroom and pulls down his pants, urinates or has a bowel movement in the potty, and dresses himself, can take time, sometimes up to three to six months. Having accidents or occasionally refusing to use the potty is normal and not considered resistance.

Early on in the training, resistance should be treated by just discontinuing training for a few weeks or a month and then trying again. In addition to a lot of praise and encouragement when he uses or even just sits on the potty, material rewards can be a good motivator. This can include stickers that he can use to decorate his potty chair or a small toy, snack or treat. You can also consider using a reward chart and getting a special treat if he gets so many stickers on his chart.

You can also give treats or rewards for staying dry. It

can help to check to make sure he hasn't had an accident between visits to the potty. If he is dry, then getting very excited and offering praise, encouragement, and maybe even a reward, can help to reinforce his not having accidents.

1.11 How to Use Positive Practice for Accidents

Another useful technique is positive practice for accidents. Dr. Schaefer describes this as what you should do when your child has an accident and wets or soils himself.

This technique involves firmly telling your child what he has done, taking him to the potty where he can clean and change himself (although you will likely need to help) and then having him practice using the potty. Dr. Schaefer recommends going through the usual steps of using the potty at least five times, starting when "the child walks to the

toilet, lowers his pants, briefly sits on the toilet (3 to 5 seconds), stands up, raises his pants, washes his hands, and then returns to the place where the accident occurred."

Although you are trying to teach him the consequences of having an accident, this should not take the form of punishment.

1.12 When to Get Help for Special Needs Kids With Potty Training Difficulties

While it may take some time and require a lot of patience, many children with special needs can be potty trained by the age of 3 to 5 years. 3 If you continue to have problems or your child is very resistant, then consider getting professional help.

In addition to your pediatrician, you might get help from an occupational therapist, especially if your child has some motor delays causing the potty training difficulty, a child psychologist, especially if your child is simply resistant to potty training and a developmental pediatrician

1.13 When it's time to begin potty training:

Choose your words. Decide which words you're going to

use for your child's bodily fluids. Avoid negative words, such as dirty or stinky.

Prepare the equipment. Place a potty chair in the bathroom or, initially, wherever your child is spending most of his or her time. Encourage your child to sit on the potty chair in clothes to start out. Make sure your child's feet rest on the floor or a stool. Use simple, positive terms to talk about the toilet. You might dump the contents of a dirty diaper into the potty chair and toilet to show their purpose. Have your child flush the toilet. Schedule potty breaks. Have your child sit on the potty chair or toilet without a diaper for a few minutes at two-hour intervals, as well as first thing in the morning and right after naps. For boys, it's often best to master urination sitting down, and then move to standing up after bowel training is complete. Stay with your child and read a book together or play with a toy while he or she sits. Allow your child to get up if he or she wants. Even if your child simply sits there, offer praise for trying — and remind your child that he or she can try again later. Bring the potty chair with you when you're away from home with your child.

Get there

Fast! When you notice signs that your child might need to use the toilet such as squirming, squatting or holding the genital area respond quickly. Help your child become familiar with these signals, stop what he or she is doing, and head to the toilet. Praise your child for telling you when he or she has to go. Keep your child in loose, easy-to-remove clothing.

Explain hygiene. Teach girls to spread their legs and wipe carefully from front to back to prevent bringing germs from the rectum to the vagina or bladder. Make sure your child washes his or her hands afterward. Ditch the diapers. After a couple of weeks of successful potty breaks and remaining dry during the day, your child might be ready to trade diapers for training pants or underwear. Celebrate the transition. Let your child return to diapers if he or she is unable to remain dry. Consider using a sticker or star chart for positive reinforcement.

Chapter 2 Getting started with toilet training

The following tips may help you get started with potty training:

If there are siblings, ask them to let the younger child see you praising them for using the toilet.

It's best to use a potty chair on the floor rather than putting the child on the toilet for training. The potty chair is more secure for most children. Their feet reach the floor and there is no fear of falling off. If you decide to use a seat that goes over the toilet, use a footrest for your child's feet. Let your child play with the potty. They can sit on it with clothes on and later with diapers off. This way they can get used to it. Never strap your child to the potty chair. Children should be free to get off the potty when they want. Your child should not sit on the potty for more than 5 minutes. Sometimes children have a bowel movement just after the diaper is back on because the diaper feels normal. Don't get upset or punish your child. You can try taking the dirty diaper off and putting the bowel movement in the potty with your child watching you. This may help your child understand that you want the bowel movement in the potty.

If your child has a normal time for bowel movements (such as after a meal), take your child to the potty at that time of day. If your child acts a certain way when having a bowel movement (such as stooping, getting quiet, going to the corner), try taking your child to potty when he or she shows it is time.

If your child wants to sit on the potty, stay next to your child and talk or read a book. It's good to use words for what your child is doing (such as potty, pee, or poop). Then your child learns the words to tell you. Remember that other people will hear these words. Don't use words that will offend, confuse, or embarrass others or your child. Don't use words such as dirty, naughty, or stinky to describe bowel movements and urine. Use a simple, matter-of-fact tone.

If your child gets off the potty before urinating or passing a bowel movement, be calm. Don't scold. Try again later. If your child successfully uses the potty, give plenty of praise such as a smile, clap, or hug. Children learn from copying adults and other children. It may help if your child sits on the potty chair while you are using the toilet.

Children often follow parents into the bathroom. This

may be one time they are willing to use the potty. Start out by teaching boys to sit down for passing urine. At first, it is hard to control starting and stopping while standing. Boys will try to stand to urinate when they see other boys standing.

Some children learn by pretending to teach a doll to go potty. Get a doll that has a hole in its mouth and diaper area. Your child can feed and "teach" the doll to pull down its pants and use the potty. Make this teaching fun for your child.

Make going to the potty a part of your child's daily routine. Do this first thing in the morning, after meals and naps, and before going to bed.

2.1 After training is started

The following tips may help you once the training is started:

Once your child starts using the potty and can tell you they need to go, taking them to the potty at regular times or reminding them too many times to go to the potty is not necessary.

You may want to start using training pants. Wearing underpants is a sign of growing up, and most children

like being a "big girl or big boy." Wearing diapers once potty training has been started may be confusing for your child.

If your child has an accident while in training pants, don't punish. Be calm and clean up without making a fuss about it.

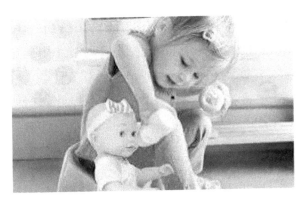

Keep praising or rewarding your child every step of the way. Do this for pulling down pants, for sitting on the potty, and for using the potty. If you show that you are pleased when your child urinates or has bowel movements in the potty, your child is more likely to use the potty next time. As children get older, they can learn to wipe themselves and wash hands after going to the bathroom. Girls should be taught to wipe from front to back so that germs from bowel movement are not wiped into the urinary area. Remember that every child is different and learns toilet training at his or her own

pace. If things are going poorly with toilet training, it's better to put diapers back on for a few weeks and try again later. In general, have a calm, unhurried approach to toilet training.

Most children have bowel control and daytime urine control by age 3 or 4. Soiling or daytime wetting after this age should be discussed with your child's healthcare provider.

Nighttime control usually comes much later than daytime control. Complete nighttime control may not happen until your child is 4 or 5 years old, or even older. If your child is age 5 or older and does not stay dry at night, you should discuss this with your child's healthcare provider.

Even when children are toilet trained, they may have some normal accidents (when excited or playing a lot), or setbacks due to illness or emotional situations. If accidents or setbacks happen, be patient. Examples of emotional situations include moving to a new house, a family illness or death, or a new baby in the house. In fact, if you know an emotional situation is going to be happening soon, don't start toilet training. Wait for a calmer time.

2.2 Potty Training Chairs

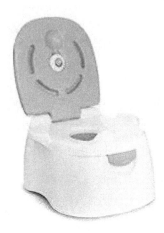

Many parents ask, "Do I need a potty training chair to be successful in potty training?" The answer to that question is "yes" and "no". For even our own kids, I used potty training chairs for two and no potty training chairs for our third child.

Now, he was an advanced child. He was doing things that the other kids never did so he never even wanted to use the potty chair. Even today as a 6-year-old in kindergarten, he doesn't like doing things that the other kindergarten kids like to do.

He calls them "babies." But I will tell you this: having a potty training chair does several things for your child. First of all, it gives them flexibility. When they have a potty training chair, more than likely it is mobile, which

means that it can be placed anywhere around the house including the TV room or the game room.

This increases the success rate of your child using the potty. The rationale? Well, as you might already know, if you're in any other room than the bathroom when you see kids doing a pee-pee dance or you realize that they've got to go, it's already too late. That pee or the bowel movement is almost on its way out the door.

But with a mobile potty chair, you can place it near their activities and in different rooms, so when the child feels the need to go, they don't have to rush all the way to the bathroom. They can simply get up and go in the vicinity of wherever they are.

Not only that, the act of running and holding for child that young is a very challenging thing. So trying to run to the bathroom from outside is almost asking for trouble. What you want to do instead is make sure that if you are going to use a potty chair, is that it's available and near. A potty chair is also great especially if you have a 2-story house and the bathroom is upstairs. You can then put the potty chair downstairs and cut out that climb. And the way potty chairs are designed today, they're colorful, they are cute and kids love them. It just

is a fun thing for them and they always get a sense of pride because it's their chair and nobody else's. What we used to do is put the potty chair in a laundry room because there was a door there. My son would be able to close the door so we couldn't see him and he would have his privacy.

2.3 Starting the process

There are three different times that you can start the training process.

Early — when the child is 2 or younger Middle — between the ages of 2 and 3, maybe 3 1/2 Later — between 3, 3 1/2 and older The optimal time for me is the age of 2.

And, I mean the day they turned 2 is when we normally like to start with potty training. With all the years that I have been in day care and all the children that I have

potty trained, I started every single one the day they turned 2. Even our own kids, we started them at the age of 2.

Now, starting at a later time is okay and that is the case with most parents. But I want to explain to you the

difference between starting at the age of 2 and starting later. The key difference in starting at the age of 2 is that the child hasn't developed all of their social skills yet and their ability to go out and have fun is limited.

At the age of 2 and somewhere between 2 and 3 is when they find their own voice. (You've heard of the terrible '2s'!?) They find their own voice and they find their own spirit and that's when they decide that they want to start doing their own thing. When you start earlier in the potty training process it is easier to get them to follow directions and it is just easier to get them to do what you want them to do versus them wanting to do what they want to do. Now, girls can start even earlier than 2. Usually girls can start about 3 or 4 months before their 2nd birthday. Girls, as we know, even later on in life, are a lot smarter than boys and men, and I will be the first to admit that.

The earliest we've seen was a little girl in my class that was only 15 months that was potty training and doing a fantastic job. But some kids can start as early as 18 or 19 months, including boys. So, potty training earlier is great because it gives you the ability to control the process versus them being in control. When you start at

that middle time frame, which is between 2 and 3 or 2 1/2 to 3 or later than that, what happens is that child goes more into the independent stage.

That's where they're able to start making to some of their decisions which happens to often include the word "no". And thus what happens as a parent is you're not only dealing with potty training but you're also dealing with behavior as the result of a child that is looking to find their self and their voice. Starting late doesn't mean you did anything wrong, and it doesn't mean that you're not going to potty train.; All it means is that it's going to be a little bit more challenging and a little bit more work. And that's okay but it just means that it's going to take a little bit more time to get the child potty trained.

Now, the other thing that you want to realize is the later you start, the more years of behavior modification you're trying to reverse and that can account for some of that difficulty. In other words, when you start the potty training at the age of 2, you only have 2 years of pooping in their diaper or potty in the diaper to reverse. Whereas the later you start, let's say at the age of 3, you've got 3, 3 1/2 years of pooping in their diaper or the potty behavior that you have to reverse. So, it's a

very big difference starting earlier than later because it's a lot more habit that has to be broken and a new habit learned.

To drive this point home, just think about how hard it is to change a behavior or a habit in yourself. If you think it's hard for yourself, think about a child that doesn't have the same cognitive ability that you have. Trying to get rid of that behavior as early as possible is better because it's less work for the child. We want to keep in mind how hard that child actually has to work to do this. The key also is that we're looking at doing this in just 3 days through consistency. So, reversing years of behavior in just 3 days is even that much more challenging the older they are.

2.4 Pre-potty training

Pre-potty training is getting the child ready for what is about to come if you really want to potty train him within 3 days, or what it is about to happen. In other words, you set a time when you're going to start potty training. It's now February and you want to start potty-training in September or something to that effect. Before

September comes around, there are things that you can

do that will make the potty training process not only easier for yourself, but also easier for the child.

The first thing you want to do is sit your child down and explain what is expected of them. Sitting down is an important component of this.

You want to sit next to them or across from them and in a very loving and caring tone, you want to say, "I am going to explain potty training to you." And you want to say, "Potty training is when you go the bathroom (tinkle, pee or poopy) in the potty." Now in terms of the words that you use, you want to be consistent. If you call it "tinkle" then you want to continue using the word "tinkle". If you call it "poopy", then continue using the word "poopy".

As a young child, too many words are going to confuse them, so staying consistent with your terminology will help you enforce the concept and they will know exactly what it means. You want to be strong and direct.

By that I mean using words like, "Mommy is going to have you potty trained, and here's what you have to do for Mommy...poopy, tinkle, etc." Or, "When you have to go potty, you have to let Mommy know, and you have to sit on the toilet and then you go potty". Then, you

physically walk them to the toilet and show them and say, "Here is where you go tinkle and poopy." This isn't being strict; it's being direct so that they know that you are in charge, and what is expected of them.

If you don't take it direct tone, kids are extremely smart. They can sense a lack of control and they might not follow your directions as well if you say, "Mommy would like" or, "It would be nice if you...""".

Take them to the bathroom and get them use to seeing you in the bathroom. Let them sit down on the toilet. Let them get used to having the toilet touch their skin as well. Many parents don't realize this, but many children have a fear of being on the toilet as opposed to just being hard to potty train. So this might help them get over that fear so when the potty training begins, you don't have to battle two things.

One thing is to start using less absorbent diapers. Today, the diapers are so absorbent the child doesn't even realize that they are wet. And most kids do not like the feeling of being wet. So when they have on a less absorbent diaper, it helps them realize the act of letting go and releasing 'number 1'. But the wet feeling also starts to psychologically or subconsciously say to them,

"When I get this feeling of letting go, I start to feel wet too, and I don't like that." You will also want to make sure that you change them frequently when they wet their diapers. This helps them get used to the feeling of being dry and staying dry. It also reinforces the feelings they have once they wet again. It is also highly encouraged that you actually consider taking your child out of diapers while they are awake a couple of months prior to the actual potty training process. So, during nap time, you will use diapers, but during their waking hours, you will want them in big boy and big girl underwear. You will also want to make sure that this whole pre-potty training process is a loving experience because you want it to subconsciously erase some of the other negative connotations and fears that your child may have. It's important that you understand pre potty training is not a necessary step. It gives you an advantage if you are starting the potty training process early, but if you are like most parents, then you might have missed the stage or the time when you could have pre-potty trained. You can still pre-potty train if you prefer, no matter at which stage you are, but it's

usually better if you can start as early as possible.

Knowing what we know and from our customers, however, most parents usually has missed this stage to the degree that they can get the most effectiveness out of it.

Chapter 3 Four stages of Potty training

In this section, I am going to teach you four stages to potty training. What you will notice and then appreciate is that these four stages can be applied to almost any other learned or practiced behavior which you are trying to alter or change.

3.1 The four stages of any behavior modification model include:

• Unconscious incompetence

• Conscious incompetence

• Conscious competence

• Unconscious competence

And now, I'll break these down to help you understand what they are and what you need to focus on during each one of these different stages.

Stage One: Unconscious Incompetence:

This is the "I do not know" stage, where your child's mind is thinking, "I do not know that going to the bathroom in my diaper is a wrong thing". In other words, the child has no idea that what they are doing is something they should not be doing. During stage one,

when they don't know the difference, this is when it becomes your responsibility to educate them and get them to understand what they are doing is not something they should be doing.

This is where you are teaching the child that they do not need to be going to the bathroom in their diaper.

Stage Two: Conscious Incompetence

At this stage, the child has reached an understanding where they know what they're doing is something they should not do, but have no idea how to correct it. During stage two you are taking it to that next level where you are reinforcing the positive behavior by showing them where they are supposed to go to the bathroom – in the potty. So, now you're teaching the child where to go, how to go, and what to do.

Stage Three: Conscious Incompetence

Here, the child knows what they are doing is something they shouldn't be doing, they know what to do about it, but they are also not that great at it. They have to think about it. That is because the process is now occurring on the conscious level. It is during stage three that the child starts to understand on their own and they start to show you the signs that they can do this on their own as well.

This is when you should be getting to the point of not having accidents anymore. Now, this is an area where most parents go wrong in that they get to stage three and they say, "My child is potty trained, there is nothing else that I have to do." In reality, this is where the real potty training begins. This is where you really want to be consistent to ensure they reach stage four and can consistently go to the potty by themselves. So, when you get to stage three, you have to make sure that you continue with consistency.

Stage Four: Unconscious Competence

And this is the fun stage. This is when the child gets to where they need to should know what they're doing and they don't have to think about it any longer. It is at stage four that your child can be officially considered 'potty trained.' Let's take a quick example to make sure the concept sinks in: If you are in stage three, you're not showing the child where to go potty anymore because they know where to go. What you're doing is being consistent with them going to the potty on a regular basis. During stage two you're not so much worried about consistency yet, you are more focused on helping them know where to go. Hopefully this description has given you a better understanding of how each stage develops and, better yet, what your actions need to be during each stage.

3.2 Potty Training as a young Mother

As a young mum who have no much experience about potty training; one of the best thing you can do to help your kid is to be a positive potty model. When you go to the bathroom, use it as an opportunity to talk your child through the process. Use words he or she can say, like pee, poop, and potty.

If you plan to start your child on a potty seat, put it in the bathroom so it becomes familiar. Make it a fun place your child wants to sit, with or without the diaper on. Have your child sit on the potty seat while you read or offer a toy.

Also, tune in to cues. Be aware of how your child behaves when he has to pee or poop. Look for a red face and listen for grunting sounds. Take notice of the time when he pees and poops during the day. Then establish a routine in which your child sits on the potty during those times, especially after meals or after drinking a lot of fluid. This helps set your child up for success.

And use plenty of praise, praise, and more praise. Is your child motivated by verbal encouragement? Stickers on a chart? Small toys or extra bedtime stories? Check in with what feels right for you and use it to reward positive potty choices. Your good attitude will come in handy, especially when "accidents" happen.

3.3 What Not to Do

Sitting on the potty should be a want-to, not a have-to. If your child isn't into it, don't force it.

Just when you think your child has nailed it, accidents happen. It's OK to be frustrated, but don't punish or shame your child -- it won't get you closer to your goal. Take a deep breath and focus on what you and your child can do better next time. Also, don't compare your son or daughter with other children. Some parents like to brag about how easy potty training went in their family. So if your neighbor says her kids potty trained themselves, smile and remember that the only right way is the one that works for you.

And if you a working mum, you juggle all your professional and personal responsibilities and, somehow, you make it look simple. Life is busy, though, and you've

got a huge task to add to the to-do list: learning how to potty-train.

Helping your little one switch from diapers to the bathroom is a tough job — regardless of whether you're a stay-at-home or working parent. Because you fall into the latter category, you have to plan the process more carefully, so you are present for the majority of the transition. As you prepare for life without diapers, here are some tips to keep in mind to make it simpler for you as you balance your professional schedule and potty-train schedule.

1. Choose the Right Time

Parenting books will probably suggest the perfect time to start potty-training, but no two children are the same. Some little ones start using the potty at as young as 24 months, but that's rare. In most cases, children begin between 24 and 36 months, and the entire process can take up to eight months to perfect after that.

Still, you should be more focused on starting the process when your child shows they are ready for it. For instance, some kids will start to show interest in their siblings' or classmates' potty behavior, which can help you ease them into using the toilet, too. Also, if your

child sleeps through nap time without wetting their diaper, they could be prepared to potty-train. To that end, staying dryer for longer also shows a little one has what it takes to wear big-kid underwear. Finally, your child might alert you when they must go, hide when they have to pee or poop, or tug at a dirty diaper.

Once you start seeing these cues, you should start thinking about beginning the process. There's no need to start too soon and put too much on your plate when you're already busy.

2. Invest in the Tools

Now that you know it's time to potty-train, you have to invest in the supplies you need to make it possible. For one thing, you'll need to pick up some underwear for your son or daughter. On a weekend or after-work trip to the store, bring your child along to help pick out their designs — they'll find it even more exciting to switch to underwear if they like the character or colors. Having the proper clothing and underwear, along with other potty-training supplies like extra bed sheets, flushable wipes, and soap you can keep your child comfortable and ready for anything.

However, mistakes happen! If they do make a mess,

teach them to not put anything other than toilet paper or flushable wipes in the toilet! By preventing the flushing of wipes and the use of too much paper, you will minimize the amount of plumbing-related issues you will experience. When clogs do occur, knowing how to effectively use a plunger and when to call in a plumber can also save you a lot of grief.

3. Work with Teachers or Nannies

You can kick off your potty-training extravaganza over the weekend but, by Monday, you'll have to go back to work. Rather than halting your progress and popping your child back into diapers, work with their nanny or preschool teacher so everyone's on the same page about the transition. Chances are, your childcare provider will be more than willing to stick to the routine you've started, as well as any rewards system you have in place. Think about it — it's beneficial for them not have to change diapers anymore, either. Make sure you pack plenty of dry clothes just in case, as accidents do happen. Then, once you pick up your child and go home, you can continue the training process yourself.

4. Reward Good Potty Habits

Experts have varying opinions on rewarding children for

their successful use of the potty. Some say it's a great way to boost their accountability, while others think the feeling of being clean and dry is reward enough. It's up to you whether or not you'll incentivize the process with treats, stickers or a potty-training chart.

No matter what, it's vital that you verbalize how proud you are of your child as they use the potty. Even if their teachers take the reins during the day, shower them with praise as soon as you pick them up and hear updates on the process. It can be frustrating if your child fusses about using the toilet or if they suffer from accidents, but you can't let them see or feel this from you. With a supportive parent helming the transition from diapers to potty, children are more likely to try.

Start and Succeed

Once you've pinpointed the right time to start, invested in the right gear and enlisted the help of your child's teachers, you're ready to potty-train. You'll be surprised how these simple steps can make it so much easier to get the job done, even while you're working. Cheer your child to the finish line both of you will be freer and happier sans diapers, which is the best benefit of all.

3.4 How to Potty Train a Child with Special Needs as a mum

If you have a child with special needs, then you know that you may not be able to rely on the "typical" signs of potty training readiness. Kristen Raney from Shifting Roots shares her experience with potty training her son.

Potty Training a Child on the Autism Spectrum First of all, don't read those stories about moms who potty train their children in three days!!! This will not work for our children and will cause you so much stress!! Remember through this process that you are a good mom doing the best you can for your child.

Most of the moms of autistic children I know were not able to potty train their children before four, many of them five, and some of them never. It just depends where your child falls on the Autism Spectrum and what their particular sensory issues are.

For context, our son would be considered to have Aspergers, but it's no longer a diagnosis and is now part of the Autism Spectrum. His body was ready to potty train around 2 1/2, but he had very intense fears about using the toilet. No bribe, game, song, or sticker chart in

the world could get him to use it. He also was terrified to pee or poo in pre-K, daycare, or anywhere in public. We started by getting him trained to pee on the potty, and he hit that milestone by 3 1/2. I don't remember how, because it was so stressful that I've erased that time from my mind. I think it involved making him pee in his diaper in the bathroom, and slowly transferring that idea to the potty. Once he got that, he had to ask for a diaper if he wanted to poo, and go in his diaper in the bathroom. To get him trained all the way, it took a 90 minute battle of wills where I told him he could poop on the potty or on the bathroom floor, it was entirely his choice. It was terrible. He chose the potty, glared at me like I was killing him. We bought him a Thomas train for the next three times he went on the potty, and a fourth one for keeping it up for a week. Yes, this sounds completely excessive and terrible, but he was 4 1/4 and we were at our wits end.

I hope your journey is much less stressful than ours, but know that you're not alone! Don't take any flack from someone with a neurotypical kid who gives you grief about not having your child trained by now. You've got this mama!

3.5 How to Potty Train a "Late" Bloomer

Here's the thing. Out of all of my mom friends, not one of our kiddos potty trained at the same age/time. In my grandparent's era, children were toilet trained early (12-18 months). This had a lot to do with the needs of the adult, however, not necessarily the readiness of the child. Most American families are now waiting until their child is at least twenty-four months or beyond to introduce potty training. Keep in mind, that times are always changing!

An article by Healthy Children.org entitled "The Right Age to Potty Train", states that there is no exact right age potty train! Research over the past several decades indicates that there is no perfect age. Parents really need to look at the physical, mental, and emotional readiness of their child and go from there. These indicators could happen at vastly different ages.

Sumer Schmitt over at Giggles, Grace, and Naptime shares her experiences with potty training on "older toddler". Her son was nearly three and a half when he was fully potty trained. She shares her story of persevering through potty training and advises:

We, as moms, have heard it a million times. Don't compare. Don't compare your child to little Suzy down the street who was potty trained at 18 months. Or the story you read online about the 6 month old baby who is already doing elimination communication. Easier said than done, right? When you're in the thick of it though, it's hard not to get stuck in the comparison game.

Trust me, I get it. But, your child will potty train in his/her own time. Chances are, by the time your child reaches kindergarten, no one is even going to be talking about this milestone anymore. Just like they no longer talk about when your child first rolled over, sat up, crawled, or started walking. Those milestones are in the past and most children will all eventually catch up to one another.

Studies actually show that sometimes potty training later is better because your child will have a better developed vocabulary. Potty training may be easier and happen faster the later the age!

3.6 How to potty train your kid as a dad

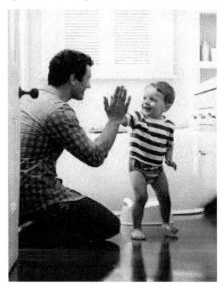

As a father, either single father or not our child is more likely to understand potty use if he's no longer wearing a nappy. Training pants are absorbent underwear worn during toilet training. They're less absorbent than nappies but are useful for holding in bigger messes like accidental poos. Once your child is wearing training pants, dress her in clothes that are easy to take off quickly.

Pull-ups are very popular and are marketed as helpful for toilet training. It isn't clear that they actually help. But you can try them to help your child get used to wearing underwear.

Generally, cloth training pants are less absorbent than

pull-ups and can feel a little less like a nappy. Pull-ups might be handier when you're going out. Wearing training pants is a big move for your child. If you celebrate it, the transition will be easier. Talk about how grown-up he is and how proud of him you are. I've heard all the tricks stickers, bribing with toys, special underpants. But you have to pick something that's consistent with your parenting style. I didn't use rewards elsewhere, so I didn't want to start here. What did work: Lots of undivided attention, positive reinforcement, love, affection and pride when my kids were successful. Making a big deal about small steps of progress is key. I didn't use any special stuff—no kiddie toilets, potty rings, or even pull-ups—because the local YMCA where my daughters attended didn't believe in them. We even had to sign a contract stating that we'd follow their potty training policy at home. I was instructed to just put the kids (they were around 2 1/2) on our regular toilet throughout the day when I thought they had to go. After a week and lots of "Yeah! You did number two!" and "Good for you! You made a wee-wee!" they were done, with barely any accidents. All told, I think they were just developmentally ready.

"The key is consistency," says James Singer, father of two, and a member of the Huggies Pull-Ups Potty Training Partners. "Whatever you do at home with your potty training plan, you also need to do elsewhere. For instance, if your child prefers to read a book while on the potty, talk to your daycare provider about sending in a favorite book. Keep in mind that daycare centers may be too busy to customize potty training to each child. In that case, ask them how they think they can help foster the success you have had at home and compromise. Then bring home something that works at daycare. If your child loves the soap they use at school, get some for home.

Boost the fun factor of using the potty with a Pee-Kaboo Reusable Potty Training Sticker. Slap a blank sticker onto the base of a portable potty, have your toddler pee in the potty, and then let him watch as an image of a train, flower, fire truck, or butterfly appears! After you empty, clean, and dry the potty, the image disappears, ready to be used again and again for up to six weeks. Too good to be true? We tested it on a formerly reluctant potty trainer, 2-year-old Gwenyth Mencel, who now shouts "Butterfly, butterfly!" when it's time to hit the potty. Are you counting down the days to the toilet transition? Or maybe you've already dabbled in a few less-than-successful attempts? Either way, we heard one thing again and again: Your kid has to be good and ready. And don't worry, he will be someday. "No child is going to graduate high school in diapers," says Carol Stevenson, a mom of three from Stevenson Ranch, California, who trained each one at a different age. "But it's so easy to get hung up and worried that your child's a certain age and not there yet, which adds so much pressure and turns it into a battle." Once you're convinced your kid's ready to ditch the diapers (watch for signs like showing an interest in the bathroom, telling you when she has to go, or wanting to be changed promptly after pooping), try any of these tricks to make it easier.

3.7 An explanation from an experience Dad

My wife, MJ, and I ran into the usual parent challenges when trying to potty-train our son. At first Will, then 2, was confused, then afraid, and next defiant. At 2 1/2 he still loved that diaper, and the mere sight of a toilet sent

him into a tantrum. The most frustrating part was that I knew he was ready. He would stay dry the entire night, wake up, and pee into his diaper while standing right in front of us, grinning. It was a not-so-subtle reminder that if Will was going to learn, it would be on his own terms.

MJ and I spent countless hours trying to make the bathroom more appealing. We brought Will's stuffed animals in there, let him flip through his books while sitting on the potty (good training for when he's older, like Dad), and even threw Cheerios in the bowl to give him a target. Nothing worked.

At last we got Will to stand on the stool, lift up the seat, pull his pants down, and loom over the toilet. But he still wouldn't go. "Dad, it's not working," he'd say in the cutest way imaginable.

At first I urged him to keep trying. No go. So I turned on the faucet, thinking the sound of running water would make him feel like peeing. But I forgot that he doesn't like noise, so this move merely upset him.

Finally I had a eureka moment. "Hey, Bud, how 'about if Dad pees with you, and we race?" I said. This clearly sparked Will's competitive spirit, because he brightened

up and agreed to the challenge. I shifted his stool to the right so I could squeeze in next to him, and we prepared for our duel. I told him we'd fire on the count of three. But my little cheater jumped the gun. I didn't even get to "two" before he let loose a stream into the toilet. Victory. Will giggled and grinned with pride, and I silently awarded myself first place in the "Best Dad in the Universe" contest for solving the potty-training riddle. I smiled broadly at father and son sharing a moment, hitting a milestone (er, Cheerio), and having some genuine fun.

A little too much fun, as it turns out. Will became so excited and began laughing so hard that he started falling in mid-spritz. I was still peeing as well, so I did my best to keep him balanced, all the while making sure we hit the porcelain bull's-eye.

Will's left foot slipped off the stool. I was able to catch him somewhat with my hip and right hand, but not before he instinctively turned toward me. Yup, that's right he sprayed me. A good father would've taken the punishment. But I'm squeamish, so I jerked my body away from his shower. That caused my own pee to hit the wall and ricochet onto my poor son's back.

We both fell to the floor, shocked and disgusted. We were silent for a moment, until Will spoke.

"Dada?" he said quizzically. "Yes, Bud?"

"You peed on me."

"To be fair, you peed on me first."

The two of us started cracking up belly laughs, guffaws, cackling, you name it - to such a degree that I would have peed myself right there if I hadn't just soaked my toddler. The racket attracted the attention of MJ, who came rushing over. When she turned the corner she stared at us: our soaked clothes, the yellow droplets slowly making their way down the wall.

I launched into an explanation. "Honey, you see, there was a pee race ..."

"I don't care," she interrupted, turning on her heels and walking away. "Just clean it up."

I did, and that day turned out to be a breakthrough. Will began using the toilet regularly (he asked me many times to race him again, but I never accepted) and was fully trained less than two months later. The bad news? He can't

resist the urge to tell anyone and everyone about the time Dad peed on him.

3.8 How to Potty train a kid as a grandpa

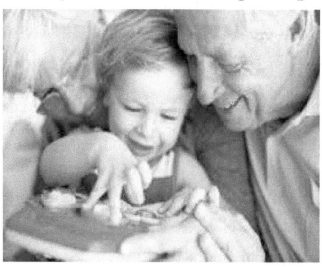

Potty training is one of the more difficult endeavors we face as old parents. Every child is different and has their own unique challenges.

Unfortunately, it's a messy, stinky destination that you'll quickly want to conquer, but will seemingly get stuck in the mud (no pun intended). So why do some grand parents struggle so much with potty training? The answer may be in the diversity, or lack there of our teachings. The way I see it, the more activities you do to promote potty usage, the better your child's chance of

success. You have to stack the deck in your favor. Some parents only do one or two things like buy pull-ups and

attempt to put their child on the potty until they get frustrated from it not working. There is a better way. In fact, several different ways which should all be used in conjunction to make potty time a little less night marish and actually more successful!

Children are typically ready to potty train around the ages of 2 or 3 but maybe earlier if there are older siblings to learn from. Look for the signs.

Look out for signs that your child is ready. These include pulling their diaper on and off, going a while or whole nap with a dry diaper, telling you they're going, showing curiosity about the potty and what goes in it, and going number 2 the same time each day.

When starting, dedicate 1-2 weeks to potty training. This includes pausing play-dates, car rides, outdoor activities, and basically anything that brings your child out of the house. Once you start, there's no turning back. Make sure you're in it for the long haul...all or nothing. Avoid pull-ups during the day as they give children a crutch to go, just like a diaper. Instead, let them be naked and

rush them to the potty if they start to go while saying, "Make sure you go pee pee in the potty."

Put them on the potty every 15 to 30 minutes. A lot of kids also have a set time of day when they do their "number 2" business. Make sure to put your child on the potty for several minutes during this time of day and encourage them to go number 2.

Make it enticing and convenient for them to go by providing a smaller, fun themed potty that's not so intimidating to a toddler. My son had a fire truck potty that he loved and we kept it in the room he would play in. Teach the process of going potty and washing hands with books! There are a ton of great books that you can read to your toddler while sitting on the potty.

Make a cool potty earning chart with fun stickers and rewards. My son received a sticker every time he went potty and after eight stickers he received a little cheap toy like a matchbox car. You can also reward with a few mini M&Ms when they're successful. Charts are a great way to be consistent. Nighttime potty training usually comes later. We put nighttime pull-ups on our toddler for a good six months after he was day time potty trained. It wasn't until he started going the entire night

without incident did we stop using them. Try your best to stay calm, use positive reinforcement, and not get angry or frustrated when they have an accident. You don't want your child to be anxious or stressed with potty time. Don't make them feel bad for having an accident. They might not tell you when it happens the next time.

As stated earlier, potty training is one of the most difficult parts of being a parent. Consistency is your friend in this situation. Don't give up. Even with hard work, regression is possible and normal. Keep working at it until your little one is a potty pro.

Chapter 4 How to potty train your kid in 3 days

The "Signs of Readiness"

I've heard people say that the child needs to show "signs of readiness" before you can potty train them for 3 days.

This is true. What most people don't understand is, "What exactly is a sign of readiness"? People often say that a sign of readiness is when the child starts showing interest in the toilet more than usual. In my opinion, this is an enormous misconception.

Children are curious creatures. As soon as they can crawl, they're out exploring their world. They inevitably find the toilet bowl and start playing in the water.

This is not "the sign" to look for (though it is if you want to prevent them from getting sick, hurt or causing other mayhem).

A necessary sign of potty training readiness is the ability for the child to frequently communicate his or her wants. I'm not talking about speech. I'm talking about gestures, behaviors, sounds, signing. If you can understand that a child wants something, and the child can direct you to the item, that is good enough.

Believe me, when a child is pulling your leg into the kitchen or bedroom, they know what they want, and they are effectively communicating with you! There is greater significance in this sign than you might think. What this behavior or attribute also means is that many children with Apraxia or speech, autism and other developmental problems can be potty trained using this method. Ultimately, the child learns that using the toilet is a good thing, something to be rewarded, and they will find a way to communicate their need to you. They like being rewarded.

A parent explained: My fifth child was diagnosed with Childhood Apraxia of Speech and was potty trained at 22 months old in under 3 days using 3

Day potty training method this is not an easy task. At the time his vocabulary consisted mainly of sounds - not actual words. If a child with apraxia can use potty at 22 month why did you think your own kid cant do that.

Secondly, your child must be able to go to bed without a bottle or cup, preferably two to three hours before bedtime.

4.1 There are a couple reasons why I say this.

1)I care about your child's dental health 2)It makes for easy potty training

What happens to you when you have a lot to drink just before going to bed? Late night visits to the bathroom! The same goes for your child. If you give them lots of fluid before bed, there's little chance they will wake up dry.

4.2 A few common questions I get from moms about this sign of readiness:

1)Our dinner is only an hour before bed, do I not give my child anything to drink? It is just fine for you to give your child something to drink with dinner. Just be sure that he's not getting tons just before he goes down for the night.

2)My child really enjoys his cup of milk before bed as it is part of our night time routine. Do I really need to stop this? No, you can continue as you have milk with your night time routine but try to decrease the amount. To do this maybe you can get him a smaller cup and then only

fill it half way full. Also be sure to follow the night time routine outlined in this eBook.

3)My child wakes often during the night needing a drink, I don't want to tell him no because it's really dry where we live.You can go ahead and let your child have his "sips" of water during the night if he really needs this but there is no need for full cups of water. Being that your child does wake for drinks, he shouldn't have a problem also getting up to go to the bathroom.

Third, in order for this method to work for children under the age of 22 months of age, your child must be waking up dry. Check for dryness within half an hour of them waking up. Don't wait until they've been up for an hour or so. By then, they will have peed and you won't get an accurate indication of readiness. If your child is over the age of 22 months old he should be waking up dry but don't worry too much if he does not. Just be sure to follow the night time method outlined in the eBook to help him with waking up dry.

4.3 A few common questions I get from moms about this sign of readiness:

1)My child is 3 years old and still wakes up with a full

diaper. Can I still potty training my child? Yes! As stated above, if your child or grandchild is over the age of 22 months and they still wake up wet, it's ok. Just be sure to follow the night time steps outlined in the eBook.

2)My first child is 5 years old and still wets the bed, I don't think my 2 year old will be able to be potty trained for nights. Can I just potty train for the days and use a pull-up or diaper for nights? Why would you want to? There is no need. You can easily potty train your child (even your older child) to wake up dry if you follow the method outlined in the eBook. It works!

3) My child is 18 months old and shows most the signs of readiness but doesn't wake up dry; can I still start potty training? Yes, just be sure to follow the steps outlined in the eBook for night time. I do recommend waiting until your child is 22 months of age because it can take longer than three days when they are younger than 22 months, but the choice is yours. It is my experience that children 22 months of age are at the ideal age to be

potty trained. It is entirely possible that a 15 month old shows these signs. For me, if my 15 month old showed these signs, I would still wait until 22 months.

4.4 The First day Journey to the 3 days potty training

Day 1 is the day that we decide to start potty training. First of all, as mentioned earlier, make sure that not only you, but also your child and anyone else who's involved, gets a good night's rest. This is extremely important. It's very difficult to accomplish something when you are not only tired but the child is tired and everyone is cranky.

It is on this day that you get rid of the diapers and the child starts wearing big boy and big girl underwear fulltime... There are no more diapers in this process... Now, some of you are saying, "Well, maybe we'll go ahead and use pull-ups or padded underwear." What I like to say is, "A diaper is a diaper no matter what you call it or what you disguise it as." And subconsciously, if you put the diaper on the child, it gives them the wrong message.

Also, seeing as that we've already explained how difficult this process is for the parents or the potty trainer as it is for the child, not having the diaper makes the parent or the potty trainer more vigilant. You will pay more attention if you know that the child does not have a diaper on.

For example, if you know the child has a diaper and you are out and about somewhere in a store or going out shopping you might say to yourself, "Well, we don't have to find a bathroom right now. We're kind of in a rush. You've got a diaper on." But note that the one time you tell that child that it's okay to go potty in that diaper; you have opened Pandora's Box. You've just told them, "its okay". And they will continue to do that and you will hit a lot of regressions. So, we start with allowing them to pick their big boy or girl underwear and put it on. (This is something you might have done during the pre-potty training process).

Then, you're going to sit down with your child and explain the process to them again. You can say, "Here's what we are doing; here is what Mommy expects; and here is what's going to happen." Then, you'll want to let them pick the spot for their potty chair.

You'll ask them, "Where do you want your potty chair?" We want to give them some control as well. If you have 2 bathrooms in the house, let them pick their favorite bathroom if they're going to be using the bathroom instead of the potty chair.

Then, you're going to take them to the bathroom. They are going to sit on the toilet and you are going to say, "Okay, Mommy wants you to use the bathroom." By this point, they should have seen you use the bathroom, so you can also say, "We want you to use the bathroom just like Mommy uses the bathroom." Don't be disappointed if nothing comes out. The act that getting them to sit there is a reward or it's an accomplishment all on its own. Once they get off the toilet, you're going to set a timer for 20 minutes.

Every 20 minutes for the first 3 days or for the first few days until they're trained, you are going to have them go and sit in the bathroom. When the timer goes off (and this is very important) it almost has to become a celebration in the house. Everybody can clap or say, "It's potty time. It's potty time. Let's go potty." And everyone can run to the bathroom.

Even with our older kids when we were potty training our youngest, would join into the celebration and run to the bathroom. And it was as if it was Cinco de Mayo or some big festivity in the house. That is very important because we're trying to make this a fun experience for the child.

Every time they go to the bathroom at those 20 minute intervals, you want to make sure they sit on the toilet for 3 to 5 minutes. This is not about them sitting on the toilet for hours; it's sitting on the toilet for 3 to 5 minutes. If they go right away and they pee or they do number 2, then they can get up right away.

Now, if they don't do either one then you want to make sure you wait the full 5 minutes with them sitting on the toilet. Note: At this point, we are not so much concerned about number 2. We want you and them to master number 1 first and then we'll move on. Now, even if they don't go, that is okay because the fact that you're getting them to sit down on the toilet is, again, an accomplishment all in its own.

But something that you want to see happen every single time they sit down on the toilet is for them to push. Even if they don't go number 2 or they don't do number 1, you want to make sure they push. So, you'll want to say, "Mommy wants to see you push. Now push." And some parents have told us, "Well, I can't tell when they're pushing." What you want to do is look at their stomach.

You can tell by the stomach muscle flexing whether they

are pushing or not. You see, with a child, it is impossible for them to hold and push at the same time. So, you're almost tricking them into using the potty by asking them to push. So, no matter what—no matter where you go, no matter what time it is—the minute they sit on the toilet you want to make sure that they push and they push every single time. Even if nothing comes out, as long as they push, that is a good thing because we want to get them used to using those muscles and pushing and moving whatever is inside of their system out. If you find they do not understand what pushing is, what you can do is just tickle their stomachs and the tickling sensation will cause them to contract their stomach muscles, which is a natural way to push.

The other thing that you want to start doing is giving them more fluids. Many people think that potty training is about not wetting themselves. That is not what potty training is about. Potty training is about recognizing when you have to go and knowing where to do it. So, one of the things that you're going to do to help them recognize that is giving them more fluids. However, you do not want to give them more juice because sometimes the sugar and starches that are in the juice can cause

constipation and other problems. Instead, you want to give them liquids like water and things that are going make them want to go potty. In addition to helping them potty, water also helps in the number 2 process as well, which we'll talk about later.

Now, sometimes what happens is that the child will sit for 5 minutes, they won't go, they'll get up and then they might wet themselves within a minute or two. So, here's what you do in that situation: shorten the amount of time that they sit on the toilet. Instead of sitting on the toilet for 5 minutes, let them sit on the toilet for 1 or 2 minutes, but you increase the frequency of how many times they go to the bathroom. So, instead of every 20 minutes, now it's every 15 minutes for 1 to 2 minutes. Another thing you'll want to do is ask them from the minute they get off the toilet and at least 3 or 4 times during that 20 minute timeframe, "Do you have to go potty? "Most of the time, they're going to tell you, "No," and that's okay.

You just want to get them used to hearing the words, "Do you have to go potty?" Then, when the 20 minutes are up and it's time to go potty, now the question is not, "Do you have to go potty?" Now, it's, "Time to potty."

One is asking and one is telling. Hopefully you see and understand the difference between the two statements. It's very, very important especially for psychologically getting the child to want to go and use the toilet.

4.5 Constipation

Alright, let's start with holding. Some children will actually hold number 2. Sometimes they will hold number 2 for a day or two days. When it finally becomes too painful they will let it all out into the diaper. First of all if you find your child is holding it that long and all the other methods are not working, and then put a diaper on to let them go. Holding bowel that long is not good for them. This is one of the rare times we recommend putting on a diaper. The thing to realize is...if they are holding it that long, then theoretically just by the nature of what potty training is, that says your child is potty trained and know what to do. For whatever reason they are afraid of the potty.

It's not an issue of potty training. It's an issue of being afraid or maybe going potty is too painful for them. If you find that their stool is hard, then it will lead to painful bowel movement. If they associate all bowels as

painful then they would rather hold the stool then to let it go. So the things that you can do are give them foods that will cause them to go to the bathroom. Give them more liquids (preferably water, not soda or juice), more liquids in their system the easier for them to go number You want to also do other things. When they're sitting on the toilet try to take their mind off the potty. Some ways to do that would be to rub their stomach or their feet. In the scientific world this is called neuro-linguistic programming. Basically you are trying to get their mind off of something that they're afraid of. So by doing something that feels good to them, you are associating the toilet with something that feels good. Now they're not afraid of that anymore. You want to tickle them. When you tickle them, it forces them to push. You've heard me use the word push over and over so it's something that I'm going to stress. Make sure they push. As long as they push you are doing good. They cannot hold and push at the same time. I cannot stress enough how important pushing is. If you feel they don't know what pushing is, then tickle their stomach and that will help them understand what pushing is. The other thing that you want to look at when it comes number 2 is constipation. There are a lot of things that cause constipation. Some causes of constipation are medical, while other causes are more mental. If you find your child is constipated, you want to do what I call the "bicycle trick". Don't ask how we had figured this out, but this works 100% of the times. What you do is you lay your child on their back. You should kneel in front of your child at the base of their feet.

Their feet should be almost touching your lap. Grab the base of their feet. Then rotate their legs as if they're riding a bicycle. Do this for about 10 minutes. Within 25 -30 minutes of doing this, the child will use the bathroom. We've told many parents to do this. Every parent I've told to try this, we've gotten a 100% success rate, whereas the child will end up using the bathroom within 30 minutes of doing the "bicycle trick".

So that is the constipation, and if you find the constipation lasting 4 or 5 days you may want to seek some form of medical attention for the child. That is not normal for them to be able to hold it for that many days.

4.6 The second day journey of the 3 days

Alright, so you've graduated from number 1. Your child

is doing very well using number 1. Now, it's time for them to start using number 2. There is not much difference between training them from number 1 to number 2. As a matter of fact, I would go so far to tell you that number 1 is a lot harder than number 2, and the reason being that when they go number 1, they have to actually take action to hold it inside.

In other words, for them not to wet themselves, they have to actually squeeze the sphincter muscle and hold the fluids inside. Whereas with number 2, they don't have to do anything to hold it. They actually have to push it out so it is an action that is a lot less difficult than holding the number 1 is. This is behaviour. They have to actually take a step. They have to be proactive to go number 2 so they have a whole lot more control in the number 2 process than they do in number 1. Now, again, one of the things that we want to make sure we do when they're sitting on the toilet is pushing. And, hopefully you understand how important the pushing strategy is. No matter how far along in the potty training process — whether they are two years old or whether they are four and a half — pushing is extremely important because that is how they are training themselves to go.

This is especially true when it comes to number 2. Now, some kids will want to go in number 2 in their diaper or a pull up. They will actually go and ask their parent for a pull up or a diaper to go number 2. Now, if this is the case for you, what you want to realize is the pull up then becomes a security blanket for the child.

In this case, what you might say is something to the effect of, "Okay, if you go number 2, then we'll put the pull up on." What that says is, "If you go number 2 first then we'll get

the pull up." Now, something else I've had parents do is actually go get the pull up, let them put the pull up on only around their ankles. That way, they have their security blanket on, and they can feel it, and they can see it, yet they're sitting on the toilet. This allows them to use the bathroom and feel comfortable.

The other thing you want is to make sure that you give them is more fluids as I explained earlier. And you will also want to make sure to track their schedule. A lot of kids will go to the bathroom for number 2 at the same time or around the same time every day. With my youngest son, it was like clockwork. Within 30 minutes of him eating anything, he would go to use the potty and

do number 2. So, we always knew after he ate that he was going to use the bathroom. Using a potty training journal is helpful.

If you don't have a potty journal and a potty chair or a potty chart, you can get yourself a potty training chart and journal to track when they go to the bathroom. Let's say you find that they go after dinner, which is around the time frame of 7:00 in the evening. Well, what happens is you're still using the same consistency as using number 1 which is every 20 minutes except now you are watching for 7 o'clock to come around because you know that they're going to be using the bathroom within a half hour.

At this point, what you want to do is time the bathroom use. You want to get them on the toilet but you also want to make sure that they stay on the toilet long enough to use the bathroom or use the bathroom to do number 2. their underwear again. It's going to help them make sure they use the bathroom the next time they go.

4.7 When they finally get it right

Alright, now you're taking them to the bathroom every

20 minutes and you go 3 days and you are not getting any accidents. Don't make the mistake that most parents make as I mentioned very early on. This is the stage when many parents decide that, "My child is potty trained and there was nothing left for me to do." This is the point in time where you want to be more consistent, more consistent, and more consistent.

This is when you want to make sure that you are still taking them to the bathroom every 20 minutes or you might change the interval from 20 minutes to 30 minutes. You might even feel comfortable waiting even longer than that - maybe 45 minutes. But don't let 45 minutes to an hour go by that you are not taking your child to the bathroom. Let me give you an example why this is. Your body has to get what's called "muscle memory." Remember at this point the child is only in stage 3 of potty training.

That's where they know what they're doing. They know what's wrong but they're thinking about it. It's not subconscious yet. At this point in time, the child is still thinking, "Should I go; should I not go? Where should I go? What should I do?" Think about it this way: Michael Jordan is one of the best basketball players that have

ever played the game, yet even when he was scoring 30, 40, 50 points a game, he was still shooting and practicing for hours a day, taking 500 to 600 foul shots every single day. Even though he was the best there was, he was still practicing harder than anybody else.

That is the difference between regular athletes and professionals. The professionals, they practice harder than anybody else because when they get into a situation, they do not have to think about it, the body automatically reacts. So, that's why when your child is finally starting to get it, you have to then make sure you maintain the consistency.

Chapter 5 Getting them to tell you

How do you get them to start telling you? Basically the question is how do we get your child from Stage 3 to Stage 4? And Stage 4 is where they can go to the bathroom themselves. They recognize on their own, they don't need you to take them to the bathroom every 20 minutes. Basically, its complete autonomy and freedom for the child and complete autonomy and freedom for you... So, the question is, "How do we get to that stage?" With consistency. You have to be consistent.

Once they start to show you they are ready, you have to make sure that you are continually being consistent. The other thing you can do is you can play the game that I call the "let's race to the potty game." All you do is sit at the table with your child and you say, "Okay, let's see who can get to the potty first and whoever wins gets a prize." So, basically it's a race between you and the child, and, of course, you're going to let the child win (but they don't know that).

Then, you pick a good reward of something that they're going to enjoy or really like. To start the race they have to say the words, "Mommy, I have to go potty." That's the cue. It's like saying "1, 2, 3, set go." But instead of

saying "1, 2, 3, set go," they say, "Mommy I have to go potty". Once they say that, the race begins, so the both of you run to the bathroom and the first one that gets to the bathroom wins the game. What this does is gets the child used to saying, "I have to go potty," and then the next steps are them going to the bathroom.

You want to practice this probably two or three times a day once you find that they are starting to be more consistent with no accidents. You don't want to start this game while they're in the potty training process because they've got enough to worry about. So, you want to start this only after you've seen that they have finally gotten it and they're starting to do pretty well on their own.

5.1 How to Use Positive Practice for Accidents

Another useful technique is positive practice for accidents. Dr. Schaefer describes this as what you should do when your child has an accident and wets or soils himself.

This technique involves firmly telling your child what he has done, taking him to the potty where he can clean and change himself (although you will likely need to

help) and then having him practice using the potty. Dr. Schaefer recommends going through the usual steps of using the potty at least five times, starting when "the child walks to the toilet, lowers his pants, briefly sits on the toilet (3 to 5 seconds), stands up, raises his pants, washes his hands, and then returns to the place where the accident occurred."

Although you are trying to teach him the consequences of having an accident, this should not take the form of punishment.

5.2 Children Tantrums

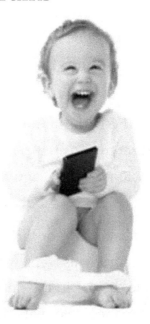

Tantrums are going to happen. A tantrum is frustration. That's the child not being able to verbally explain or talk about their emotion. So, the only way they know how to do that is through screaming and pitching a fit. Here's how you handle a tantrum... What you don't want to do is make potty training a battle. It's not a battle between you and the child, but the child is trying to battle you.

The child is trying to be in charge, and you're trying to be in charge at the same time. So, sometimes the way that you handle that is to totally ignore the tantrum. If your child is throwing a tantrum, you can walk away and say, "Mommy is not listening to you. Mommy will talk to you when you are calmed down," or "Mommy is not listening to you when your voice is louder than Mommy's." So you can turn around and use reverse psychology by turning the tables on your child. Once they have calmed down, you will want to say in a very strong and direct voice, "Mommy did not appreciate that," or "Grandma did not appreciate that," or "Daddy did not appreciate that behavior.

We expect better things. Let's go and try again." So, now you go right back to the basics and you take the child back to the bathroom and say, "We are going to use the bathroom and here's what we expect." If they throw a tantrum again, you walk away.Mind you, while

that tantrum is going on, do not give them any rewards. Do not allow them to play with their toys. They are not allowed to do any of that fun stuff that they normally would want to do because you want to associate that tantrum with a bad behavior that results in loosing something.

So, the most important thing I can tell you is to ignore the tantrum, don't pay attention to it because as the laws of physics say, "For every action, there's an equal and opposite reaction." If you react to that tantrum, they are going to react to you. Once you react, they react. You react again, they react and it's going to escalate even more.

So, the easiest way to squash it is not to put in the energy toward that tantrum. Once the child feels and sees that they're not getting energy out of you, then they realize that they're getting nothing by throwing this tantrum and there's nothing to be gained from it.

5.3 Regression in potty Training

What is a regression? A regression is a child that was potty trained, they were doing well, or they were starting to do well and for whatever reasons, they have

done an about-face. Now, they are wetting themselves or they are soiling their diapers with poop. The question is "What really is the regression? What are the cause and the root of that regression?" These are the issues that need to be dealt with. Usually a regression is not so much an issue with potty training, but it's an emotional issue. The child will regress as a way to get attention or as a way of expression.

So, most parents deal with regression by dealing with potty training, but the reality is the best way to deal with a regression is to try to find the underlying root cause. It could be one of many things causing the regression. A new baby being born, you've moved, a friend has moved, a family member might have passed away... Something has happened in that child's life and they don't know how to express it except through regression.

Something that a lot of parents have asked is, "When it comes to potty training, we've got a new baby on the way, should I wait to have the baby or will they regress if I potty train them and then we have the baby?" The best thing to do is to potty train them now. It is a lot easier to retrain a child that has been trained and has

gone through a regression than it is to try to train a child that has never been trained. In addition to that as a parent, if you are having a new baby coming, you do not want to have a new baby and potty training duties at the same time. That's very, very, difficult. What I always tell parents is that they'll only need two to three days to get the child to Stage 3. Stage 4 is what will take you a couple of days from there. Some kids even get to Stage 4 in one day.

But the key is, take the two or three days, get your child to Stage 3, then through consistency, work toward getting them to Stage 4. When the new baby comes, or whatever that activity is—whether it's a vacation or a move—if they do regress, they've already been trained. Getting them back and reversing the regression is going to be a lot easier than if you had never started at all. So what you want to do when your child does regress is you go back to the basics. This includes them being on the toilet every 20 minutes for 3-5 minutes. They will continue to do that until they stop the regressive behavior.

The only time our youngest had a regression, I went on a business trip with Greg. Lorenzo had been fully potty

trained for about three months both day and night. Then I went on that business trip with my husband, and Lorenzo went to stay at Grandma's. We only were gone Thursday, Friday, and Saturday and came back on Sunday. When we returned, it was as if this child had never seen a potty chair or had been potty trained in his life. Now I have no idea what happened in those four days. Maybe Grandma had let him do whatever he wanted, I do not know. Or maybe he just said, "You know what? You guys left me, and I'm going to fix you guys." Basically, we took him back to the basics, went back to every 20 minutes with him on the toilet. And within about a day, he was back to normal. But it was a little scary seeing that happen.

5.4 Addressing fear in the kids

What you want to do is separate the difference between a fear of the toilet and potty training. Many of the parents that we have worked with have lumped the two into one category by saying that the fear of the toilet is a potty training problem. The reality is that a fear of the toilet has nothing to do with potty training, and, in most cases, it is a fear of the toilet as we noted earlier. So

what you have to do is address that fear by sitting and asking your child. Don't be afraid to do this. Just ask them what they are afraid of. Sometimes it might not be the potty training, but something else. One of the things that you can do to help your child if there is a fear of the toilet is get yourself a potty chair or potty seat insert. An insert is actually put into the toilet and the child can sit on that toilet instead of the adult seat, which is especially helpful if the child is a little bit smaller.

They are usually colorful and have giraffes on them and dinosaurs. There is also a handle so the child can hold on to the handle and balance themselves. This will help them feel safe and comfortable without the fear of falling into the toilet. Placing a step stool under their feet will also assist them in this area. But, if you find that they have a fear of the toilet, then a potty training chair will be the way to go instead of the insert.

Now the question is this, if there's a fear of the toilet, what is the cause of that fear? Sometimes it can be pain that the child has when they are going to the bathroom. This is especially true with number 2. So the question is, have they ever had diarrhea or have they ever had a diaper that was on too long which caused a skin

irritation? They are now associating the toilet and potty with that pain.

It might possibly be constipation. As an adult, constipation can be very painful. So, think about the child. It also might not be actual constipation, but some kids naturally have hard stools and letting that go can be extremely painful for them. If that is the case, you want to make sure that you take a look when your child does use the bathroom more if they are in their diaper. Is their stool harder or is it soft? Was there any illness like the stomach virus or anything that caused them some pain? These are all the things that can cause the child to be not only fearful of the toilet, but can also cause a child to regress. So you want to be careful about this and ask yourself whether any of this has happened.

If you find the child has hard stool, one of the things that you can do is start giving the child more water, less sugar, and less starchy items, which will help them become hydrated. When the body becomes dehydrated, it will start to pull any fluids that it can get wherever it can get it. One of the places that it pulls the fluid from is going to be the stomach and the intestines. And once those fluids are pulled out, the result is hardened stool.

Once that stool becomes hard it's going to be very difficult and very painful for that child to go to the bathroom. So having fluids in the system will help give him or her softer stool. Something else that you can do if there is a fear of the toilet is calling it by a different name. Instead of calling it "potty," you can give it another name that doesn't bear a negative connotation. Something simple might be, "Let's go push."

Another thing that will help you make the experience more enjoyable for the child is to place books by the toilet. You should also have some toys in the bathroom or let them

bring some toys with them so that it's a comfortable environment and something that is more fun for them. Again, the key is making it a loving time and not a stressful time. If you can read to them or let them look at picture books, it turns into more of an enjoyable process and a less stressful process.

5.5 Potty training Twins or multiple children

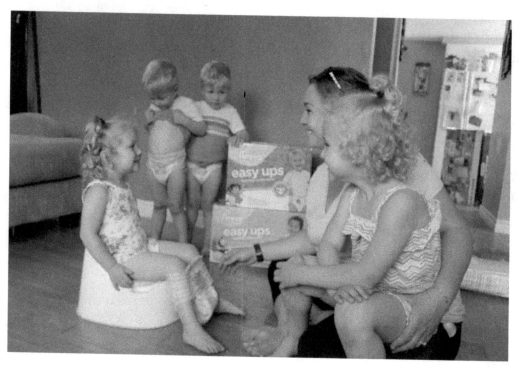

I have many parents with twins or multiples ask if this method can work for them. I also have parents with children at two different ages ask if the children can be potty trained simultaneously. The answer to both of these situations is "YES". You can potty train twins, multiples and two or more children at the same time. It's more demanding on you, and may take a few extra days, but it can be done.

If I, personally, had to choose between potty training multiples simultaneously or doing it one-at-a-time, I

would bite the bullet and do them all at the same time; "just be done with it." Having someone to help out is by far the best way. Be sure they read the guide. Discuss with them how you want situations handled. The two of you need to handle things identically. You can go it alone if you need to. Just be mentally prepared for some extra work. Also, the children must be right by your side at all times. If one child needs to use the restroom, ask the other child to come with. The underlying principle for potty training two or more children simultaneously is that you need to treat each child as an individual. Ideally, each child should have their own potty chair. They should each have their own underclothes and their own favorite treats and favorite drinks. Be sure to not use one's successes against the other child or children. Don't say things like, "See, Johnny can do it. Now you need to too." Just because one child might catch on right away doesn't mean that the other child / children will get it the first day or two. Keep in mind that they are individuals and that they may catch on at different times.

5.6 Help from daycare provider

If your child is in daycare be sure to discuss with your

daycare providers your plan a day or two before you start. Explain to them that when your child returns to daycare that they are not to put a pull-up or diaper on the child. They may come back to you and say that if the child has an accident, they will put a diaper on the child.

Gently remind them about the importance of being consistent, about how that would send mixed signals to the child, and could undo all the progress you've worked so hard to achieve, and that you greatly appreciate their support. Maybe even offer a pair of movie tickets. You or your spouse may need to take Friday or Monday off from work to give this method the best possible chance for success. Do not put your child in daycare during the three days. It's just too soon.

Day 4 is the earliest that I recommend returning your child to daycare.

Sometimes you may just have to play it by ear. At the end of day 3, if the whole toilet thing has not "clicked" with your child, you may need to take the next day off from work. The "clicking" or "getting it" needs to occur before the child returns to daycare. If your daycare provider is not on board with you then you might have a set back or two. I've never had my kids in daycare but

many of the moms that I've helped potty train have kids in daycare.

There are many wonderful daycare providers out there and they are willing to work with the parents but there are some that want nothing to do with helping the parents out. They want the child in a pull-up or diaper until they leave for school. If your daycare provider is one that isn't willing to support you during this training you might need to spend an extra day or two at home to make sure that there are no more accidents and that the child is confident in his new skill. You may need to be firm with your daycare provider with regards to your "no diaper" position.

If you are concerned about your daycare provider putting a pull-up or diaper back on your child, you might want to try Pods. Pods are little thin strips you place in your little ones underwear. These strips will absorb any accident your child has so he doesn't make a "mess" on the floor. Your child will feel the strips turn to a cold jell like substance and asked to go to the bathroom. The daycare provider can then just replace the strip. Pods can be the solution for those hard to work with daycare providers.

5.7 Travelling and Errands during potty Training

Alright, let's face the fact. You are a busy Mom or busy Dad or a busy Grandparent or a busy potty trainer. But you don't want to be stuck in the house during that potty training process. And yes —for a day or two you might be. But don't let potty training keep you from enjoying life and having fun and doing the things that you got to do.You may have shopping to do and errands to run. You might have a family to take care of. You've got things that you need to do. So here are some tips that will help you have a more successful potty training experience especially when you have things that you need to do.

First of all, you want to get yourself a spill-proof travel potty. If you don't have one, try to get one online travel and get yourself a spill-proof travel potty. Basically, it is a simple little potty chair which has a spill-proof lid. With that, you can keep it in the car so instead of having to be home to go to the bathroom every 20 minutes. You can be in the mall, you can be at the grocery store, you can be out shopping, and your child can still use the potty without the fear of having accidents. When you are

travelling or you're going to run errands, what you want to do is just like with the day care scenario, you want to use the bathroom before you leave. You will also want to plan your day and where you will be going so you'll be prepared about whether or not those places have bathrooms.

In other words, if you are going to place A and they have a bathroom and place B, does not have a bathroom, then you want to go to place B first right when you leave the house because your child has just gone. Once we would get to a location like a grocery store or a mall, especially if this is a grocery store or a mall that you've never been to, we would find the bathroom. So now, let's say we are out in the middle of shopping and Lorenzo had to go to the bathroom. It's wasn't a problem.

As soon as he said he had to go to the bathroom or we said, "Lorenzo, do you have to go to the bathroom?" and he said, "Yes," we knew where the bathrooms were. Most parents don't take that one step so what happens is the child says, "I have to go to the bathroom," the parents are in a state of panic to find the bathrooms. So, when we first got to the store, we would find the

bathroom and then go to the bathroom. We would then get our most important stuff done first because we knew we just went to the bathroom and had more free time now than we might later. So, the smaller, less important things could wait. Back to the travel potty, these are really great because they will also help you out when you are going to take a long road trip. If you don't have one, you know that stopping frequently is going to be an issue.

When Lorenzo was 2 years and 2 weeks, we had him fully potty trained and we took a trip to Florida. Back then, we were at Code Orange, and the government said it wasn't a good idea to fly. So, we decided to take a bus with three kids from Connecticut to Florida. It was a thirty-hour bus ride with a child that just finished potty training. To tell you it was a challenge is an understatement. Back then, there weren't spill-proof potty chairs so we didn't have one to bring, so we bought a huge 2 litre bottle. Every 20 minutes on the bus, we would hide in the corner or go into to the back and say, "Okay Lorenzo, pee into the bottle," and that's what he did. When he had to go number 2 luckily for us, was during a rest stop. But we didn't let the fact that he

had the potty train keep us from doing what we had to do.

Chapter 6 Naptime and Nighttime Training

6.1 Naptime

Yes it's ok to put your child down for a nap during training. I personally have found that most kids will not have an accident if you have them go pee before the nap and then just as they wake up. Make sure you stay close though so you know when your child wakes.

6.2 Nighttime

Do not give your child anything to drink when they are getting ready for bed. In fact, it's best to stop the liquids 2 to 3 hours beforehand. Take them to the toilet at least twice before tucking them in to bed for the night. If nothing happens in the bathroom, maybe read a book together for a few minutes and try again. Remember what I said about "trying" don't keep them on the toilet. Having them clear their bladder is important. Once your child has released twice you can put them in bed. Do not use a diaper (you shouldn't have any).

If your child has a hard time waking up dry and they are older than 22 months, the following procedure may help:

• Wake the child 1 hour after he or she has gone to sleep

• Take them to the toilet and return them to bed

• In the morning, wake the child 1 hour before they normally arise

Take them to the toilet This helps the child realize two things:

1)It is ok to get up to go pee

2)It is also expected If your child is in a crib, you can still follow these steps.

You just need to keep an ear open for them. If you hear your child stirring, or whimpering, they may need to pee. You do not need to do the above steps if your child usually wakes up dry. Your child may wet the bed at night. Don't be alarmed or upset.

This is halfway to be expected – we're giving them lots of liquid. Don't make a big deal of it – don't reprimand or scold. Just change the sheets. Remind the child to tell you when he needs to go pee, and that they need to keep their underwear dry. Again, don't be negative; don't say "Bad, No," etc.

This will be the end of a busy and perhaps frustrating day. Do not worry. It will click; your child will "get it", if

not tomorrow, then on the third day. Be sure to keep a positive and loving attitude with your child, even if you have to change sheets in the middle of the night.

A tip for parents with older children: To help your child to go to the bathroom before bed and to stay dry during the night you can try using a chart system with the following on it:

6.3 Bedtime Routine:

- go pee

- put on night clothes

- read a book

- brush teeth

- go pee again

- keep bed dry all night

Let your child know that if he gets a star by each one he will get a prize in the morning.

Remind him that he's got to get up and go pee if he's got to go. A special tip, that works for even the hardest of cases. The following has been used even with long time bed-wetters to help them overcome bed wetting... Once your child goes to sleep, make a bed up on the

floor without him knowing. Now throughout the night you will say to him "be sure to tell mommy when you

have to go pee". Anytime during the night when you hear him start to move and stir around, say to him "Do you have to go pee? Make sure tell mommy when you have to go pee".

What this does is allows you to see how often your child is stirring in his bed and will help him remember that he's suppose to pee in the potty not in his bed.

6.4 Toddler discipline and proper upbringing

Have you ever found yourself in deep negotiations with your 2-year-old over whether she can wear her princess costume to preschool for the fifth day in a row? Have you taken the "walk of shame" out of the local supermarket after your toddler threw a temper tantrum on the floor? There may be comfort in knowing you're not alone, but that doesn't make navigating the early years of discipline any easier.

Toddlerhood is a particularly vexing time for parents because this is the age at which children start to become

more independent and discover themselves as individuals. Yet they still have a limited ability to communicate and reason.

Child development specialist Claire Lerner, director of parenting resources for the nonprofit organization Zero to Three, says, "They understand that their actions matter -- they can make things happen. This leads them to want to make their imprint on the world and assert themselves in a way they didn't when they were a baby. The problem is they have very little self-control and they're not rational thinkers. It's a very challenging combination."

What do you do when your adorable toddler engages in not-so-adorable behavior, like hitting the friend who snatches her toy, biting Mommy, or throwing her unwanted plate of peas across the room? Is it time for...timeout?

Timeout -- removing a child from the environment where misbehavior has occurred to a "neutral," unstimulating space -- can be effective for toddlers if it's used in the right way, says Jennifer Shu, MD, an Atlanta pediatrician, editor of Baby and Child Health and co-author of Food Fights: Winning the Nutritional

Challenges of Parenthood Armed With Insight, Humor, and a Bottle of Ketchup and Heading Home With Your Newborn: From Birth to Reality.

"Especially at this age, timeout shouldn't be punitive. It's a break in the action, a chance to nip what they're doing in the bud."

Timeouts shouldn't be imposed in anger, agrees Elizabeth Pantley, president of Better Beginnings, a family resource and education company in Seattle, and author of several parenting books, including The No-Cry Discipline Solution. "The purpose of timeout is not to punish your child but to give him a moment to get control and reenter the situation feeling better able to cope." It also gives you the chance to take a breath and step away from the conflict for a moment so you don't lose your temper.

6.5 Timeouts is Not for Every Kid

Some experts insist that timeouts work for all, but Shu and Pantley disagree. "For some kids who just hate to be alone, it's a much bigger punishment than it's worth, especially with young toddlers," says Shu. "They get so upset because you're abandoning them that they don't remember why they're there, and it makes things worse." She suggests holding a child with these fears in a bear hug and helping her calm down.

You can also try warding off the kind of behavior that might warrant a timeout with "time-in." That means noticing when your children's behavior is starting to get out of hand and spending five or 10 minutes with them before they seriously misbehave. "It's like a preemptive strike," Shu says. "Once they've gotten some quality time with you, you can usually count on reasonably OK behavior for a little while."

6.6 Toddler Discipline Dos & Don'ts

Shu says a good stage to initiate timeouts is when your toddler is around age 2. Here are a few guidelines.

Do remove your child from the situation. Do tell him what the problem behavior was.

Use simple words like "No hitting. Hitting hurts."

Don'tberateyourchild.

Do place her in a quiet spot -- the same place every time, if possible. For young toddlers, this may have to be a play yard or other enclosed space.

Don't keep him there long — the usual rule of thumb is one minute per year of age. Do sit down with your child after timeout is over and reassure her with a hug while you "debrief" by saying something like, "We're not going to hit anymore, right?" Don't belabor what the child did wrong. Instead, ask her to show you how she can play nicely.

6.7 Commandments Discipline for Toddler

Children aren't born with social skills it's human nature for them to start out with a survival-of-the-fittest mentality. That's why you need to teach your toddler how to act appropriately and safely -- when you're around and when you're not. In a nutshell, your job is to implant a "good citizen" memory chip in her brain (Freud called this the superego) that will remind her how she's supposed to behave. It's a bit like breaking a wild horse, but you won't break your child's spirit if you do it correctly. The seeds of discipline that you plant now will blossom later, and you'll be very thankful for the fruits of your labor. (Just don't expect a tree to grow overnight.) Here are the commandments you should

commit to memory.

1. Expect rough spots. Certain situations and times of the day tend to trigger bad behavior. Prime suspect

   number 1: transitions from one activity to the next (waking up, going to bed, stopping play to eat dinner). Give your child a heads-up so he's more prepared to switch gears ("After you build one more block tower, we will be having dinner").

2. Pick your battles. If you say no 20 times a day, it will lose its effectiveness. Prioritize behaviors into large, medium, and those too insignificant to bother with. In Starbucks terms, there are Venti, Grande, and Tall toddler screwups. If you ignore a minor infraction -- your toddler screams whenever you check your e-mail -- she'll eventually stop doing it because she'll see that it doesn't get a rise out of you.

3. Use a prevent defense. Sorry for the football cliche, but this one is easy. Make your house kid-friendly, and have reasonable expectations. If you clear your Swarovski crystal collection off the end table, your child won't be tempted to fling it at the TV set. If you're taking your family out to dinner, go early so you won't have to wait for a table.

4. Make your statements short and sweet. Speak in brief sentences, such as "No hitting." This is much more effective than "Chaz, you know it's not nice to hit the dog." You'll lose Chaz right after "you know."

5. Distract and redirect. Obviously, you do this all day. But when you try to get your child interested in a different activity, she'll invariably go back to what she was doing -- just to see whether she can get away with it. Don't give up. Even if your child unrolls the entire toilet-paper roll for the 10th time today, calmly remove her from the bathroom and close the door.

6. Introduce consequences. Your child should learn the natural outcomes of his behavior -- otherwise known as cause and effect. For example, if he loudly insists on selecting his pajamas (which takes an eternity), then he's also choosing not to read books before bed. Cause: Prolonged picking = Effect: No time to read. Next time, he may choose his pj's more quickly or let you pick them out.

7. Don't back down to avoid conflict. We all hate to be the party pooper, but you shouldn't give in just to escape a showdown at the grocery store. If you decide

that your child can't have the cereal that she saw on TV, stick to your guns. Later, you'll be happy you did.

8. Anticipate bids for attention. Yes, your little angel will act up when your attention is diverted (making dinner,

talking on the phone). That's why it's essential to provide some entertainment (a favorite toy, a quick snack). True story: My son once ate dog food while I was on the phone with a patient. Take-home lesson: If you don't provide something for your toddler to do when you're busy, she'll find something -- and the results may not be pretty.

9. Focus on the behavior, not the child. Always say that a particular behavior is bad. Never tell your child that he is bad. You want him to know that you love him, but you don't love the way he's acting right now.

10. Give your child choices. This will make her feel as if she's got a vote. Just make sure you don't offer too many options and that they're all things that

you want to accomplish, such as, "It's your choice: You can put your shoes on first, or your coat."

11. Don't yell. But change your voice. It's not the volume, but your tone that gets your point across.

Remember The Godfather? Don Corleone never needed to yell.

12. Catch your child being good. If you praise your child when he behaves well, he'll do it more often -- and he'll be less likely to behave badly just to get your attention.

Positive reinforcement is fertilizer for that superego.

13. Act immediately. Don't wait to discipline your toddler. She won't remember why she's in trouble more than five minutes after she did the dirty deed.

14. Be a good role model. If you're calm under pressure, your child will take the cue. And if you have a temper tantrum when you're upset, expect that he'll do the same. He's watching you, always watching.

15. Don't treat your child as if she's an adult. She really doesn't want to hear a lecture from you and won't be able to understand it. The next time she throws her spaghetti, don't break into the "You Can't Throw Your Food" lecture. Calmly evict her from the kitchen for the night.

16. Use time-outs -- even at this age. Call it the naughty chair or whatever you like, but take your child away from playing and don't pay attention to him for one

minute for each year of age. Depriving him of your attention is the most effective way to get your message across. Realistically, kids under 2 won't sit in a corner or on a chair -- and it's fine for them to be on the floor kicking and screaming. (Just make sure the time-out location is a safe one.) Reserve time-outs for particularly inappropriate behaviors -- if your child bites his friend's arm, for example -- and use a time-out every time the offense occurs.

17. Don't negotiate with your child or make promises. This isn't Capitol Hill. Try to avoid saying anything like, "If you behave, I'll buy you that doll you want." Otherwise, you'll create a 3-year-old whose good behavior will always come with a price tag. (Think Veruca Salt from Charlie and the Chocolate Factory.)

18. Shift your strategies over time. What worked beautifully when your child was 15 months probably isn't going to work when he's 2. He'll have read your playbooks and watched the films.

19. Don't spank. Although you may be tempted at times, remember that you are the grown-up. Don't resort to acting like a child. There are many more effective ways of getting your message across. Spanking your child for

hitting or kicking you, for example, just shows him that it's okay to use force. Finally, if your toddler is pushing your buttons for the umpteenth time and you think you're about to lose it, try to take a step back. You'll get a better idea of which manipulative behaviors your child is using and you'll get a fresh perspective on how to change your approach.

20. Remind your child that you love her. It's always good to end a discipline discussion with a positive comment. This shows your child that you're ready to move on and not dwell on the problem. It also reinforces the reason you're setting limits -- because you love her.

6.8 Disciplining Your Toddler to make the right choice

As a 2-year-old, Nathaniel Lampros of Sandy, Utah, was fascinated with toy swords and loved to duel with Kenayde, his 4-year-old sister. But inevitably, he'd whack her in the head, she'd dissolve in tears, and Angela, their mother, would come running to see what had happened. She'd ask

Nathaniel to apologize, as well as give Kenayde a hug and make her laugh to pacify hurt feelings. If he resisted, Angela would put her son in

time-out.

"I worried that Nathaniel would never outgrow his rough behavior, and there were days when I'd get so frustrated with him that I'd end up crying," recalls Lampros, now a mother of four. "But I really wanted Nathaniel to play nicely, so I did my best to teach him how to do it."

For many mothers, doling out effective discipline is one of the toughest and most frustrating tasks of parenting, a seemingly never-ending test of wills between you and your child. Because just when your 2-year-old "gets" that she can't thump her baby brother in the head with a doll, she'll latch on to another bothersome behavior — and the process starts anew.

How exactly does one "discipline" a toddler? Some people equate it with spanking and punishment, but that's not what we're talking about. As many parenting experts see it, discipline is about setting rules to stop your little one from engaging in behavior that's aggressive (hitting and biting), dangerous (running out in the street), and inappropriate (throwing food). It's also about following through with consequences when he breaks the rules — or what Linda Pearson, a Denver-based psychiatric nurse practitioner who specializes in

family and parent counseling, calls "being a good boss." Here are seven strategies that can help you set limits and stop bad behavior.

1. Pick Your Battles

"If you're always saying, 'No, no, no,' your child will tune out the no and won't understand your priorities," says

Pearson, author of The Discipline Miracle. "Plus you can't possibly follow through on all of the nos.'" Define what's important to you, set limits accordingly, and follow through with appropriate consequences. Then ease up on little things that are annoying but otherwise fall into the "who cares?"

category—the habits your child is likely to outgrow, such as insisting on wearing purple (and only purple).

"Keeping a good relationship with your child—who is of course in reality totally dependent upon you—is more important for her growth than trying to force her to respond in ways that she simply is not going to respond," says Elizabeth Berger, M.D., child psychiatrist and author of Raising Kids with Character. You may worry that "giving in" will create a spoiled monster, but Dr. Berger says this common anxiety isn't justified.

For Anna Lucca of Washington, D.C., that means letting her 2-1/2-year-old daughter trash her bedroom before she dozes off for a nap. "I find books and clothes scattered all over the floor when Isabel wakes up, so she must get out of bed to play after I put her down," Lucca says. "I tell her not to make a mess, but she doesn't listen. Rather than try to catch her in the act and say,

'No, no, no,' I make her clean up right after her nap." Lucca is also quick to praise Isabel for saying please and sharing toys with her 5-month-old sister. "Hopefully, the positive reinforcement will encourage Isabel to do more of the good behavior—and less of the bad," she says.

2. Know Your Child's Triggers

Some misbehavior is preventable—as long as you can anticipate what will spark it and you create a game plan in advance, such as removing tangible temptations. This strategy worked for Jean Nelson of Pasadena, California, after her 2-year-old son took delight in dragging toilet paper down the hall, giggling as the roll unfurled behind him. "The first two times Luke did it, I told him, 'No,' but when he did it a third time, I moved the toilet paper to a high shelf in the bathroom that he couldn't reach," Nelson says. "For a toddler, pulling toilet paper is

irresistible fun. It was easier to take it out of his way than to fight about it."

If your 18-month-old is prone to grabbing cans off grocery store shelves, bring toys for him to play with in the cart while you're shopping. If your 2-year-old won't share her stuffed animals during playdates at home, remove them from the designated play area before her pal arrives. And if your 3-year-old likes to draw on the walls, stash the crayons in an out-of-reach drawer and don't let him color without supervision.

3. Practice Prevention

Some children act out when they're hungry, overtired, or frustrated from being cooped up inside, says Harvey Karp, M.D., creator of the DVD and book The Happiest Toddler on the Block. If your child tends to be happy and energetic in the morning but is tired and grumpy after lunch, schedule trips to the store and visits to the doctor for when she's at her best. Prepare her for any new experiences, and explain how you expect her to act.

Also prepare her for shifting activities: "In a few minutes we'll need to pick up the toys and get ready to go home." The better prepared a child feels, the less likely she is to make a fuss.

4. Be Consistent

"Between the ages of 2 and 3, children are working hard to understand how their behavior impacts the people around them," says Claire Lerner, LCSW, director of parenting resources with Zero to Three, a nationwide nonprofit promoting the healthy development of babies and toddlers. "If your reaction to a situation keeps changing—one day you let your son throw a ball in the house and the next you don't—you'll confuse him with mixed signals."

There's no timetable as to how many incidents and reprimands it will take before your child stops a certain misbehavior. But if you always respond the same way, he'll probably learn his lesson after four or five times. Consistency was key for Orly Isaacson of Bethesda, Maryland, when her 18-month-old went through a biting phase. Each time Sasha chomped on

Isaacson's finger, she used a louder-than-usual voice to correct her—"No, Sasha! Don't bite! That hurts Mommy!"—and then handed her a toy as a distraction. "I'm very low-key, so raising my voice startled Sasha and got the message across fast," she says. A caveat: by age 2, many kids learn how to make their parents lose resolve just by

being cute. Don't let your child's tactics sway you—no matter how cute (or clever) they are.

5. Don't Get Emotional

Sure, it's hard to stay calm when your 18-month-old yanks the dog's tail or your 3-year-old refuses to brush his teeth for the gazillionth night in a row. But if you scream in anger, the message you're trying to send will

get lost and the situation will escalate, fast.

"When a child is flooded with a parent's negative mood, he'll see the emotion and won't hear what you're saying," advised the late William Coleman, M.D., professor of pediatrics at the University of North Carolina Medical School in Chapel Hill. Indeed, an angry reaction will only enhance the entertainment value for your child, so resist the urge to raise your voice. Take a deep breath, count to three, and get down to your child's eye level. Be fast and firm, serious and stern when you deliver the reprimand.

Trade in the goal of "controlling your child" for the goal of "controlling the situation," advises Dr. Berger. "This may mean re-adjusting your ideas of what is possible for a time until your daughter's self-discipline has a chance to grow a little more," she says. "You may need to lower

your expectations of her patience and her self-control somewhat. If your goal is to keep the day going along smoothly, so that there are fewer opportunities for you both to feel frustrated, that would be a constructive direction."

6. Listen and Repeat

Kids feel better when they know they have been heard, so whenever possible, repeat your child's concerns. If she's whining in the grocery store because you won't let her open the cookies, say something like: "It sounds like you're mad at me because I won't let you open the cookies until we get home. I'm sorry you feel that way, but the store won't let us open things until they're paid for. That's its policy." This won't satisfy her urge, but it will reduce her anger and defuse the conflict.

7. Keep It Short and Simple

If you're like most first-time parents, you tend to reason with your child when she breaks rules, offering detailed explanations about what she did wrong and issuing detailed threats about the privileges she'll lose if she doesn't stop misbehaving. But as a discipline strategy, overt-talking is as ineffective as becoming overly

emotional, according to Dr. Coleman. While an 18-month-old lacks the cognitive ability to understand complex sentences, a 2- or 3-year-old with more developed language skills still lacks the attention span to absorb what you're saying.

Instead, speak in short phrases, repeating them a few times and incorporating vocal inflections and facial expressions. For example, if your 18-month-old swats

your arm, say, "No, Jake! Don't hit Mommy! That hurts! No hitting." A 2-year-old can comprehend a bit more: "Evan, no jumping on the sofa! No jumping. Jumping is dangerous—you could fall. No jumping!" And a 3-year-old can process cause and effect, so state the consequences of the behavior: "Ashley, your teeth need to be brushed. You can brush them, or I can brush them for you. You decide. The longer it takes, the less time we'll have to read Dr. Seuss."

8. Offer Choices

When a child refuses to do (or stop doing) something, the real issue is usually control: You've got it; she wants it. So, whenever possible, give your preschooler some control by offering a limited set of choices. Rather than

commanding her to clean up her room, ask her, "Which would you like to pick up first, your books or your blocks?" Be sure the choices are limited, specific, and acceptable to you, however. "Where do you want to start?" may be overwhelming to your child, and a choice that's not acceptable to you will only amplify the conflict.

9. Watch Your Words

It helps to turn "you" statements into "I" messages. Instead of saying, "You're so selfish that you won't even

share your toys with your best friend," try "I like it better when I see kids sharing their toys." Another good technique is to focus on do's rather than don'ts. If you tell a 3-year-old that he can't leave his trike in the hallway, he may want to argue. A better approach: "If you move your trike out to the porch, it won't get kicked and scratched so much."

Make sure your tone and words do not imply that you no longer love your child. "I really can't stand it when you act like that" sounds final; "I don't like it when you try to pull cans from the store shelves," however, shows your child that it's one specific behavior—not the whole person—that you dislike.

10. Teach Empathy

It's rarely obvious to a 3-year-old why he should stop doing something he finds fun, like biting, hitting, or grabbing toys from other children. Teach him empathy instead: "When you bite or hit people, it hurts them"; "When you grab toys away from other kids, they feel sad because they still want to play with those toys." This helps your child see that his behavior directly affects other people and trains him to think about consequences first.

11. Give a Time-Out

If repeated reprimands, redirection, and loss of privileges haven't cured your child of her offending behavior, consider putting her in time-out for a minute per year of age. "This is an excellent discipline tool for kids who are doing the big-time no-nos," Dr. Karp explains.

Before imposing a time-out, put a serious look on your face and give a warning in a stern tone of voice ("I'm counting to three, and if you don't stop, you're going to time-out. One, two, THREE!"). If she doesn't listen, take her to the quiet and safe spot you've designated for time-outs, and set a timer. When it goes off, ask her to

apologize and give her a big hug to convey that you're not angry. "Nathaniel hated going to time-out for hitting his sister with the plastic sword, but I was clear about the consequences and stuck with it," says Angela Lampros. "After a few weeks, he learned his lesson." Indeed, toddlers don't like to be separated from their parents and toys, so eventually, the mere threat of a time-out should be enough to stop them in their tracks.

12. Talk Options

When you want your child to stop doing something, offer alternative ways for him to express his feelings: say, hitting a pillow or banging with a toy hammer. He needs to learn that while his emotions and impulses are acceptable, certain ways of expressing them are not. Also, encourage your child to think up his own options. Even 3-year-olds can learn to solve problems themselves. For instance, you could ask: "What do you think you could do to get Tiffany to share that toy with you?" The trick is to listen to their ideas with an open mind. Don't shoot down anything, but do talk about the consequences before a decision is made.

13. Reward Good Behavior

It's highly unlikely that your child will always do whatever you say. If that happened, you'd have to think about what might be wrong with her! Normal kids resist control, and they know when you're asking them to do something they don't want to do. They then feel justified in resisting you. In cases in which they do behave appropriately, a prize is like a spoonful of sugar: It helps the medicine go down.

Judicious use of special treats and prizes is just one more way to show your child you're aware and respectful of his feelings. This, more than anything,

gives credibility to your discipline demands.

14. Stay Positive

No matter how frustrated you feel about your child's misbehavior, don't vent about it in front of him. "If people heard their boss at work say, 'I don't know what to do with my employees. They run the company, and I feel powerless to do anything about it,' they'd lose respect for him and run the place even more," says Pearson. "It's the same thing when children hear their parents speak about them in a hopeless or negative

way. They won't have a good image of you as their boss, and they'll end up repeating the behavior."

Still, it's perfectly normal to feel exasperated from time to time. If you reach that point, turn to your spouse, your pediatrician, or a trusted friend for support and advice.

Ages & Stages

Effective discipline starts with understanding where your child falls on the developmental spectrum. Our guide: At 18 months your child is curious, fearless, impulsive, mobile, and clueless about the consequences of her actions—a recipe for trouble. "My image of an 18-month-old is a child who's running down the hall away from his mother but looking over his shoulder to see if she's there and then running some more," said Dr. Coleman.

"Though he's building a vocabulary and can follow simple instructions, he can't effectively communicate his needs or understand lengthy reprimands. He may bite or hit to register his displeasure or to get your attention. Consequences of misbehavior must be immediate. Indeed, if you wait even 10 minutes to react, he won't remember what he did wrong or tie his action to the consequence, says nurse practitioner Pearson.

At age 2 your child is using her developing motor skills to test limits, by running, jumping, throwing, and climbing. She's speaking a few words at a time, she becomes frustrated when she can't get her point across, and she's prone to tantrums. She's also self-centered and doesn't like to share. Consequences should be swift, as a 2-year-old is unable to grasp time. But since she still lacks impulse control, give her another chance soon after the incident, says Lerner of Zero to Three.

At age 3 your child is now a chatterbox; he's using language to argue his point of view. Since he loves to be with other children and has boundless energy, he may have a tough time playing quietly at home. "Taking a 3-

year-old to a gym or karate class will give him the social contact he craves and let him release energy," says Dr. Karp. "At this age, kids need that as much as they need affection and food." He also knows right from wrong, understands cause and effect, and retains information for several hours. Consequences can be delayed for maximum impact, and explanations can be more detailed. For example, if he hurls Cheerios at his sister, remind him about the no-food-throwing rule and explain that if he does it again, he won't get to watch Blues

Clues. If he continues to throw food, take it away from him. When he asks to watch TV, say, "Remember when

Mommy told you not to throw cereal and you did anyway? Well, the consequence is no Blues Clues today."

Chapter 7 Toddler timing and Developmental Milestones

Skills such as taking a first step, smiling for the first time, and waving "bye-bye" are called developmental milestones. Developmental milestones are things most children can do by a certain age. Children reach milestones in how they play, learn, speak, behave, and move (like crawling, walking, or jumping).

During the second year, toddlers are moving around more, and are aware of themselves and their surroundings. Their desire to explore new objects and people also is increasing. During this stage, toddlers will show greater independence; begin to show defiant behavior; recognize themselves in pictures or a mirror; and imitate the behavior of others, especially adults and older children. Toddlers also should be able to recognize the names of familiar people and objects, form simple phrases and sentences, and follow simple instructions and directions.

7.1 Positive Parenting Tips

Following are some of the things you, as a parent, can do to help your toddler during this time:

Mother reading to toddler

Read to your toddler daily.

Ask her to find objects for you or name body parts and objects.

Play matching games with your toddler, like shape sorting and simple puzzles. Encourage him to explore and try new things.

Help to develop your toddler's language by talking with her and adding to words she starts. For example, if your toddler says "baba", you can respond, "Yes, you are right—that is a bottle."

Encourage your child's growing independence by letting him help with dressing himself and feeding himself.

Respond to wanted behaviors more than you punish unwanted behaviors (use only very brief time outs). Always tell or show your child what she should do instead.

Encourage your toddler's curiosity and ability to recognize common objects by taking field trips together to the park or going on a bus ride.

7.2 Child Safety First

Because your child is moving around more, he will come across more dangers as well. Dangerous situations can happen quickly, so keep a close eye on your child. Here are a few tips to help keep your growing toddler safe:

Do NOT leave your toddler near or around water (for example, bathtubs, pools, ponds, lakes, whirlpools, or the ocean) without someone watching her. Fence off backyard pools. Drowning is the leading cause of injury and death among this age group.

Block off stairs with a small gate or fence. Lock doors to dangerous places such as the garage or basement.

Ensure that your home is toddler proof by placing plug covers on all unused electrical outlets.

Keep kitchen appliances, irons, and heaters out of reach of your toddler. Turn pot handles toward the back of the stove.

Keep sharp objects such as scissors, knives, and pens in a safe place.

Lock up medicines, household cleaners, and poisons.

Do NOT leave your toddler alone in any vehicle (that means a car, truck, or van) even

for a few moments.

Store any guns in a safe place out of his reach.

Keep your child's car seat rear-facing as long as possible. According to the National

Highway Traffic Safety Administration, it's the best way to keep her safe. Your child should remain in a rear-facing car seat until she reaches the top height or weight limit allowed by the car seat's manufacturer. Once your child outgrows the rear-facing car seat, she is ready to travel in a forward-facing car seat with a harness.

7.3 The right Healthy Bodies for your Kids

Give your child water and plain milk instead of sugary drinks. After the first year, when your nursing toddler is eating more and different solid foods, breast milk is still an ideal addition to his diet.

Your toddler might become a very picky and erratic eater. Toddlers need less food because they don't grow as fast. It's best not to battle with him over this. Offer a selection of healthy foods and let him choose what she wants. Keep trying new foods; it might take time for him to learn to like them.

Limit screen time and develop a media use plan for your family.external icon For children younger than 18 months of age, the AAP recommends that it's best if toddlers not use any screen media other than video chatting.

Your toddler will seem to be moving continually—running, kicking, climbing, or jumping. Let him be active—he's developing his coordination and becoming strong.

Make sure your child gets the recommended amount of sleep each night: For toddlers 1-2 years, 11–14 hours per 24 hours (including naps)

7.4 The proper height and Weight for your children

Baby growth charts for boys and girls are an important tool health providers use when it comes to comparing your child's growth to other kids her age. But for the average parent, they can be a little confusing to decipher.

To make it easier for you to get informed, we had experts breakdown the information you really want to

know about your child's physical development. Here's a simple look at average height and weight growth at every age:

7.5 Baby Height and Weight Growth

Birth to 4 Days Old

The average newborn is 19.5 inches long and weighs 7.25 pounds. Boys have a head circumference of about 13.5 inches and girls measure in at 13.3 inches, according to the National Center for Health Statistics.

A baby drops 5 to 10 percent of his total body weight in his first few days of life because of the fluid he loses through urine and stool, says Parents advisor Ari Brown, M.D., author of Baby 411.

5 Days to 3 Months

Babies gain about an ounce a day on average during this period, or half a pound per week, and they should be back to their birthweight by their second-week visit. Expect a growth surge around 3 weeks and then another one at 6 weeks.

3 Months to 6 Months

A baby should gain about half a pound every two weeks.

By 6 months, she should have doubled her birthweight.

7 Months to 12 Months

A child is still gaining about a pound a month. If you're nursing, your baby may not gain quite this much, or he may dip slightly from one percentile to another on the growth chart.

"At this point, babies may also burn more calories because they're starting to crawl or cruise," says Tanya Altmann, M.D., a Los Angeles pediatrician and author of Mommy Calls. Even so, by the time he reaches his first birthday, expect him to have grown 10 inches in length and tripled his birthweight and his head to have grown by about 4 inches.

Toddler Height and Weight Growth

Age 1

Toddlers will grow at a slower pace this year but will gain about a half a pound a month and will grow a total of about 4 or 5 inches in height.

Age 2

A kid will sprout about 3 more inches by the end of her third year and will have quadrupled her birthweight by gaining about 4 more pounds. By now, your pediatrician

will be able to make a fairly accurate prediction about her adult height.

7.6 Preschooler Height and Weight Growth (Ages 3-4)

A preschooler will grow about 3 inches and gain 4 pounds each year.

You may also find that your child starts to shed the baby fat from his face and looks lankier, since kids' limbs grow more by the time they are preschoolers, says Daniel

Rauch, M.D., associate professor of pediatrics at Mount Sinai School of Medicine, in New York City.

7.7 Kids Height and Weight Growth (Ages 5+)

Starting at 5 years old, kids will begin to grow about 2 inches and gain 4 pounds each year until puberty (usually between 8 and 13 for girls and 10 and 14 for boys). Girls often reach their full height about two years after their first period. Boys usually hit their adult height around age 17.

7.8 How to keep your little toddler always happy and joyful

What Makes a Child Happy?

We all want the same things for our kids. We want them to grow up to love and be loved, to follow their dreams, to find success. Mostly, though, we want them to be happy. But just how much control do we have over our children's happiness?

Happy toddlers don't just happen...they're molded by parents who care!

Bubbling giggles, chubby feet and colorful facial expressions all make-up a happy toddler!

It thrills my soul to see a content, obviously well-loved toddlers, explore their new world.

Their enthusiasm about daily life is contagious

But some toddlers don't enjoy the blessings of a home that's filled with encouraging words, bundles of hugs and wheelbarrels full of kisses. Instead, they face daily criticism and harshness.

Have you ever heard a mother or father yell "Shut-up!" to their toddler?

Unfortunately I have. I absolutely shutter and my teeth

clench when I hear those anger-filled words. Instead of tearing toddlers down, we should be encouraging them!

Our focus should be creating happy toddlers — not creating sad, frustrated, misunderstood toddlers! I'll admit it.

Sometimes it is crazy-easy to snap at toddler because you're trying to get other work done and they interrupt you once again.

Be present in your toddler's life. Don't push your munchkin away when you are answering an email. Instead take a few moments and address her needs or wants. Take time to play with your toddler every day. Make tents together, color pictures, go on walks, bake together, try these simple toddler activities or whatever your child enjoys doing — do it! My youngest child enjoys swinging on our large patio swing. I try to make a "date" with him everyday for this special time. We are making memories!

Set goals. Are you making dinner soon? Ask your toddler to help set the table. Do you clean your room in the morning? Ask your little one to help you make your bed. By giving toddlers responsibilities you are letting them know they have an important place

in the family. When a child successfully completes a goal, like chores, he begins to develop security and an "I can do it!" attitude.

It is my three-year-old son's task to open the door for visitors after they leave our home. He enjoys it so much! When he runs back to us, he always has an upbeat spirit and can't wait to help out in another area!

Establish boundaries. Definite boundaries help a child understand what is acceptable in your home and what is not. If she does not know the rules, she can become paranoid and insecure of messing up. Make your rules reasonable and make sure you stick to them! If rules are not enforced, they are worthless.

Examples of acceptable rules for toddlers: λ No whining or screaming.

λ Say "please" and "thank-you."

λ Pick up your toys after you play.

λ Do not open the refrigerator.

As your child obeys these rules, she will feel confident that she is able to obey "house ules."

By establishing clear boundaries, you are promoting even more security for your toddler!

Praise often. Criticism and negativity comes from

everywhere in the outside world. Create a haven in your home by praising your toddler for jobs well-done, good attitudes or any positive characteristics you observe. Praising a child always adds extra dashes of happiness to the soul! Use eye contact. When praising or correcting, get down on your toddler's eye level and speak one-on-one together. You are letting him know she is the focus of your thoughts and energy. When he asks for a drink, squat down and ask him if he want juice or milk. Take these special short conversations to interact with your child in order to build his confidence in your unbiased love.

Smile often. It's so easy to lose our smile when we're busy in daily tasks and life, isn't it? But a toddler finds much happiness in seeing a smile on mom's face. When a toddler sees that smile, the entire world seems like a peaceful, happy place...and the toddler knows that mom really does love and care for him! Our face speaks a thousand words!

Listen. Nothing says, "You don't really matter," like someone not listening to what you are saying. When your toddler gets excited about something and wants to show and tell you about this new discovery, really listen

and pay attention. Comment on their discovery. Don't just say, "Uh...yeah. That's neat. Now, go and play!" Your toddler knows when you're really listening and when you're just trying to shoo her away.

Laugh!. Go ahead, let your hair down and be super silly with your toddler. Sing silly songs with them, talk in funny voices — anything to get a smile or laugh from your kiddos. Adding some silliness and fun to your toddler's day is the perfect way to build them up!

Celebrate victories! Did your toddler finally get the potty-training deal?! :) Did your toddler learn to successfully and routinely nap?! Those are HUGE milestones and should be celebrated! Celebrate with just an ice cream cone, a trip to the park or some stickers! Keep it simple so it's always convenient to celebrate a new milestone in your munchkin's life.

If your toddler is struggling with napping successfully, we have an awesome super-loaded course for that! Yay for a toddler naps ,right?!

Chapter 8 Montessori toddler discipline techniques

"The first idea that the child must acquire, in order to be actively disciplined, is that of the difference between good and evil; and the task of the educator lies in seeing that the child does not confound good with immobility, and evil with activity, as often happens in the case of the old-time discipline." Maria Montessori

A Montessori approach to discipline consists of a delicate balance between freedom and discipline. Like any part of Montessori education, it requires respect for the child.

I'd like to share some Montessori articles that give more insight into Montessori discipline, which by nature is a form of gentle/positive discipline. As a parent, your greatest ally is the child's own desire to grow, to learn, to master her own emotions, and to develop her own character. By keeping calm and respecting your child and her desires, you can help her on her own quest for inner discipline. By setting clear expectations and supporting your child's active thought and reflection, you can support the sense of personal autonomy she is naturally seeking as she follows her

own unique path to physical, emotional, and intellectual independence.

8.1 Validate a child's emotions.

Of course, sometimes a child is going to want to take an action that is not permissible. A preschool-age child doesn't always understand why he is allowed to make some choices, but not others. Why can he choose what he has for dinner, but not when he has dinner? Why can he choose what to wear to school, but not whether he has to go to school in the first place? As an adult, you can help the child master himself in these frustrating moments by acknowledging his emotions. "You really wanted to wear your boots today! You are not in the mood for shoes! You're sad and mad about it." Be sure to allow your child time to experience the disappointment, and remember to save any reasoning or discussion until the initial emotion has run its course.

Montessori also encouraged teachers to talk with children about their behavior. To quote Dr. Montessori herself:

...if he shows a tendency to misbehaves, she will check him with earnest words...

Many people misinterpret the Montessori method to be a permissive method that allows children unlimited freedom. In reality, the freedom is within limits that are carefully enforced through guidance by the teacher. Common consequences in a Montessori classroom include:

λ Putting a material away that's not being used properly λ Cleaning up a mess or a spill

λ Staying close to the teacher

You can use these same consequences in your home.

Natural Consequences

When it comes to discipline, parents often feel the need to impose consequences and punishments on the child, rather than letting things run their course. However, this teaches your child to fear getting caught by a parent, teacher or authority figure rather than learning the natural consequences of their actions.

But, what are natural consequences?

In part, it's helping your child see what will happen as a result of their choices and actions, and letting it happen. Like what? For example, your child chooses to skip lunch. You allow them to skip lunch, but save their plate for later and when they ask for a snack, they can finish

their lunch. Or your child leaves toys out and doesn't want to clean up. You can explain that leaving toys on the floor is dangerous for others because they might step on them and the family needs a clean place to live. Then, you can clean up the toys together, ensuring your child helps. Rather than feeling threatened with punishment, your child learns to see how their actions affect themselves and others.

An easy way to implement this technique is by narrating what you see and helping your child predict the future. This also works well with aggressive behaviors like biting and hitting, and of course tantrums. You can say for example "I see you're angry. You want to hit me." However, in these cases, you may need to intervene to prevent children from getting hurt and say things like "I won't let you hurt your brother".

Montessori encouraged the use of control of error in materials and classroom activities. Natural consequences are the control of error of life. For example, Montessori encouraged the use of real glass dishes so that if children weren't careful or had an accident, the dishes would break. She believed this natural consequence was valuable for children to experience so that they could

change their behavior in the future.

8.2 Best way to make your kids grow faster

Most parents would love for their children to be tall and strong, as it has been widely regarded as a sign of good health. Parents usually go to great lengths to ensure that their children grow up healthily, and their height is treated as an indication of their overall health condition by most parts of the society.

Genes have the most say in determining the height of the child – however, it is not the only factor which influences it. Many external factors, like living conditions and a healthy diet, can influence the height of children quite a lot. Therefore, it is possible for parents to improve the chances of their children grow up to be tall and strong, through simple methods. Let us take a look at the top 10 ways to make your child grow taller.

8.3 How to Increase the Height of a Child

There are many ways a parent can influence the height of their child, and here's a list of the top ten ways.

1. A Balanced Diet

The most important aspect of how to increase your kid's height is to ensure that he gets proper nutrition. The food he consumes has to be healthy so that he grows up to be tall. A balanced diet has to include proteins, carbohydrates, fat and vitamins in the correct proportion – loading up on only one of these can have a detrimental effect. You must also ensure that the child keeps away from junk food most of the time – this includes food like burgers, aerated sweetened drinks and fried items in general. Lean proteins have to be had aplenty, along with leafy vegetables and items rich in minerals like calcium and potassium. Simple carbs like pizza and cakes have to be avoided for the most part. Zinc has been found to have a huge effect on the growth of the child, so zinc-rich foods like squash seeds and peanuts must also be added to their diet. A balanced diet not only provides the right nutrients to increase your child's height but it will also make him stronger in every sense.

2. Stretching Exercises

Stretching exercises, even if they are simple ones, can have a huge impact on the height of your child. Introducing your child to stretching exercises from a

young age will facilitate the process of height growth. Stretching helps elongate the spine and also improves the posture of your child at all times. The exercises can be simple ones. Make him stand on his toes with his back against the wall and stretch the muscles in his leg while reaching up simultaneously. Another simple exercise for stretching involves the child sitting on the floor with his legs wide apart, and reaching to touch the toes of both legs with his arms. Stretching exercises to grow taller

3. Hanging

Hanging has been recommended for decades now, for parents who want their children to be taller. Hanging from bars also helps the spine elongate, which is an important part of becoming taller. Apart from regular hanging, you can also encourage your child to do pull-ups and chin-ups. Both make the muscles of the arm and the back stronger and are great exercises to help him keep fit.

4. Swimming

Swimming is another healthy habit, one which helps your child stay active and enjoy it, too. Swimming is a full-body exercise, meaning that it works all the muscles

in the body to great effect. Swimming for a long time can help your child lose any extra fat present, making him healthier as a whole. The exercise involves a lot of stretching forward, which strengthens the spine and lays the groundwork for a tall, healthy body. Swimming is also a highly enjoyable activity- no child has ever said no to playing in the water!

5. Jogging

Jogging is an amazing exercise, not just for children- it has a range of benefits for grown-ups too. Jogging strengthens the bones in the leg and also increases the quantity of HGH, the growth hormone, which is required for any growth in the body. To make it even more fun, you can maybe join in with your child and make jogging be an activity you do together!

6. Sleep

The importance of sleep can never be stressed upon enough, not just for children – for adults, too. Skipping sleep occasionally does not affect the growth of your child in the long term- however, you have to ensure that the child gets a good 8 hours of sleep on most nights, in order for him to be taller and stronger. This is because the growth hormone in children, HGH, is released only when the child sleeps. This plays a direct role in making your child taller, so skipping sleep constantly is definitely a bad idea.

7. Posture

To increase your child's height, it is integral that he has a proper posture. Slumping or slouching can put unnecessary stress on the spine which can have many negative affects on the body. Additionally, poor posture can alter the shape of your child's spine which can compromise his growth. Make sure that your child practices good posture not only to increase his height but also to prevent any long term health issues. Remind him to sit and stand up straight every time you see him slouching.

There are many ways to make your child grow taller, but all of them work only when complemented by the other activities on the list. A good diet must be accompanied by regular exercise and sound sleep- else, you do not get what you want. Therefore, take care of your child the right way, and make him grow tall and strong.

8.4 How to keep your toddler busy and Happy at the same time

We all know that watching TV and playing video games isn't good for our kids. No parent is proud of how much time their kids spend in front of a screen but what are we supposed to do?

Sometimes, we just need to get things done. We need to clean the house or cook food or just take a few minutes for ourselves. It's hard to think of other things that could keep a kid distracted long enough to actually accomplish anything.

There are options, though. Sure, they take a bit more energy than just plopping a child in front of a screen, but encouraging your child to do something constructive just might be worth the extra effort.

We all know that watching TV and playing video games isn't good for our kids. No parent is proud of how much time their kids spend in front of a screen – but what are we supposed to do?

Sometimes, we just need to get things done. We need to clean the house or cook food or just take a few minutes for ourselves. It's hard to think of other things that could

keep a kid distracted long enough to actually accomplish anything. There are options, though. Sure, they take a bit more energy than just plopping a child in front of a screen, but encouraging your child to do something constructive just might be worth the extra effort.

Create a game box

Fill a box full of things your child can play with alone – things like coloring books, playing cards, or easy puzzles. When you need to keep your kids busy, give them the box. They might resist at first, but the more you do it, the more they'll accept "game box time" as part of their routine.

8.5 Have them make their own cartoon

Instead of watching cartoons, have your children make their own. Give them a piece of paper and some crayons, and ask them to draw you a hero and a bad guy. When they're done, let them come back and tell you their hero's story.

8.6 Let them help you

If you're cooking or cleaning, let your kids help. Give

them a job they can handle. For young kids, that might be stringing beans or setting the table. For older kids, that might be slicing vegetables, sweeping the house, or taking out the recycling.

8.7 Give them an important mission

Give your child a task, and make it a really big deal. Tell them they need to draw a picture for Dada, or that they need to make a block fort for Grandma. If they think it's an important job, they won't complain about working on it independently.

8.8 Generate an idea box

Brainstorm ideas with your children about what they can do to overcome boredom. Write down their suggestions, and put them in an empty box. Then, the next time they're bored, have them pick out one of their own suggestions. Given that it was their idea, they'll be more willing to actually do it.

8.9 Offer creative toys

Any toy that lets a child create is sure to keep them distracted for a long time. Invest in Legos, puzzles, and

Play-Dough. Not only will your child be able to play with them for hours, but they'll build up their spatial reasoning, too.

8.10 Design a treasure hunt

Hide something like a coin or a sticker somewhere in the house. Give your kids a clue, and let them run wild trying to find it. If you make it a bit tricky to find, you'll build up their resilience – and their ability to find things without begging for your help.

8.11 Let them play outside

Don't forget how your parents kept you busy. Just give your child a ball and a stick, and let them run wild. If you're worried about their safety, just keep them in sight of the window. They'll be fine.

8.12 Send them to a friend's house

Work out a deal with another parent on your street. When you need some time, send your kid over to play with their kid. To be fair, you'll have to let them send their kid over sometimes, too. When two kids play together, they keep themselves distracted.

8.13 Build a fort

Give your child a few pillows and a blanket, and challenge them to turn the couch into a fort. No child will turn down the chance to make a secret base – and they'll be much more likely to play independently once they're inside.

8.14 Make a sculpture

Give your child a few pipe cleaners and a piece of Styrofoam – or any other child-friendly items you might have on hand – and ask them to make a sculpture. Anything will do, but favorite heroes are a winning suggestion.

8.15 Listen to an audiobook

If your child's too young to read independently, pick up audio versions of their favorite books. Let them sit down and turn the pages while listening to a friendly voice read to them. Or, if you can't find a recording, use your phone to make one yourself.

Play with locks and bolts

Hand your child a lock and a key or a nut and bolt and let them play with it. Young kids, especially, will be

mesmerized by the act of unlocking something – and they'll develop their motor skills while they're at it. Give them a mixed bag, and see if they can figure out which lock goes with which key.

Conclusion

Congratulations! You have made it to the end and I want to personally thank you for trusting us with this very important stage in your child's life. I want to wish you all the luck so that you are successful in potty training. You have taken the necessary steps that many have not. You have taken the steps to getting the information so that you know what you need to do to be successful.

Remember, you want to be consistent. Consistency is one of the most important things that you can do right now for your child to help them be successful in potty training. If there is anything that you learn from us today, please let that be that consistency is crucial. Secondly is the 'push.' Every time your child sits on that toilet, make sure they are pushing. Once they push they can get up even if they have not done anything on the toilet, as long as they have pushed it is okay for them to get up. Remember that you are in charge. You are the parent and you have to set the stage. You are pulling the strings, so remember that as your child is trying to push the boundaries you have set. As a parent and as a human this process maybe frustrating. This process maybe tough and we understand that, and so

we're telling you to be parents and be human. You're going to be frustrated, you're going to be mad, and you might even yell a couple times.

But don't let that keep you from saying to yourself, "I'm not a good parent." You are human, it's going to happen, so you have to be yourself and do how you normally do things and be yourself and be happy and true to yourself. Most importantly, as we said, get some rest because you don't want to be stressed during this process. You want to have as much energy as possible. That not only will increase the chances for your child success, but help you maintain your sanity and increase your own success as well. We wish you good luck and lots of fun. Be strong!

9 781802 247510